BREAST RECONSTRUCTION – CURRENT TECHNIQUES

Edited by **Marzia Salgarello**

Breast Reconstruction – Current Techniques
Edited by Marzia Salgarello

Published by InTech

Janeza Trdine 9, 51000 Rijeka, Croatia

Publishing Process Manager Ivana Zec

Technical Editor Teodora Smiljanic

Cover Designer InTech Design Team

Additional hard copies can be obtained from orders@intechopen.com

Breast Reconstruction – Current Techniques, Edited by Marzia Salgarello
p. cm.
ISBN 978-953-307-982-0

For EU product safety concerns:
IN TECH d.o.o., Prolaz Marije Krucifikse Kozulić 3, 51000 Rijeka, Croatia,
info@intechopen.com or visit our website at intechopen.com.

Meet the editor

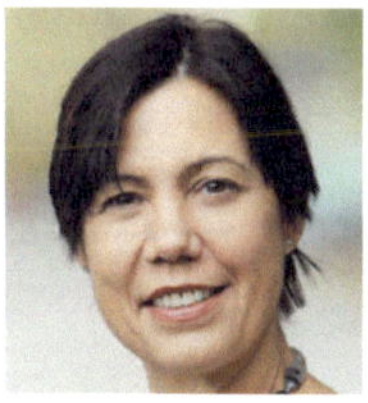

Dr Marzia Salgarello was born in Rovigo, Italy in 1959. She graduated in 1983 from the Catholic University of "Sacro Cuore", Rome, Italy and, in 1988, she began to specialize in plastic surgery. She is now an Assistant Professor of Plastic Surgery at the Department of Plastic and Reconstructive Surgery and is in charge of the microsurgery teaching program at the University Hospital "Agostino Gemelli", Catholic University of "Sacro Cuore", Rome, Italy. She currently focuses her activity on breast reconstruction and aesthetics, and post-oncologic reconstructive microsurgery. She is author of about 70 peer-reviewed articles and of chapters in six books. She has given presentations at national and international plastic surgery meetings, covering all aspects of breast reconstruction and aesthetic breast surgery. She is the section editor for reconstructive plastic surgery for the Aesthetic Plastic Surgery Journal and is a member of the Italian Society of Plastic, Reconstructive and Aesthetic Surgery, the Italian Society of Microsurgery, and of the International Society of Aesthetic Plastic Surgery.

Contents

Preface XI

Part 1 Oncology and Breast Reconstruction 1

Chapter 1 **Oncological Considerations for Breast Reconstruction 3**
Grant W. Carlson

Part 2 Prosthetic Breast Reconstruction 21

Chapter 2 **Implant and Implant Assisted Breast Reconstructions 23**
Sarah S.K. Tang and Gerald P.H. Gui

Chapter 3 **One-Stage Immediate Breast Reconstruction with Implants in Conservative Mastectomies 49**
Marzia Salgarello, Giuseppe Visconti and Liliana Barone-Adesi

Chapter 4 **The Effect of Breast Reconstruction on Maintaining a Proper Body Posture in Patients After Mastectomy 83**
Sławomir Cieśla and Małgorzata Bąk

Part 3 Autogenous Breast Reconstruction 103

Chapter 5 **Modified Extended Latissimus Dorsi Myocutaneous Flap with Added Vascularised Chest Wall Fat in Immediate Breast Reconstruction After Conservative (Sparing) Mastectomies 105**
Adel Denewer and Omar Farouk

Chapter 6 **Breast Reconstruction with DIEP and S/IGAP 129**
Maria M. LoTempio, Grace Lucta Gerald and Robert J. Allen

Chapter 7 **Preoperative Computed Tomographic Angiogram for Deep Inferior Epigastric Artery Perforator Flap for Breast Reconstruction: The Imaging Mapping Era 159**
Jaume Masia, Carmen Navarro, Juan A. Clavero and Xavier Alomar

Chapter 8 **The Superficial Inferior Epigastric Artery (SIEA) Flap and Its Applications in Breast Reconstruction 171**
Zachary Menn and Aldona Spiegel

Chapter 9 **Double-Pedicle DIEP and SIEA Flaps and Their Application in Breast Reconstruction 177**
Marzia Salgarello, Liliana Barone-Adesi and Giuseppe Visconti

Chapter 10 **The Omentum Flap 195**
Sirlei dos Santos Costa and Rosa Maria Blotta

Part 4 Fat Graft in Breast Reconstruction 215

Chapter 11 **Autologous Fat Transplantation – A Paradigm Shift in Breast Reconstruction 217**
Daniel Del Vecchio and Hetal Fichadia

Part 5 Breast Reconstruction After Conservative Treatment 241

Chapter 12 **Breast Reconstruction Approach to Conservative Surgery 243**
Egidio Riggio and Valentina Visintini Cividin

Preface

Breast reconstruction is an evolving art that challenges surgeons to combine reconstructive and aesthetic principles in the search for the best results possible.

The goal of breast reconstruction after mastectomy and after conservative treatment, is to restore the appearance of the breast and to improve a woman's psychological health after cancer treatment. Similarly, rebuilding the breast after severe breast malformation such as Poland syndrome, is similar to breast reconstruction after oncologic treatment. In this way the book joins together breast reconstruction after cancer treatment, and after a serious congenital condition that may even result in the absence of the breast and the deformity of the homo-lateral chest. Although the technical strategies for breast reconstruction are getting increasingly sophisticated, the two main options can still be summarized as autogenous and/or prosthetic, both now reaching a high standard of results. Having this in mind, the purpose of this book is to examine many of the modern techniques for breast reconstruction, and also giving some insight into specific topics.

The text consists of five sections. The first is an introduction to the oncologic aspects of breast reconstruction. In brief, this chapter introduces the issue of immediate breast reconstruction, of which the main benefit is superior aesthetic results compared to those of delayed reconstruction, together with a gain in psychological, social, and sexual well-being, and a significant cost reduction. The book goes on to examine the topic of detection and treatment of local recurrences after breast reconstruction, and the relationship between immediate breast reconstruction and adjuvant therapies. This chapter also provides significant information on the safety of conservative mastectomies. Section two focuses on prosthetic breast reconstruction, which contains chapters for two-stage and one-stage implant-assisted reconstruction together with a chapter examining the effect of mastectomy and implant breast reconstruction on the maintenance of proper body posture after surgery. Section three is about autogenous breast reconstruction, and has several chapters covering the main topics from latissimus dorsi and abdominal flaps to omentum flap. Section four analyzes breast reconstruction with the use of a fat graft. Finally, section five covers the current approaches to breast reshaping after conservative treatment, mainly modified reduction mammaplasty, and adjacent tissue rearrangement.

Dr. Marzia Salgarello
University Hospital "Agostino Gemelli",
University of "Sacro Cuore",
Rome,
Italy

Part 1

Oncology and Breast Reconstruction

1

Oncological Considerations for Breast Reconstruction

Grant W. Carlson
Emory University School of Medicine, Winship Cancer Institute, Atlanta, GA, USA

1. Introduction

Fifteen percent of women treated for breast cancer with total mastectomy receive immediate or early breast reconstruction [1, 2]. The percentage is higher in young women and those treated in tertiary care medical centers. Immediate breast reconstruction (IBR) has several advantages [3, 4]. It can prevent some of the negative psychological and emotional sequelae seen with mastectomy. The aesthetic results of immediate reconstruction are superior to those seen after delayed reconstruction. IBR also reduces hospital costs by reducing the number of procedures and length of hospitalization. Immediate breast reconstruction has the potential to impact the treatment of breast cancer. It could affect the delivery of adjuvant therapy and the detection and treatment of recurrent disease. Chemotherapy and radiation therapy could also impact the complication rates of reconstruction. The oncological considerations of breast reconstruction are outlined in this chapter.

2. Local recurrence after skin sparing and nipple sparing mastectomy

Women with breast cancer who undergo immediate breast reconstruction do not have a worse survival than those not undergoing breast reconstructions. A review of a large National Cancer Institute database of 51,702 breast cancer patients identified 8,645 (16.7%) who underwent immediate breast reconstruction [5]. Patients treated by mastectomy and IBR had a lower hazard of death (HR 0.62) compared to those treated by mastectomy alone ($p<0.001$). The study was controlled for age, race, income, and tumor stage. Potential compounding factors like obesity, smoking, and underlying chronic disease were not accounted for.

Skin sparing mastectomy (SSM) has markedly improved the aesthetic results of immediate breast reconstruction (Figure 1). Preservation of the native skin envelope and the inframammary fold reduces the amount of tissue necessary for reconstruction [6]. Breast symmetry can often be achieved without operating on the contralateral breast and the periareolar incisions are inconspicuous in clothes.

There have been concerns that the skin, nipple and inframammary fold preservation reduce the effectiveness of total mastectomy. There is a large body of evidence that the local recurrences (LRs) after SSM are comparable to non-skin sparing mastectomy (Table 1) [7-9]. Care must be taken however, in patients with superficial cancers or diffuse DCIS to assure adequate surgical margins.

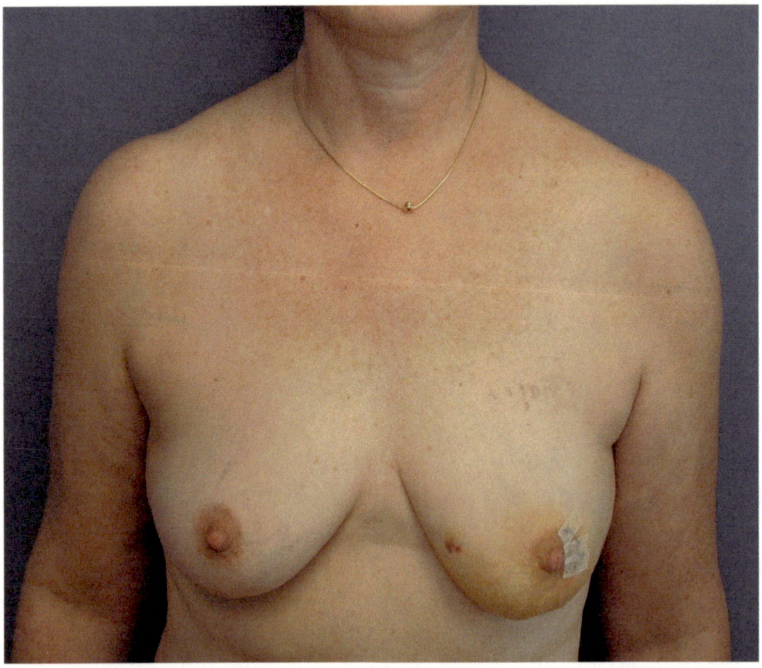

(a)

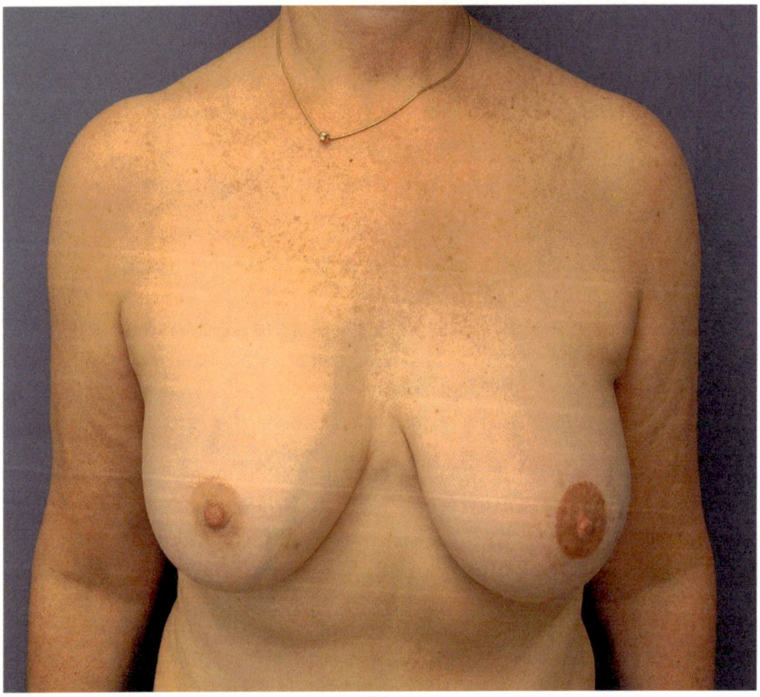

(b)

Fig. 1. (a) Preoperative photograph (b) Postoperative photograph after skin sparing mastectomy and TRAM flap reconstruction

Author	*Followup (Months)*	*SSM (N)*	*LR in SSM (%)*	*Non-SSM (N)*	*LR in Non-SSM (N)*
Newman [81]	50	437	6.2	437	7.4
Carlson [7]	41.3	187	4.8	84	9.5
Kroll [8]	72	114	7.0	40	7
Simmons [9]	15.6-32.4	77	3.9	154	3.2
Rivadeneira [82]	49	71	5.6	127	3.9
Medina-Franco [83]	73	176	4.5	-	-
Carlson [84]	64.6	565	5.5	-	-
Slavin [85]	44.8	51	3.9	-	-
Toth [86]	51.5	50	0	-	-
Spiegel [87]	117.6	221	4.5	-	-
Foster [88]	49.2	25	4.0	-	-

SSM skin sparing mastectomy
LR local recurrence
Non-SSM non skin sparing mastectomy

Table 1. Published series of local recurrence of breast cancer after skin sparing and non-skin sparing mastectomy

Nipple sparing mastectomy (NSM) is growing in popularity because of its perceived aesthetic benefits (Figure 2). Patient satisfaction with nipple-areolar reconstruction following SSM can be disappointing [10]. Data regarding the oncological safety of NSM is hampered by small sample size, varying indications and surgical techniques, and short follow-up (Table 2). There are limited oncological and reconstructive indications to perform NSM. Large tumors and those located in the central breast have an increased incidence of nipple involvement. Larger, more ptotic breasts are not good candidates for the procedure. Nipple elevation cannot be achieved without preservation of a dermoglandular pedicle which impacts the completeness of mastectomy. The ideal candidate for a NSM has small to moderate sized breasts with minimal ptosis.

3. Detection of local recurrence after breast reconstruction

The role of postreconstruction imaging after the treatment of breast cancer remains controversial. There is a paucity of data that addresses the issue and there no established guidelines [11]. The incidence of local recurrence of breast cancer is related to tumor stage. Most LRs after total mastectomy are in the skin and subcutaneous tissue and are readily detected by physical examination [12]. A flap or implant could potentially delay the discovery of chest wall recurrences.

Systemic relapse is not inevitable following local recurrence, especially after the treatment of DCIS [13, 14]. This argues that early detection of local recurrences may have a potential survival impact. All forms of mastectomy leave residual breast tissue. The differences are in terms of the microscopic breast tissue left behind in the skin and inframammary fold which are largely preserved after SSM. Torresan et al evaluated residual glandular tissue in the skin flaps that would have been preserved after SSM [15]. They found that 60% contained residual glandular tissue and it correlated with skin flap thickness.

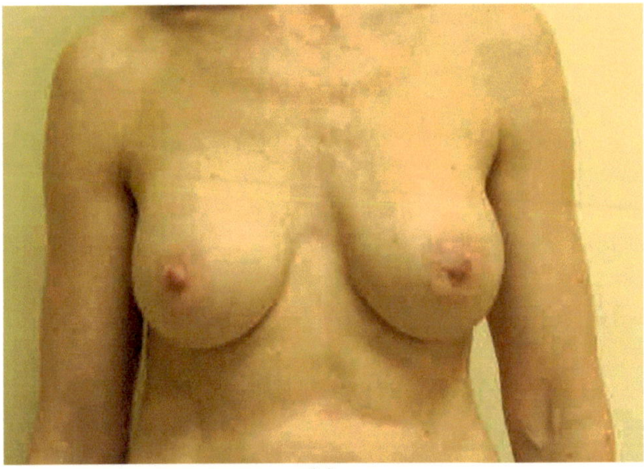

(a)

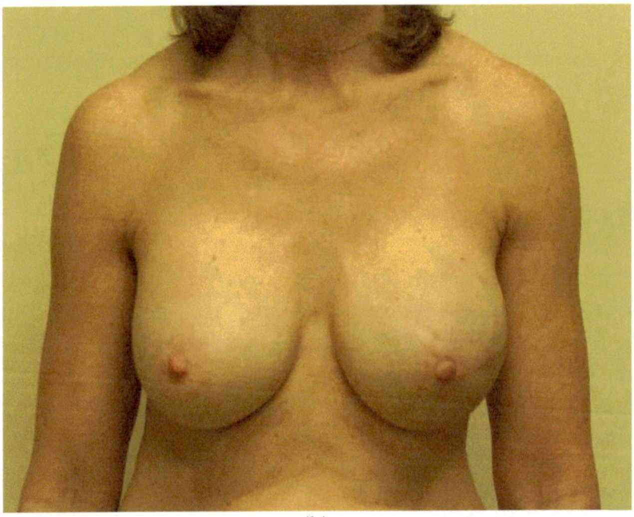

(b)

Fig. 2. (a) Preoperative photograph (b) Postoperative photograph after nipple sparing mastectomy and implant reconstruction

The completeness of mastectomy is important in the treatment of DCIS because most cases of recurrence represent unexcised residual disease. Several authors have reported LR of DCIS treated by SSM and IBR [13, 16, 17]. They found that the majority of LRs were invasive carcinomas. This suggests that postreconstruction mammography can have a role in the early detection of recurrences prior to the development of invasive carcinoma.

Physical examination of implant reconstruction is relatively easy. There is minimal soft tissue covering the implant except along the inframammary fold and in the axillary tail. Deep chest wall recurrences are extremely unlikely because the implants are placed in the submuscular plane. Conventional mammographic evaluation has limited utility because the implants obscure soft tissue visualization. MRI, which has been used extensively to evaluate the integrity of silicone gel implants, may have a role in the selective surveillance after implant reconstruction [18-21].

Study	N	LR (%)	NAC Recurrence (%)	Follow-up (months)
Gerber [89]	60	6 (10)	1 (1)	101
Caruso [90]	50	6 (12)	1 (2)	66
Sacchini [91]	68	2 (2.9)	0 (0)	26.4
Voltura [92]	32	2 (6.3)	0 (0)	18
Benediktsson [93]	169	48 (28.4)	0 (0)	156
Kim [94]	152	3 (9.1)	2 (1.3)	60

Table 2. Local recurrences after nipple sparing mastectomy

The sensitivity of physical examination of autologous reconstruction is lower than that seen with implant reconstruction. Deep chest wall recurrences often avoid detection until symptoms develop. Autologous reconstruction causes less impairment of mammographic tissue visualization [22]. Benign mammographic findings after TRAM flap reconstruction include fat necrosis, lipid cysts, calcifications, lymph nodes, and epidermal inclusion cysts (Figure 3) [23]. Breast cancer recurrences in autologous tissue reconstruction are mammographically similar to that of primary tumors (Figure 4) [24, 25]. Proponents of surveillance mammography feel that screening breast cancer patients with autologous reconstructions can detect nonpalpable recurrences before clinical examination.

Helvie et al evaluated surveillance mammography in 113 patients after TRAM flap reconstruction [26]. Six patients underwent biopsy for suspicious mammographic findings and two local recurrences were detected. Two patients in the study group went on to develop recurrences that were detected by physical examination. There was one false-negative mammogram resulting in a sensitivity of 67% and specificity of 98% for surveillance mammography after TRAM flap reconstruction.

There is a paucity of data regarding the efficacy of MRI of the breast following autogenous breast reconstruction [27, 28]. Breast MRI has been shown to clearly delineate autogenous flaps from residual mammary adipose tissue. The absence of contrast medium uptake during breast MRI precludes recurrent carcinoma to a high probability. Fat necrosis in a TRAM flap will show early postoperative contrast enhancement but this resolves within six to twelve months. Rieber et al evaluated MRI of the breast in the follow-up of forty-one patients who had undergone autogenous tissue breast reconstruction [29]. MRI was able to distinguish flaps from surrounding residual breast tissue in all cases. It excluded disease recurrence in 4 patients with suspicious mammographic or sonographic findings. It returned false-positive findings in three cases.

The potential indications for postreconstruction imaging include patients with close surgical margins and patients with diffuse DCIS treated by SSM. Its routine use after autologous reconstruction after SSM for invasive carcinoma warrants further study. The low detection rate and specificity does not justify the routine use of MRI in the follow-up of patients postreconstruction. MRI is most useful in patients with abnormal findings on physical examination or mammography and ultrasound. It is also helpful to delineate the extent of local disease recurrence.

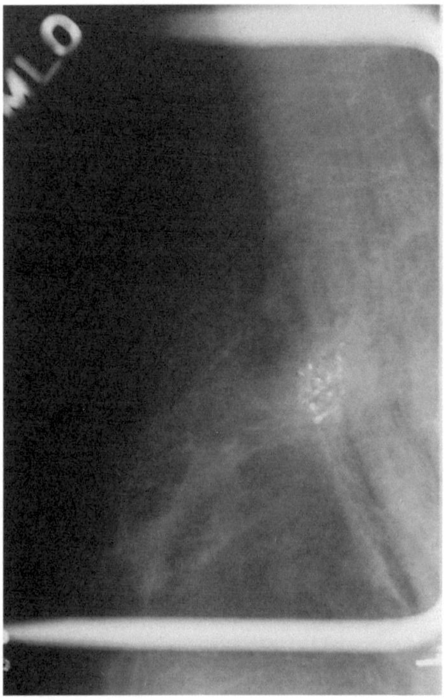

Fig. 3. Mammographic appearance of fat necrosis in a TRAM flap reconstruction

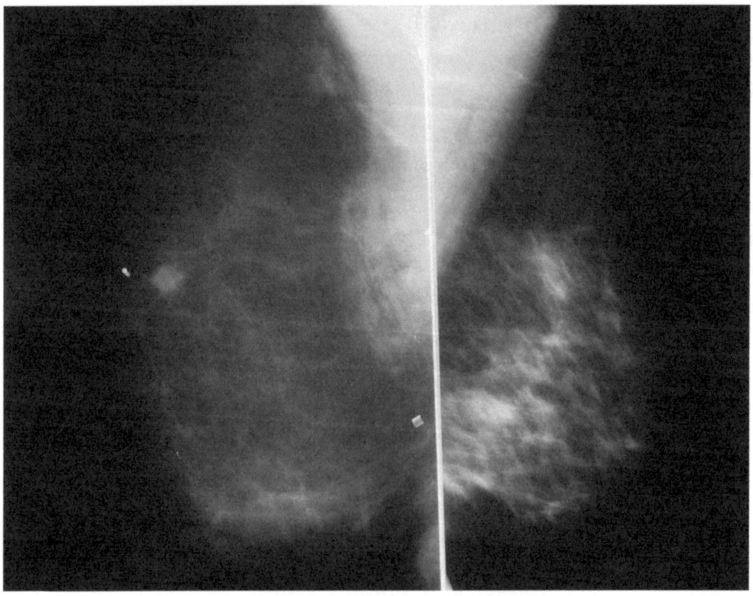

Fig. 4. Mammographic appearance of local recurrence in TRAM flap (L), opposite breast (R)

4. Breast reconstruction and adjuvant therapy

4.1 Chemotherapy

There are concerns that immediate breast reconstruction may delay the administration of adjuvant chemotherapy. A survey of 376 consultant breast surgeons in the United Kingdom and Ireland found that the majority (57%) preferred delayed reconstruction because of these concerns [30]. Breast reconstruction does have a high complication rate especially in patients who are obese, smoke tobacco, or have a history of chest wall irradiation. Alderman et al performed a multi-institutional study of complication rates after tissue expander or TRAM flap reconstruction [31]. They reported a 52% complication rate, with major complications occurring in 30% of patients.

It seems logical that the high complication rate of IBR could potentially delay the administration of adjuvant therapy. Studies comparing onset of chemotherapy after IBR and control group treated with mastectomy alone have failed to show significant differences [32-35]. Alderman et al performed a multi-institutional cohort study of 3643 breast cancer patients [35]. They found that IBR did not lead to an omission of adjuvant chemotherapy but was associated with a modest delay in initiating treatment. Wound complications after IBR must be treated aggressively to remove necrotic, potentially infected tissue. Patients with clean, open wounds can receive chemotherapy with minimal compromise in wound healing. These patients must be followed closely detect early signs of infection.

Patients with locally advanced, Stage III breast cancer are generally treated with chemotherapy followed by total mastectomy and adjuvant radiation. The five-year survival is 50%-80%, and patients with a poor response to chemotherapy have an especially bad prognosis. It may be preferable to delay reconstruction until after mastectomy and adjuvant radiation in these patients. This avoids the potential problems with radiation delivery and the adverse effects of postmastectomy radiation therapy on immediate reconstruction. These issues will be discussed in detail later in the chapter.

Neo-adjuvant chemotherapy may impact the complication rate of immediate breast reconstruction and delay adjuvant radiation. Mitchem et al evaluated the impact of neo-adjuvant chemotherapy on tissue expander reconstruction [36]. Eleven (32%) of 34 expanders required removal with infection accounting for 82% of implant losses. Deutsch et al reported a 55% complication rate in 31 patients after immediate TRAM flap reconstruction who received neo-adjuvant chemotherapy [37]. Six percent had a delay in resumption of chemotherapy because of complications. Sultan et al found a 14% complication rate in 21 patients who received neo-adjuvant chemotherapy and underwent IBR [38]. The mean interval between surgery and resumption of chemotherapy was 19 days and there was no delay in any patients. Mehrara et al found that neo-adjuvant chemotherapy was an independent predictor of overall complications in free flap breast reconstruction [39]. Zweifel-Schlatter et al compared 47 patients undergoing immediate free flap breast reconstruction after neo-adjuvant chemotherapy with 52 patients who did not receive preoperative therapy and found no delay in beginning adjuvant therapy [40].

4.2 Radiation therapy

Postmastectomy radiotherapy (PMRT) is increasing utilized in the adjuvant treatment of breast cancer. The current recommendations for PMRT include patients with 4 or more positive axillary lymph nodes, locally advanced cancer, tumors 5 cm. or larger and positive margins. It is considered for medial quadrant tumors, tumors with lymphovascular invasion, and in patients with 1-3 metastatic lymph nodes. Two randomized trials have shown a survival benefit for post-mastectomy radiotherapy in patients with 1-3 metastatic lymph nodes [41, 42]. These studies were criticized because of high rate of regional failure in the non-irradiated group which was felt the result of inadequate axillary surgery and the use of non-anthracycline based chemotherapy. A survey of radiation oncologists found that only 58% would use PMRT in patients with 1-3 metastatic lymph nodes but 95% would recommend it for patients with 4 or more metastatic nodes [43].

There are technical problems related to irradiation of the reconstructed breast. Distortion of the chest wall anatomy means that radiotherapy portals need to be modified. The treatment is more difficult, particularly irradiating the internal mammary lymph nodes. This may result changing the depth of tangential fields resulting in increased volume of irradiated lung or heart. Motwani et al examined the effect of immediate autologous breast reconstruction on the technical delivery of PMRT [44]. Two radiation oncologists reviewed radiotherapy plans in 110 patients. These were compared to matched controls that had mastectomy alone. A scoring system was used that evaluated chest wall coverage, treatment of the internal mammary lymph node chain, minimization of lung exposure, and avoidance of the heart. They found that 52% of the immediate reconstruction patients had compromise of their radiotherapy plans compared to 7% of controls. If coverage of the internal mammary lymph nodes was eliminated, 23% of the IBR group had compromised plans. M.D. Anderson Cancer Center recommends deflating tissue expanders prior to the administration of PMRT to overcome potential dosimetry compromise [45]. Most institutions feel that the potential interference of breast implants with can overcome with alteration in treatment planning.

Radiation therapy has a negative impact on all forms of breast reconstruction. A meta-analysis of over 1,000 patients showed that patients undergoing PMRT and breast reconstruction were more likely to suffer morbidity compared to patients not receiving PMRT [46]. It also showed that autologous reconstruction was associated with less morbidity than implant reconstruction when PMRT was administered. There are three clinical scenarios that are encountered: immediate reconstruction in patients, who have received preoperative radiation, delayed reconstruction after PMRT, and immediate reconstruction in patients who will receive PMRT. Berry et al, reviewed 1037 cases of immediate breast reconstruction (expander 559 and autologous 478) [47]. Radiation whether administered preoperatively or postoperatively significantly increased the complication rate in expander reconstruction but had no significant impact on autologous reconstruction.

Chest wall irradiation after expander / implant reconstructions results in an increase incidence of capsular contraction and implant exposure. Because of this, many authors feel that implant reconstruction is contraindicated when postmastectomy radiation is planned. Krueger et al performed a prospective evaluation of tissue expander reconstruction in 81 patients, including 19 patients who received radiation [48]. Patients receiving radiation had a two fold increase in complications ($p=0.006$) and a four fold increase in reconstruction failure ($p=0.005$). The addition of autologous tissue such as the latissimus flap may reduce the risk of complications seen with the use of implants in the setting of radiation [49].

Radiation also has a deleterious effect on TRAM flap reconstruction as evidenced by increased incidence of fibrosis, fat necrosis, and revisional surgery [50-52]. There is an unpredictable volume, contour, and symmetry loss that is seen with pedicled TRAM flaps, free TRAM flaps, and DIEP flaps. Tran et al reviewed the M.D. Anderson Cancer Center experience of TRAM flap irradiation [52]. The review included 41 TRAM flaps (free TRAM 32, pedicled TRAM 9). Ten patients (24%) required an additional flap to correct radiation induced contracture. Nine patients (22%) maintained normal breast volume and palpable fat necrosis was noted in 34% of flaps. The paper by Rogers and Allen has demonstrated similar deleterious effects of radiation on DIEP flap reconstruction [51]. They reported a 23.3% incidence of fat necrosis in the radiated group vs. 0% incidence in the control group. Radiation fibrosis was seen in 56.7% of cases with 5 (16.7%) requiring surgical revision.

5. The treatment of local recurrence after breast reconstruction

Surgical options following LR after breast reconstruction depend on the location and number of metastatic deposits and previous treatment. Imaging of the reconstructed breast and body scans are necessary to delineate the extent of tumor involvement (Figure 4). Isolated local recurrences can be treated with removal of as much reconstructed tissue as necessary to achieve negative margins. Adjuvant chest wall radiation is usually administered (Figure 5).

In cases of implant reconstruction, it may be necessary to remove a portion of the implant capsule necessitating implant removal in some cases [53]. Howard et al reviewed 16 cases of LR after TRAM flap reconstruction [54]. Eight recurrences occurred in the skin and were detected on physical examination. Eight recurrences occurred in the chest wall and were symptomatic, being detected on physical examination or diagnostic imaging. Twelve were felt amenable to surgical resection and three required removal of the entire TRAM flap.

6. Oncological considerations in partial mastectomy reconstruction

Oncoplastic surgery combines the principles of oncologic surgery (breast conserving therapy) and plastic surgery (breast reconstruction). It has the potential for better tumor free margins and enhancement of the cosmetic outcome [55]. Reconstruction can be performed via parenchymal rearrangement or volume replacement with local or distant flaps [56, 57].

Studies suggest these techniques are associated with low local recurrence but the long term oncological safety of these procedures is not clearly defined [58]. Young patients, especially those with diffuse high grade DCIS; do not appear to be good candidates because of the increase in margin involvement and LR. Follow-up mammographic evaluation does not appear to be significantly impacted by onco-plastic reconstruction.

6.1 Sentinel lymph node biopsy and breast reconstruction

Sentinel lymph node biopsy has replaced axillary dissection as the standard of care for axillary node sampling. The sensitivity of intraoperative pathological SLN analysis is 68%-91% [59-61]. It is related to the size of the metastatic deposits which is related to tumor size. False negative intraoperative diagnoses of sentinel lymph node metastases present unique problems in breast cancer patients after immediate breast reconstruction. The standard of care for patients with tumor positive SLNs is a completion axillary lymph node dissection. This procedure can be technically demanding if a latissimus dorsi flap reconstruction has been performed or the thoracodorsal vessels have been used for microvascular reconstruction [62]. Fortunately, the internal mammary vessels have become the vessels of choice for microsurgical breast reconstruction. They are easier to access and permit early postoperative arm mobilization without risk of injury to the flap vascular pedicle. Vessel location facilitates placement and the latissimus dorsi muscle blood supply is preserved if salvage surgery is necessary. Internal mammary lymph nodes can sometimes be encountered at the time of vessel dissection [63]. Involvement of these lymph nodes has prognostic significance and should be biopsied when they are discovered.

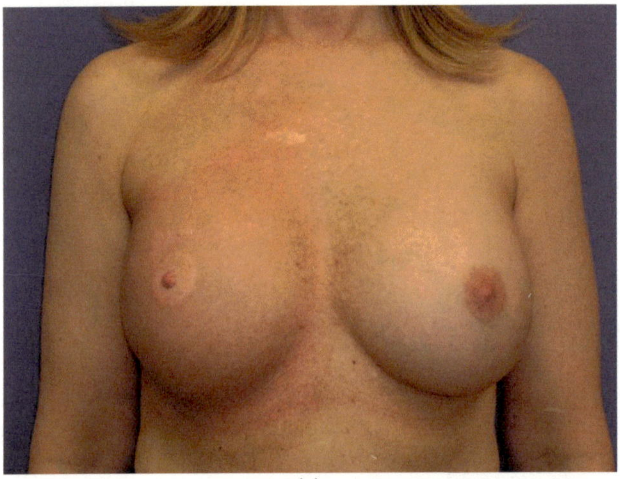

(a)

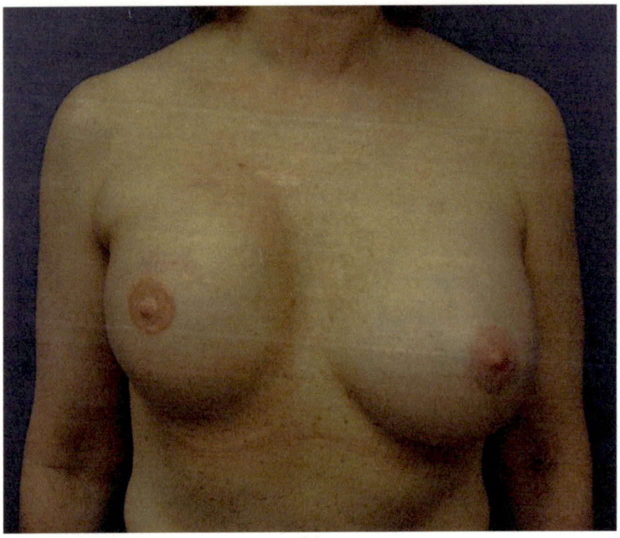

(b)

Fig. 5. (a) Photograph tissue expander reconstruction of the right breast immediately after completing radiation (b) Appearance 12 months after completing radiation

A few studies have suggested SLN biopsy prior to mastectomy and IBR to avoid potential complications seen with PMRT [64-66]. This could facilitate decision making regarding immediate breast reconstruction and avoid a second operation in cases of FNG SLN biopsies. McGuire et al found that SLN biopsy before mastectomy and IBR changed the operative strategy in 62% of patients [67].

7. Contralateral prophylactic mastectomy

More women are choosing to have a contralateral prophylactic mastectomy (CPM) at the time of treatment of their unilateral breast cancer. Tuttle et al used SEER data to evaluate the treatment of unilateral breast cancer from 1998-2003 [68]. They found the rate of CPM in women undergoing total mastectomy more than doubled in the six year period. The use of CPM is associated with younger patient age, a family history of breast cancer, the use of immediate breast reconstruction, the use of breast MRI at the time of diagnosis, non-invasive histology, and prior attempts at breast conservation [68-73].

Contralateral prophylactic mastectomy at the time of total mastectomy and IBR has two main advantages: it reduces the risk of developing a new cancer and it facilitates breast reconstruction. Women with unilateral breast cancer have an increased risk of developing a second cancer in the contralateral breast. The annual incidence of new breast cancer has been reported to be 0.7% - 1.8% [74-76]. Adjuvant hormonal therapy has been shown to reduce this risk. Despite the high incidence of cancer development, most patients will not experience a survival benefit from a CPM. The risk of systemic metastases from the index cancer exceeds the risk of contralateral cancers, which tend to be lower in stage. Younger women with stage I and II estrogen receptor negative cancer have been shown to benefit from CPM [70].

The Society of Surgical Oncology updated their position statement on prophylactic mastectomy in 2007 [77]. It detailed potential indications in patients with current or previous diagnosis of breast cancer to include:

- Patients at high risk of contralateral breast cancer (BRCA mutation, strong family history)
- Patients with mammographically dense breasts or those with diffuse indeterminate microcalcifications
- Patients with unilateral breast cancer treated by total mastectomy and IBR who desire improved symmetry or have a desire for bilateral reconstruction

A CPM and bilateral reconstruction is especially useful in cases of implant based reconstruction (Figure 6). The contralateral breast frequently requires remedial surgery to achieve symmetry with an implant reconstructed breast. Clough et al found that the cosmetic outcome of unilateral implant reconstruction deteriorated with time [78]. They attributed this asymmetry largely to ptosis of the native breast seen with aging. Bilateral reconstruction would prevent this asymmetry development.

The majority of women are satisfied with their decision to undergo CPM [79]. The most common reasons for regret appear to be poor cosmetic outcome and a diminished sense of sexuality [80].

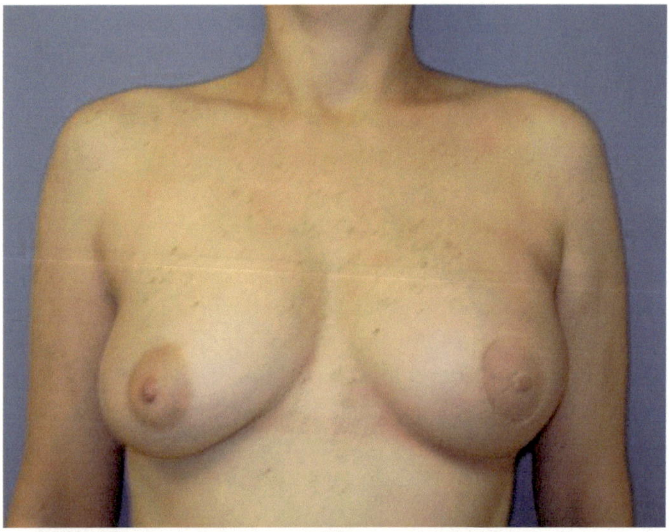

(a)

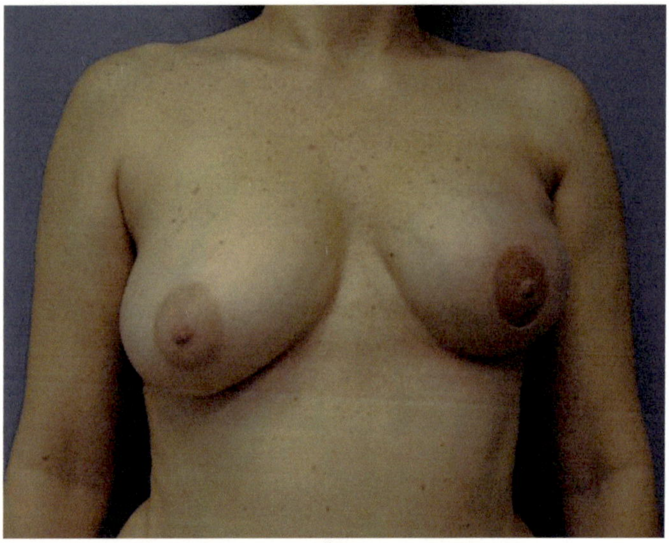

(b)

Fig. 6. (a) Photograph after left TRAM flap reconstruction (b) Appearance 12 months after completing radiation.

8. References

[1] Alderman, AK, McMahon, L, Jr., and Wilkins, EG, *The national utilization of immediate and early delayed breast reconstruction and the effect of sociodemographic factors. Plast Reconstr Surg*, 2003. 111(2): p. 695-703; discussion 704-5.

[2] Polednak, AP, *How frequent is postmastectomy breast reconstructive surgery? A study linking two statewide databases. Plast Reconstr Surg*, 2001. 108(1): p. 73-7.

[3] DeBono, R, Thompson, A, and Stevenson, JH, *Immediate versus delayed free TRAM breast reconstruction: an analysis of perioperative factors and complications. Br J Plast Surg,* 2002. 55(2): p. 111-6.

[4] Schain, WS, Wellisch, DK, Pasnau, RO, et al., *The sooner the better: a study of psychological factors in women undergoing immediate versus delayed breast reconstruction. Am J Psychiatry,* 1985. 142(1): p. 40-6.

[5] Agarwal, S, Liu, JH, Crisera, CA, et al., *Survival in breast cancer patients undergoing immediate breast reconstruction.* Breast J, 2010. 16(5): p. 503-9.

[6] Carlson, GW, Skin sparing mastectomy: anatomic and technical considerations. Am Surg, 1996. 62(2): p. 151-5.

[7] Carlson, GW, Bostwick, J, 3rd, Styblo, TM, et al., *Skin-sparing mastectomy. Oncologic and reconstructive considerations.* Ann Surg, 1997. 225(5): p. 570-5; discussion 575-8.

[8] Kroll, SS, Khoo, A, Singletary, SE, et al., *Local recurrence risk after skin-sparing and conventional mastectomy: a 6-year follow-up.* Plast Reconstr Surg, 1999. 104(2): p. 421-5.

[9] Simmons, RM, Fish, SK, Gayle, L, et al., *Local and distant recurrence rates in skin-sparing mastectomies compared with non-skin-sparing mastectomies. Ann Surg Oncol,* 1999. 6(7): p. 676-81.

[10] Zhong, T, Antony, A, and Cordeiro, P, *Surgical outcomes and nipple projection using the modified skate flap for nipple-areolar reconstruction in a series of 422 implant reconstructions. Ann Plast Surg,* 2009. 62(5): p. 591-5.

[11] Barnsley, GP, Grunfeld, E, Coyle, D, et al., *Surveillance mammography following the treatment of primary breast cancer with breast reconstruction: a systematic review. Plast Reconstr Surg,* 2007. 120(5): p. 1125-32.

[12] Langstein, HN, Cheng, MH, Singletary, SE, et al., *Breast cancer recurrence after immediate reconstruction: patterns and significance.* Plast Reconstr Surg, 2003. 111(2): p. 712-20; discussion 721-2.

[13] Carlson, GW, Page, A, Johnson, E, et al., *Local recurrence of ductal carcinoma in situ after skin-sparing mastectomy.* J Am Coll Surg, 2007. 204(5): p. 1074-8; discussion 1078-80.

[14] Carlson, GW, Styblo, TM, Lyles, RH, et al., *Local recurrence after skin-sparing mastectomy: tumor biology or surgical conservatism?* Ann Surg Oncol, 2003. 10(2): p. 108-12.

[15] Torresan, RZ, dos Santos, CC, Okamura, H, et al., *Evaluation of residual glandular tissue after skin-sparing mastectomies.* Ann Surg Oncol, 2005. 12(12): p. 1037-44.

[16] Rubio, IT, Mirza, N, Sahin, AA, et al., *Role of specimen radiography in patients treated with skin-sparing mastectomy for ductal carcinoma in situ of the breast. Ann Surg Oncol,* 2000. 7(7): p. 544-8.

[17] Slavin, SA, Love, SM, and Goldwyn, RM, *Recurrent breast cancer following immediate reconstruction with myocutaneous flaps.* Plast Reconstr Surg, 1994. 93(6): p. 1191-204; discussion 1205-7.

[18] Bone, B, Aspelin, P, Isberg, B, et al., *Contrast-enhanced MR imaging of the breast in patients with breast implants after cancer surgery. Acta Radiol,* 1995. 36(2). p. 111-6.

[19] Gorczyca, DP, Sinha, S, Ahn, CY, et al., *Silicone breast implants in vivo: MR imaging.* Radiology, 1992. 185(2). p. 407-10.

[20] Harms, SE, Flamig, DP, Evans, WP, et al., *MR imaging of the breast: current status and future potential.* AJR Am J Roentgenol, 1994. 163(5): p. 1039-47.

[21] Heywang, SH, Hilbertz, T, Beck, R, et al., *Gd-DTPA enhanced MR imaging of the breast in patients with postoperative scarring and silicon implants. J Comput Assist Tomogr*, 1990. 14(3): p. 348-56.

[22] Lindbichler, F, Hoflehner, H, Schmidt, F, et al., *Comparison of mammographic image quality in various methods of reconstructive breast surgery. Eur Radiol*, 1996. 6(6): p. 925-8.

[23] Hogge, JP, Robinson, RE, Magnant, CM, et al., *The mammographic spectrum of fat necrosis of the breast.* Radiographics, 1995. 15(6): p. 1347-56.

[24] Eidelman, Y, Liebling, RW, Buchbinder, S, et al., *Mammography in the evaluation of masses in breasts reconstructed with TRAM flaps.* Ann Plast Surg, 1998. 41(3): p. 229-33.

[25] Helvie, MA, Wilson, TE, Roubidoux, MA, et al., *Mammographic appearance of recurrent breast carcinoma in six patients with TRAM flap breast reconstructions. Radiology*, 1998. 209(3): p. 711-5.

[26] Helvie, MA, Bailey, JE, Roubidoux, MA, et al., *Mammographic screening of TRAM flap breast reconstructions for detection of nonpalpable recurrent cancer. Radiology*, 2002. 224(1): p. 211-6.

[27] Ahn, CY, Narayanan, K, Gorczyca, DP, et al., *Evaluation of autogenous tissue breast reconstruction using MRI.* Plast Reconstr Surg, 1995. 95(1): p. 70-6.

[28] Kurtz, B, Audretsch, W, Rezai, M, et al., *[Initial experiences with MR-mammography in after-care following surgical flap treatment of breast carcinoma].* Rofo Fortschr Geb Rontgenstr Neuen Bildgeb Verfahr, 1996. 164(4): p. 295- 300.

[29] Rieber, A, Schramm, K, Helms, G, et al., *Breast-conserving surgery and autogenous tissue reconstruction in patients with breast cancer: efficacy of MRI of the breast in the detection of recurrent disease. Eur Radiol*, 2003. 13(4): p. 780-7.

[30] Callaghan, CJ, Couto, E, Kerin, MJ, et al., *Breast reconstruction in the United Kingdom and Ireland.* Br J Surg, 2002. 89(3): p. 335-40.

[31] Alderman, AK, Wilkins, EG, Kim, HM, et al., *Complications in postmastectomy breast reconstruction: two-year results of the Michigan Breast Reconstruction Outcome Study. Plast Reconstr Surg*, 2002. 109(7): p. 2265-74.

[32] Allweis, TM, Boisvert, ME, Otero, SE, et al., *Immediate reconstruction after mastectomy for breast cancer does not prolong the time to starting adjuvant chemotherapy. Am J Surg*, 2002. 183(3): p. 218-21.

[33] Caffo, O, Cazzolli, D, Scalet, A, et al., *Concurrent adjuvant chemotherapy and immediate breast reconstruction with skin expanders after mastectomy for breast cancer. Breast Cancer Res Treat*, 2000. 60(3): p. 267-75.

[34] Taylor, CW, Horgan, K, and Dodwell, D, *Oncological aspects of breast reconstruction.* Breast, 2005. 14(2): p. 118-30.

[35] Alderman, AK, Collins, ED, Schott, A, et al., *The impact of breast reconstruction on the delivery of chemotherapy.* Cancer, 2010. 116(7): p. 1791-800.

[36] Mitchem, J, Herrmann, D, Margenthaler, JA, et al., *Impact of neoadjuvant chemotherapy on rate of tissue expander/implant loss and progression to successful breast reconstruction following mastectomy. Am J Surg*, 2008. 196(4): p. 519-22.

[37] Deutsch, MF, Smith, M, Wang, B, et al., *Immediate breast reconstruction with the TRAM flap after neoadjuvant therapy.* Ann Plast Surg, 1999. 42(3): p. 240-4.

[38] Sultan, MR, Smith, ML, Estabrook, A, et al., *Immediate breast reconstruction in patients with locally advanced disease.* Ann Plast Surg, 1997. 38(4): p. 345-9; discussion 350-1.

[39] Mehrara, BJ, Santoro, TD, Arcilla, E, et al., *Complications after microvascular breast reconstruction: experience with 1195 flaps.* Plast Reconstr Surg, 2006. 118(5): p. 1100-9; discussion 1110-1.

[40] Zweifel-Schlatter, M, Darhouse, N, Roblin, P, et al., *Immediate microvascular breast reconstruction after neoadjuvant chemotherapy: complication rates and effect on start of adjuvant treatment. Ann Surg Oncol,* 2010. 17(11): p. 2945-50.

[41] Ragaz, J, Jackson, SM, Le, N, et al., *Adjuvant radiotherapy and chemotherapy in node-positive premenopausal women with breast cancer [see comments]. N Engl J Med,* 1997. 337(14): p. 956-62.

[42] Overgaard, M, Hansen, PS, Overgaard, J, et al., *Postoperative radiotherapy in high-risk premenopausal women with breast cancer who receive adjuvant chemotherapy. Danish Breast Cancer Cooperative Group 82b Trial* [see comments]. *N Engl J Med,* 1997. 337(14): p. 949-55.

[43] Ceilley, E, Jagsi, R, Goldberg, S, et al., *Radiotherapy for invasive breast cancer in North America and Europe: results of a survey.* Int J Radiat Oncol Biol Phys, 2005. 61(2): p. 365-73.

[44] Motwani, SB, Strom, EA, Schechter, NR, et al., *The impact of immediate breast reconstruction on the technical delivery of postmastectomy radiotherapy.* Int J Radiat Oncol Biol Phys, 2006. 66(1): p. 76-82.

[45] Kronowitz, SJ, Hunt, KK, Kuerer, HM, et al., *Delayed-immediate breast reconstruction.* Plast Reconstr Surg, 2004. 113(6): p. 1617-28.

[46] Barry, M and Kell, MR, *Radiotherapy and breast reconstruction: a meta-analysis.* Breast Cancer Res Treat, 2011. 127(1): p. 15-22.

[47] Berry, T, Brooks, S, Sydow, N, et al., *Complication rates of radiation on tissue expander and autologous tissue breast reconstruction. Ann Surg Oncol.* 17 Suppl 3: p. 202-10.

[48] Krueger, EA, Wilkins, EG, Strawderman, M, et al., *Complications and patient satisfaction following expander/implant breast reconstruction with and without radiotherapy. Int J Radiat Oncol Biol Phys,* 2001. 49(3): p. 713-21.

[49] Chang, DW, Barnea, Y, and Robb, GL, *Effects of an autologous flap combined with an implant for breast reconstruction: an evaluation of 1000 consecutive reconstructions of previously irradiated breasts. Plast Reconstr Surg,* 2008. 122(2): p. 356-62.

[50] Carlson, GW, Page, AL, Peters, K, et al., *Effects of radiation therapy on pedicled transverse rectus abdominis myocutaneous flap breast reconstruction. Ann Plast Surg,* 2008. 60(5): p. 568-72.

[51] Rogers, NE and Allen, RJ, *Radiation effects on breast reconstruction with the deep inferior epigastric perforator flap.* Plast Reconstr Surg, 2002. 109(6): p. 1919-24; discussion 1925-6.

[52] Tran, NV, Evans, GR, Kroll, SS, et al., *Postoperative adjuvant irradiation: effects on tranverse rectus abdominis muscle flap breast reconstruction.* Plast Reconstr Surg, 2000. 106(2): p. 313-7; discussion 318-20.

[53] McCarthy, CM, Pusic, AL, Sclafani, L, et al., *Breast cancer recurrence following prosthetic, postmastectomy reconstruction: incidence, detection, and treatment. Plast Reconstr Surg,* 2008. 121(2): p. 381-8.

[54] Howard, MA, Polo, K, Pusic, AL, et al., *Breast cancer local recurrence after mastectomy and TRAM flap reconstruction: incidence and treatment options. Plast Reconstr Surg,* 2006. 117(5): p. 1381-6.

[55] Clough, KB, Thomas, SS, Fitoussi, AD, et al., *Reconstruction after conservative treatment for breast cancer: cosmetic sequelae classification revisited. Plast Reconstr Surg,* 2004. 114(7): p. 1743-53.

[56] Clough, KB, Kroll, SS, and Audretsch, W, *An approach to the repair of partial mastectomy defects.* Plast Reconstr Surg, 1999. 104(2): p. 409-20.

[57] Kat, CC, Darcy, CM, O'Donoghue, JM, et al., *The use of the latissimus dorsi musculocutaneous flap for immediate correction of the deformity resulting from breast conservation surgery. Br J Plast Surg,* 1999. 52(2): p. 99-103.

[58] Asgeirsson, KS, Rasheed, T, McCulley, SJ, et al., *Oncological and cosmetic outcomes of oncoplastic breast conserving surgery.* Eur J Surg Oncol, 2005. 31(8): p. 817-23.

[59] Chao, C, Wong, SL, Ackermann, D, et al., *Utility of intraoperative frozen section analysis of sentinel lymph nodes in breast cancer. Am J Surg,* 2001. 182(6): p. 609-15.

[60] Dupont, EL, Kuhn, MA, McCann, C, et al., *The role of sentinel lymph node biopsy in women undergoing prophylactic mastectomy. Am J Surg,* 2000. 180(4): p. 274-7.

[61] Khalifa, K, Pereira, B, Thomas, VA, et al., *The accuracy of intraoperative frozen section analysis of the sentinel lymph nodes during breast cancer surgery. Int J Fertil Womens Med,* 2004. 49(5): p. 208-11.

[62] Kronowitz, SJ, Chang, DW, Robb, GL, et al., *Implications of axillary sentinel lymph node biopsy in immediate autologous breast reconstruction. Plast Reconstr Surg,* 2002. 109(6): p. 1888-96.

[63] Hofer, SO, Rakhorst, HA, Mureau, MA, et al., *Pathological internal mammary lymph nodes in secondary and tertiary deep inferior epigastric perforator flap breast reconstructions. Ann Plast Surg,* 2005. 55(6): p. 583-6.

[64] Brady, B, Fant, J, Jones, R, et al., *Sentinel lymph node biopsy followed by delayed mastectomy and reconstruction. Am J Surg,* 2003. 185(2): p. 114-7.

[65] Klauber-Demore, N, Calvo, BF, Hultman, CS, et al., *Staged sentinel lymph node biopsy before mastectomy facilitates surgical planning for breast cancer patients. Am J Surg,* 2005. 190(4): p. 595-7.

[66] Schrenk, P, Woelfl, S, Bogner, S, et al., *The use of sentinel node biopsy in breast cancer patients undergoing skin sparing mastectomy and immediate autologous reconstruction. Plast Reconstr Surg,* 2005. 116(5): p. 1278-86.

[67] McGuire, K, Rosenberg, AL, Showalter, S, et al., *Timing of sentinel lymph node biopsy and reconstruction for patients undergoing mastectomy.* Ann Plast Surg, 2007. 59(4): p. 359-63.

[68] Tuttle, TM, Habermann, EB, Grund, EH, et al., *Increasing use of contralateral prophylactic mastectomy for breast cancer patients: a trend toward more aggressive surgical treatment. J Clin Oncol,* 2007. 25(33): p. 5203-9.

[69] Arrington, AK, Jarosek, SL, Virnig, BA, et al., *Patient and surgeon characteristics associated with increased use of contralateral prophylactic mastectomy in patients with breast cancer. Ann Surg Oncol,* 2009. 16(10): p. 2697-704.

[70] Bedrosian, I, Hu, CY, and Chang, GJ, *Population-based study of contralateral prophylactic mastectomy and survival outcomes of breast cancer patients. J Natl Cancer Inst.* 102(6): p. 401-9.

[71] Jones, NB, Wilson, J, Kotur, L, et al., *Contralateral prophylactic mastectomy for unilateral breast cancer: an increasing trend at a single institution. Ann Surg Oncol,* 2009. 16(10): p. 2691-6.

[72] King, TA, Sakr, R, Patil, S, et al., *Clinical management factors contribute to the decision for contralateral prophylactic mastectomy. J Clin Oncol*, 2011. 29(16): p. 2158-64.

[73] Tuttle, TM, Jarosek, S, Habermann, EB, et al., *Increasing rates of contralateral prophylactic mastectomy among patients with ductal carcinoma in situ. J Clin Oncol*, 2009. 27(9): p. 1362-7.

[74] Hankey, BF, Curtis, RE, Naughton, MD, et al., *A retrospective cohort analysis of second breast cancer risk for primary breast cancer patients with an assessment of the effect of radiation therapy. J Natl Cancer Inst*, 1983. 70(5): p. 797-804.

[75] Peralta, EA, Ellenhorn, JD, Wagman, LD, et al., Contralateral prophylactic mastectomy improves the outcome of selected patients undergoing mastectomy for breast cancer. Am J Surg, 2000. 180(6): p. 439-45.

[76] Rosen, PP, Groshen, S, Kinne, DW, et al., *Contralateral breast carcinoma: an assessment of risk and prognosis in stage I (T1N0M0) and stage II (T1N1M0) patients with 20-year follow-up. Surgery*, 1989. 106(5): p. 904-10.

[77] Giuliano, AE, Boolbol, S, Degnim, A, et al., *Society of Surgical Oncology: position statement on prophylactic mastectomy. Approved by the Society of Surgical Oncology Executive Council, March 2007. Ann Surg Oncol*, 2007. 14(9): p. 2425-7.

[78] Clough, KB, O'Donoghue, JM, Fitoussi, AD, et al., *Prospective evaluation of late cosmetic results following breast reconstruction: I. Implant reconstruction. Plast Reconstr Surg*, 2001. 107(7): p. 1702-9.

[79] Frost, MH, Slezak, JM, Tran, NV, et al., *Satisfaction after contralateral prophylactic mastectomy: the significance of mastectomy type, reconstructive complications, and body appearance. J Clin Oncol*, 2005. 23(31): p. 7849-56.

[80] Montgomery, LL, Tran, KN, Heelan, MC, et al., *Issues of regret in women with contralateral prophylactic mastectomies.* Ann Surg Oncol, 1999. 6(6): p. 546-52.

[81] Newman, LA, Kuerer, HM, Hunt, KK, et al., *Presentation, treatment, and outcome of local recurrence afterskin- sparing mastectomy and immediate breast reconstruction. Ann Surg Oncol*, 1998. 5(7): p. 620-6.

[82] Rivadeneira, DE, Simmons, RM, Fish, SK, et al., *Skin sparing mastectomy with immediate breast reconstruction: a critical analysis of local recurrence. Cancer J, 2000.* 6(5): p. 331-5.

[83] Medina-Franco, H, Vasconez, LO, Fix, RJ, et al., *Factors associated with local recurrence after skin-sparing mastectomy and immediate breast reconstruction for invasive breast cancer. Ann Surg*, 2002. 235(6): p. 814-9.

[84] Carlson, GW, Styblo, TM, Lyles, RH, et al., *Local recurrence after skin-sparing mastectomy: tumor biology or surgical conservatism?* Ann Surg Oncol, 2003. 10(2): p. 108-12.

[85] Slavin, SA, Schnitt, SJ, Duda, RB, et al., *Skin-sparing mastectomy and immediate reconstruction: oncologic risks and aesthetic results in patients with early-stage breast cancer. Plast Reconstr Surg*, 1998. 102(1): p. 49-62.

[86] Toth, BA, Forley, BG, and Calabria, R, *Retrospective study of the skin-sparing mastectomy in breast reconstruction.* Plast Reconstr Surg, 1999. 104(1): p. 77-84.

[87] Spiegel, AJ and Butler, CE, *Recurrence following treatment of ductal carcinoma in situ with skin-sparing mastectomy and immediate breast reconstruction. Plast Reconstr Surg*, 2003. 111(2): p. 706-11.

[88] Foster, RD, Esserman, LJ, Anthony, JP, et al., *Skin-sparing mastectomy and immediate breast reconstruction: a prospective cohort study for the treatment of advanced stages of breast carcinoma. Ann Surg Oncol*, 2002. 9(5): p. 462-6.

[89] Gerber, B, Krause, A, Dieterich, M, et al., *The Oncological Safety of Skin Sparing Mastectomy With Conservation of the Nipple-Areola Complex and Autologous Reconstruction: An Extended Follow-Up Study. Ann Surg*, 2009.

[90] Caruso, F, Ferrara, M, Castiglione, G, et al., *Nipple sparing subcutaneous mastectomy: sixty-six months follow-up.* Eur J Surg Oncol, 2006. 32(9): p. 937-40.

[91] Sacchini, V, Pinotti, JA, Barros, AC, et al., *Nipple-sparing mastectomy for breast cancer and risk reduction: oncologic or technical problem? J Am Coll Surg*, 2006. 203(5): p. 704-14.

[92] Voltura, AM, Tsangaris, TN, Rosson, GD, et al., *Nipple-sparing mastectomy: critical assessment of 51 procedures and implications for selection criteria. Ann Surg Oncol*, 2008. 15(12): p. 3396-401.

[93] Benediktsson, KP and Perbeck, L, *Survival in breast cancer after nipple-sparing subcutaneous mastectomy and immediate reconstruction with implants: a prospective trial with 13 years median follow-up in 216 patients. Eur J Surg Oncol*, 2008. 34(2): p. 143-8.

[94] Kim, HJ, Park, EH, Lim, WS, et al., *Nipple areola skin-sparing mastectomy with immediate transverse rectus abdominis musculocutaneous flap reconstruction is an oncologically safe procedure: a single center study. Ann Surg*, 2010. 251(3): p. 493-8.

Part 2

Prosthetic Breast Reconstruction

2

Implant and Implant Assisted Breast Reconstructions

Sarah S.K. Tang and Gerald P.H. Gui
Royal Marsden NHS Trust,
United Kingdom

1. Introduction

The number of women in the USA with breast implants is now estimated at over 6 million based on national surveys. This is numerically in excess of 5% of the female adult population. The majority of these women had cosmetic augmentations but 20-30% had implant based post-mastectomy breast reconstructions or correction of congenital abnormalities. In 2010, 296203 breast augmentations were performed in the USA and silicone implants were used in 60% of cases (American Society of Plastic Surgeons [ASPS], 2010). 93083 breast reconstructions were performed for congenital or postmastectomy defects. Of these 67% were performed using tissue expander and implant techniques. The significant majority of implants used in breast reconstruction were silicone (73%). Reconstructions using autologous tissue formed a small percentage of overall reconstructions (transverse rectus abdominus myocutaneous flaps (TRAM) 7%, latissimus dorsi (LD) flaps 7% and deep inferior epigastric perforator flaps (DIEP) 5%).

RECONSTRUCTIVE PROCEDURES	TOTAL PROCEDURES	13-19	20-29	30-39	40-54	55 AND OVER
Breast reconstruction	93,083	555	2,466	11,203	47,155	31,704
Saline Implants	18,334	-	-	-	-	-
Silicone Implants	50,559	-	-	-	-	-
Implant alone	9,452	-	-	-	-	-
Tissue expander and implant	62,081	-	-	-	-	-
TRAM flap	6,758	-	-	-	-	-
DIEP flap	5,118	-	-	-	-	-
Latissimus Dorsi Flap	6,335	-	-	-	-	-
Breast reduction	83,241	4,645	13,464	19,950	30,251	14,931
Breast implant removals (Reconstructive patients only)	14,991	134	1,031	2,870	6,779	4,177

Table 1. Breakdown of breast reconstruction procedures performed in 2010 according to procedure type and age range (ASPS, Report of the 2010 Plastic Surgery Statistics)

The history of implant based breast reconstruction spans five decades when the first silicone breast implants became available. The last 20 years have seen rapid advances in expander and implant technology such that the era in which implant reconstructions aimed at simply producing the appearance of a breast mound in clothing has transitioned into the current era in which in appropriately selected patients an implant based reconstruction has the potential to resemble a natural breast in contour, projection and a well-defined inframammary crease.

A common misconception is that breast reconstructions with autologous tissue are necessarily superior in quality compared to reconstructions with implants. Patient selection and a full discussion on rewards versus risks enable patient choice in making an informed decision about the reconstructive options available. The longer complex procedures to harvest autologous donor material, often involving microvascular surgery, are associated with donor site healing and scars with a longer period of recovery compared with implant based breast reconstruction. Excellent outcomes can be achieved with implant based reconstruction, optimising the implant pocket where necessary with staged surgery, acellular dermal matrices, fat transfer techniques but with the more likely need for maintenance surgery in the longer term. Breast reconstruction surgery is a process and often involves secondary procedures, whether the primary reconstruction is autologous or implant based.

Implant based breast reconstruction is technically challenging and great care and attention to detail is necessary to achieve the best results. With autologous breast reconstruction, if sufficient amounts of skin and fat can be brought to the site of the mastectomy, it is relatively simple to shape this tissue to achieve an attractive result with the breast reconstruction. Implant based breast reconstruction requires careful assessment to determine suitability for one-stage or two-stage surgery; fixed volume, expandable implants or tissue expanders; shaped or round devices; pocket enhancement techniques or the incorporation of implant plus autologous tissue flaps. The process can be a complex algorithm based on multifactorial parameters that may be patient and surgeon dependent.

The backbone of two-stage implant based reconstructions is tissue expansion. The placement of an expander can be performed in either an immediate or delayed setting following mastectomy for breast cancer. Tissue expansion is often a pre-requisite in the delayed setting while a choice of tissue expansion, the insertion of a permanent fixed volume or expandable implant is available in the immediate setting. Immediate reconstructions have the advantage that patients wake up from surgery with a reconstructed breast, limiting some of the psychological sequelae experienced by patients following mastectomy. This is of particular relevance in patients undergoing risk reducing surgery who are usually young women undergoing bilateral procedures who should not require adjuvant therapy and would desire a rapid return to normal life. However, there are some advantages to delaying reconstruction in an oncologic setting. The delayed insertion of a tissue expander is less technically challenging. As the post-mastectomy skin-flaps have been allowed time to heal, there is a reduced risk of skin flap ischaemia and wound healing complications. Delaying reconstruction also eliminates the uncertainty of postoperative chest wall radiotherapy and allows more flexibility with operating theatre scheduling. Returning to surgery for the implant exchange allows pocket revision to optimise the reconstructed breast form.

Initial expander and implant devices were rudimentary and cosmetic outcomes were limited. These early devices had smooth elastomer surfaces and were associated with high rates of capsular contracture and device displacement. Aesthetic outcome was less predictable and in many cases, it was necessary to perform multiple adjustments to improve implant position, projection, or inframammary fold definition. In other cases, patients were expected to live with reconstructions that simply produced the impression of a breast mound in clothing. The unpredictability and inconsistency of expander-implant reconstructions drove the development of alternative strategies to reconstruct the breast, namely autologous tissue options (initially the TRAM and LD flaps, and later the DIEP flaps), initially as replacements or salvage techniques and later as the primary approach to breast reconstruction. Autologous tissue reconstructions have become popular with some surgeons as a satisfactory breast mound can usually be achieved in a single operative procedure with more predictable long-term results and lower complication rates when compared with tissue expansion and implant techniques (Beasley &Ballard, 1990; Rosen et al., 1990). It is possible to combine tissue expansion with autologous tissue flap procedures, although an often cited advantage of autologous reconstruction is to avoid the disadvantages associated with the use of an implant. The main advantages that expander-implant reconstructions have over autologous muscle flap techniques include the shorter surgical time and quicker recovery, avoiding the use of donor tissue and associated donor site morbidity with relatively short scars to complement the minimal access approach of skin-sparing mastectomy. The need for secondary procedures to refine the reconstructed breast, the contralateral breast or the trunk is common to all reconstruction types. Several generations of silicone implants have been developed since 1963, with a gradual progression to improved surface texturing, gel consistencies, range of sizes and shapes. The availability of these newer and improved devices has enabled surgeons to obtain more consistent and aesthetically pleasing results. Within the limitations of each individual's chest wall anatomy, soft tissue characteristics and opposite breast contour, a realistic implant based breast reconstruction is now achievable.

2. Types of implants

2.1 Silicone

Silicone refers to a group of polymers, based on the element silicon. Silicon dioxide (sand) is one of the most abundant compounds on Earth. The silicone polymer polydimethylsiloxane (PDMS) is abundantly used in medical applications from indwelling catheters, extended wear contact lenses, pacemakers, syringes and pharmaceuticals to name but a few. Silicone is ideally suited for medical use because of its thermal and oxidative stability, chemical and biological inertness, hydrophobic nature and sterilization capability. Silicone polymers may be produced in a variety of forms, including oil, gels or elastomers (rubber). The physical state is determined by the degree of chemical cross-linking. Cross-linking occurs between vinyl and hydrogen groups on silicon atoms. Silicone oils are straight chains of PDMS without cross-linking and are insoluble in water. Silicon gels consist of cross-linked PDMS chains, together with variable amounts of PDMS liquid. Elastomers of silicone have high degrees of cross-linking and almost no PDMS oil. Common to all implants is the outer shell made out of silicone elastomer reinforced with silica. The shell can be single or double layered, smooth or textured, barrier coated and/or covered with polyurethane foam.

2.1.1 A short history of silicone implants

The modern silicone breast implant as we know it was released to the open market in 1963. It has gone through intense phases of development which have improved the initially primitive and limited devices to current day devices which exhibit a tremendous range of surface textures, sizes, gel consistencies and anatomical shapes.

2.1.2 First generation (1960s)

The original silicone gel implant was developed by Cronin and Gerow and was named the Silastic 0. These implants had envelops of thick smooth walled silicone elastomer made in 2 sections and filled with viscous silicone gel material. The shell halves were then glued together. By the end of the 1960s the shell was cast as a single unit and sealed with a small patch. Fixation patches were introduced in the early part of this period because it was felt that scar and tissue ingrowth was necessary to fix the implant and prevent migration. These fixation patches were made out of Dacron mesh, perforated silicone or polyurethane foam. Not only were the patches found to be generally unnecessary, they also increased the rupture rate by creating stress points in the envelope.

2.1.3 Second generation (1970s)

A new generation of thinner shells and less viscous gels were released in the mid-1970s as attempts to reduce capsular contractures. Unfortunately not only were capsular contracture rates unchanged, these fragile devices were more prone to rupture.

2.1.4 Third generation (1980s)

This period saw significant advances in silicone technology and the implants produced during this era form the backbone of our current devices. Stronger shells reduced the amount of silicone oil "bleed" into adjacent tissues. The gel content was made more viscous and cohesive. Expandable implants with subcutaneous ports were also developed. In 1989 textured-surface envelopes became available. These were felt to reduce capsular contracture rates. Polyurethane coating of implants was first introduced in the 1960s but did not gain popularity until the 1980s. The reduction in capsular contracture seen with polyurethane coated devices was attributed to its open cell structure which allowed tissue in-growth and prevented a regular circumferential deposition of collagen.

In the early 1990s the modern silicone implant was affected by a substantial negative media publicity campaign over the apparent danger of breast implants resulting in a marked drop in the use of silicone implants for all indications. Safety issues centred around silicone oil leakage locally and systemically and the use of polyurethane coating that had become popular towards the end of 1980s. Polyurethane was shown to undergo a degradation process in vivo that produced toluenediamine (TDA). This chemical was a known carcinogen in rats. At that time, the risk to humans was unknown but has been since shown to be extremely low. Further, the polyurethane coating was found to completely delaminate from the underlying silicone shell after several years in vivo. This resulted in loss of implant form. The devices were voluntarily removed from the market in the early 1990s. There has since been extensive research proving the safety of silicone and breast implants. Evidence is widely available disproving any correlation between implants (or silicone) and carcinogenesis, delayed cancer detection, autoimmune disease, neurological disease, teratogenecity and TDA toxicity.

2.1.5 Fourth and fifth generation implants

The adverse publicity seen in the 1990s resulted in stricter manufacturing standards. Current implants of the fourth and fifth generations are essentially refined 3rd generation devices. These devices include cohesive gel products in which, instead of cross linkage of only 20% of gel contents (and therefore the remaining 80% being oil), the cross linking is 40% of the contents. The resulting gel is much stiffer and maintains its shape even when cut therefore controlling spread of gel contents in the event of shell rupture. Larger incisions are however required to accommodate these less flexible implants. In an effort to reduce gel bleed from silicone-filled devices, phenyl or triflouropropyl groups are bonded to the shell to decrease the shell permeability to PDMS oil. These low bleed implant shells with barrier coating are characteristic of current third, fourth and fifth generation implants.

2.2 Saline

These devices are inserted empty and are filled with saline at surgery. Each size has a recommended fill range provided by the manufacturer. Overfilling produces a firm device and under filling risks early rupture from a process called "fold flaw" which results in increased rubbing of the membrane at that point. Any breach of the shell results in instant deflation and harmless absorption of the saline over the next day or two.

2.3 Textured versus smooth surfacing

There are several commercially manufactured varieties of textured silicone elastomer shells. Mentor have developed the Siltex pattern which results as a negative contact imprint of a texturing foam This process produces many fine nodules on the surface of the shell in a regular distribution. Allergan's Biocell surface is produced through a lost salt technique. The implant shell is coated with finely graded salt under light pressure. The salt crystals are subsequently lost through the manufacturing process, leaving many fine depressions on the surface of the shell. True tissue in-growth with textured surfaces only occurs reliably when the implant is placed in a snug pocket or in the tissue expansion environment. These textured surfaces may reduce the rate of capsular contracture but this effect has only been seen in silicone implants and not in saline filled devices. Texturing to provide adhesion of the implant to the surrounding tissue is an important consideration with shaped devices to prevent rotation but may impact negatively on implant scalloping of the overlying skin.

2.4 Expandable implants

Permanent expandable implants combine an outer chamber of factory prefilled silicone with an inner chamber that allows post-operative filling with saline. In current practice the 2 relevant implant valve types are the Becker self-sealing valve which closes on removal of the filling tube and port and the Allergan 150 valve which is plugged when the fill tube is removed. These implants permit gradual and temporary over inflation to create an ample pocket and then can be left in as a permanent implant after the size has been adjusted satisfactorily.

2.5 Shaped versus round implants

Implants can be either shaped or round. Shaped implants can also be referred to as tear dropped, contoured or anatomical. Shaped implants have greater fullness in the lower half and less fullness in the upper half. Some surgeons feel that these implants provide a more natural breast shape particularly in women with extremely little or no breast tissue as these women would appear too full in the upper pole if a round implant was inserted. Others feel that the shaped implant makes no difference to the final result and compensate for upper pole fullness in small breasted women by lowering the position of the implant. Further, because the silicone gel or saline component of the round implant gravitates to the lower pole of the implant when a woman stands, the lower pole naturally becomes fuller, and some argue that this negates the need for a shaped implant. The disadvantage of shaped implants is that post-surgery rotation would result in an obvious sideways appearance to the breast requiring revisional surgery, a problem that does not arise with a round implant. In order to reduce the risk of rotation, shaped implants are textured to reduce the risk of rotation. Shaped implants are generally more expensive than rounded implants.

3. Patient selection

Important factors that should be considered during the patient selection process include patient features (breast volume, breast shape, the contralateral breast, chest wall, body mass index, lifestyle including work and sport, and co-morbid factors), patient understanding (of the procedure, complications, implications and of the device), and the oncologic features (skin sparing mastectomy versus traditional mastectomy, systemic therapy needs and adjuvant radiotherapy). Conventional teaching stipulates that the ideal woman for an implant based reconstruction has small to moderate sized breasts without significant ptosis. Bilateral breast reconstructions for cancer or risk reduction may also be ideal because it provides an optimum scenario for achieving symmetry. Patients undergoing unilateral mastectomies may require a contralateral procedure for symmetrisation by augmentation, mastopexy or breast reduction. Women who rely on upper limb strength for work or sport may be directed towards an implant reconstruction or muscle sparing autologous abdominal option as this would avoid the potential functional morbidity experienced that may follow an LD flap reconstruction.

Women with large or ptotic breasts may still be suitable for implant reconstruction by utilization of a skin-sparing volume reducing approach. A Wise pattern approach allows reduction of the skin envelope. The de-epithelialized lower flap facilitates lower pole implant cover and often allows for pseudo-ptosis with careful positioning of the inframammary crease. The nipple may be preserved on the superior mastectomy skin flap. Caution may need to be exercised in women with a generous subcutaneous adipose covering as implant projection may be compromised by the depth of the rib cage below the fat layer.

There are relative contraindications which would make some patients less suited to an implant based reconstruction. Aside from the usual medical conditions that would increase the risk of anaesthesia or infection, a significant contraindication is unrealistic expectation. Patients with large or advanced breast cancers and clinically involved axillary lymph nodes are likely to require adjuvant radiotherapy. Radiotherapy either prior to implant insertion or following implant insertion can result in hardened and thickened soft tissues and initiate or exacerbate capsular contraction.

4. Preparing a patient for an implant breast reconstruction

4.1 Biodimensional planning

Biodimensional planning involves taking a few detailed chest measurements, including the sternal-notch nipple, inframammary crease nipple and midline nipple distances. The attributes of the existing breast form should be measured, namely the transverse breast width, vertical breast height and projection. These measurements along with pre-operative photographs form an essential part of the medical records of the pre-operative state on which post-operative evaluation can be compared. Careful assessment should be made of the patient's chest wall, general predisposition and soft tissue properties.

	Implant reconstruction	Autologous reconstruction
Anatomy and patient physique	Small to moderate sized breasts with minimal ptosis are best suited for implant reconstruction Implant reconstruction for large, ptotic breasts can still be achieved by performing a Wise-pattern skin-sparing volume reducing mastectomy Body habitus/BMI: excessive subcutaneous adiposity risks compromising implant projection	Larger, ptotic breasts may be better reconstructed using autologous tissue
Attitude and anxieties	Patient wants a shorter procedure with a more rapid post-operative recovery period Does not mind the presence of a device	Patient is willing to invest time and effort in a longer and more complex operation Can accept the additional potential complications associated with the donor site Does not want reconstruction using a device
Stage of disease	Earlier disease with a lesser chance of adjuvant chest wall radiotherapy with its associated increased risk of capsulation A temporizing implant can be used to maintain the skin envelope. This can be deflated if radiotherapy is required to optimize delivery of external beam therapy. If radiotherapy is not required, prompt implant exchange can be performed to avoid delay to other adjuvant therapies	More advanced disease with a higher chance to chest wall radiotherapy becoming necessary. Radiotherapy will still affect autologous tissues but capsulation is avoided
General health	A patient who would benefit from a shorter operation and more rapid post-operative recovery period i.e. a person with a greater number of comorbidities and is at higher anaesthetic risk	Low anaesthetic risk
Muscle function	Relies on upper limb function for work or sport and therefore should avoid a latissimus dorsi flap. Increased use of abdominal wall in sport or work, may be at higher risk of abdominal wall herniation if TRAM is performed	Loss of muscle function or effect of long scars should not have profound effect on work, activities of daily living or sport
Bilateral procedures	Ideally suited to implant reconstructions as provides the greatest opportunity to achieve symmetry	Increases the complication and anaesthetic risks associated with these longer and more complex procedures

Table 2. Description of patient characteristics that may influence the type of breast reconstruction chosen

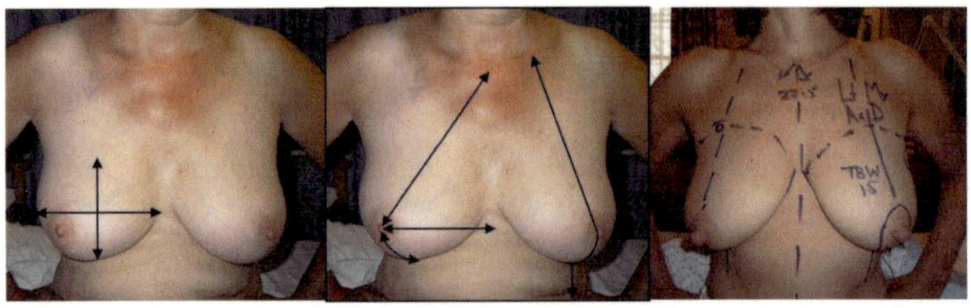

Transverse breast width
Vertical breast height

Midline to nipple
Sternal notch to nipple
Nipple to inframammary fold
Breast meridian

Fig. 1. Measurement of the existing breast form are taken as part of biodimensional planning

These factors contribute to the choice of surgical technique and aid implant selection so that the optimum breast reconstruction is achieved for that individual. Both round and shaped implants are available in a range of base widths, heights and profiles. The main determinant of implant selection is breast width. This takes account of the patient's chest wall characteristics and is an essential consideration in order to avoid placing a narrow implant on a wide chest wall or conversely a wide implant on a narrow chest wall. Once the base width is established the appropriate height can be selected. Patients who have less ptosis will have a fuller upper pole and would therefore benefit from a rounded implant or taller height implant whereas a more ptotic breast would be better reconstructed using a shaped implant with a shorter height. The profile refers to the amount of forward projection of the implant from the chest wall and range from low to ultra-high projections. Profile selection can be guided by comparison to the contralateral breast or by patient's desire for projection, adjusting the contralateral breast as appropriate. In patients with extremely wide chest walls and excessive subcutaneous tissue, achieving adequate projection is a challenge and these patients are therefore less suited to an implant only reconstruction.

4.2 Marking up

With the patient sitting or standing up, the midline, the breast meridian, inframammary folds, lateral border and upper extents of both breasts should be marked. The breast meridian can be taken from a point 5cm lateral to the medial end of the clavicle to the centre of the nipple and the line extended to the inframammary crease. Mark the meridian beyond the inframammary crease as the marking often washes out during the surgery. The skin incision should also be indicated. In many cases of immediate breast reconstruction, a skin-sparing approach is suitable but may sometimes need to be modified to take into account pre-existing scars. The choice of skin incision is extremely variable and dependent on each individual case and the surgeon's preference. Common skin incisions include the circumareolar incision, circumarealor incision with a lateral or vertical extension and the inframammary fold incision. It is best to avoid extending the incision into the superior and medial sectors of the breast. The incision should be planned to allow preservation of the most favourable blood supply to the mastectomy skin flaps.

If skin excision is to form part of the mastectomy, commonly used patterns include the circumareolar to excise the nipple areolar complex with a range of extensions, most commonly lateral or vertical. The nipple areolar complex could also be incorporated into a number of skin excision patterns including the oblique ellipse, transverse ellipse, vertical ellipse, inverted T shape, mastopexy and Wise pattern excisions. This wide variation could also be modified for nipple preservation in suitable cases. Ultimately the goal is to leave sufficient amounts of well-vascularized skin while excising the maximum amount of breast tissue.

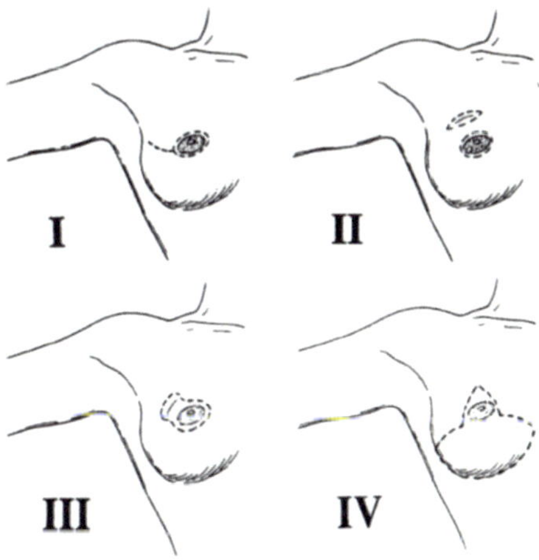

Type	Classification
I	Only nipple-areola removed
II	Nipple-areola removed, skin overlying superficial tumours and previous biopsy incision removed without intervening skin
III	Nipple-areola, skin overlying superficial tumours and previous biopsy incision removed in continuity with nipple-areola
IV	Nipple-areola removed with an inverted or reduction pattern skin incision

Fig. 2. Classification of skin sparing mastectomy (Carlson, 1997)

Good cover of the implant or the tissue expander should be obtained such that the desired breast shape is created without undue laxity or tension and without skin necrosis from ischaemic flaps. When the plan for reconstruction includes the addition of a flap, the surgical excision can be designed such that the planned skin paddle of the transposed myocutaneous flap accurately replaces the area of removed native breast skin.

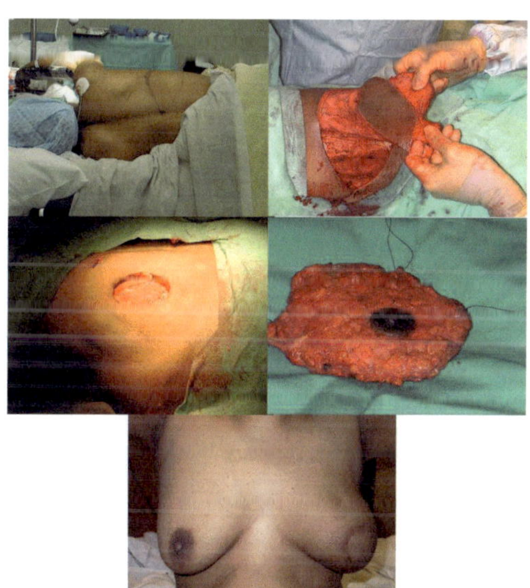

Fig. 3. An implant assisted LD breast reconstruction following a skin sparing mastectomy. The planned skin paddle of the LD flap accurately replaces the removed nipple-areolar complex

4.3 Positioning

Most surgeons would perform the mastectomy on a supine patient with both arms out on a board to add access to the lateral extent of the breast incision, to allow access to the axillary nodes and to enable comparison with the contralateral breast. Adequate exposure should be provided when draping the patient to view the collar bones, lateral extents of both breasts and the lower chest. Creation of the submuscular pocket, reshaping of the mastectomy space and device insertion can be done with the patient supine initially, and the patient can be moved into a sitting position intra-operatively to allow for positional variation. Further adjustments to the pocket can then be performed. These stages of the breast reconstruction can be performed on patients at 45 degrees or in a complete upright sitting position. Appropriate operating table choice and positioning is essential prior to draping.

5. Reconstruction options

5.1 Immediate reconstruction

The options for immediate implant based reconstruction are as follows:

- One stage using a permanent implant
- One stage using an expandable implant
- Two stage using a tissue expander and subsequent implant exchange

The replacement of mammary tissue with an implant immediately after a mastectomy has been refined over the years and usually implies the use of an expandable implant as a planned one stage procedure or the insertion of a tissue expander prior to the subsequent placement of a permanent fixed volume implant. Occasionally an adequate submuscular pocket can be created for a fixed volume implant at the primary procedure. Unless oncologic criteria determine otherwise, a skin-sparing mastectomy is commonly performed in association with an immediate breast reconstruction.

5.1.1 Implant reconstruction in small breasts with minimal ptosis

This forms the classic group of patients in whom implant based breast reconstruction is often described. Tissue expansion can usually be avoided in patients with small breasts who require reconstruction of a non-ptotic breast of similar or slightly larger size. In such patients, an increase in the desired reconstructed breast size usually requires the use of an expandable implant as a planned one stage procedure in the presence of an adequate pocket. A significant increase in size is best addressed as a two stage procedure. If nipple preservation is being considered, this can usually be maintained attached to the mastectomy flap via the periareolar extension, with or without extensions for access.

5.1.2 Implant reconstruction in moderate sized breasts

The place of implant breast reconstruction in this patient is also established. For women with moderate sized breasts and no or minimal ptosis, total submusculo-fascial cover may not be achieved and it is not the authors' preference to have incomplete implant cover. Such cases may be best addressed as a two stage tissue expansion procedure, inserting a tissue expander into the submusculo-fascial pocket and expanding over an interval in outpatients, before a two stage implant exchange.

The use of acellular dermal matrices (vide infra) has extended the role of one stage implant reconstruction in this group of patients. An implant assisted latissimus flap also provides for excellent long term implant cover in this patient group. The acceptance of nipple preservation in some patient subgroups in conjunction with use of an acellular dermal matrix has renewed interest in the inframammary crease approach, preserving the nipple in its normal anatomical position and draping the lower pole of the retained skin envelope over the acellular dermal matrix sheet interpositioned between the lower freed border of pectoralis major and the surgically created inframammary crease. Nipple preservation if appropriate can also be maintained via the periareolar incision with or without extension for access. The larger the increase in size from the original breast envelope the more unpredictable the final nipple position on the reconstructed breast. Great care needs to be taken in surgical planning to maintain the nipple position at the appropriate height in the breast meridian that needs to coincide with the projected new midline nipple distance, that requires to match the contralateral side.

5.1.3 Implant reconstruction in women with larger breasts

In women with larger and ptotic breasts, the use of a Wise pattern approach provides excellent access to perform a mastectomy despite the breast size. The lower mastectomy-skin flap is de-epithelialized and used to provide lower pole implant cover. This approach usually results in a smaller breast mound that corrects for ptosis and is considered a skin-sparing volume reducing technique. The implant reconstruction can usually be performed with a fixed volume device or expandable implant as a one stage procedure. Planning a two stage procedure has some advantages of returning to optimize the pocket but may not be an essential second step as excellent pocket control can be achieved with this surgery. The procedure is well suited to bilateral cases and in unilateral cases, the contralateral breast will require a reduction mammaplasty for symmetry. Nipple preservation is possible with this technique if oncologic parameters allow, usually based on the superior skin flap. The ability to use the de-epithelialized lower flap often negates the requirement for an acellular dermal matrix in this type of operation.

5.2 Skin sparing mastectomy

Many access incisions for skin-sparing mastectomy have been described. Fiberoptic lighting or headlamps are very useful to visualize dissection through minimal access incisions. Great care must be taken to avoid trauma by distension and diathermy injury to the skin flaps. Insulated instruments are helpful when diathermy dissection is used. After mastectomy, careful haemostasis is essential.

If the nipple is to be preserved, intra-operative frozen sections of the nipple base or nipple core to confirm a clear nipple margin of resection can be helpful. Histologically proven cancer extension into the nipple zone at the time of surgery is best treated by primary nipple resection. Preservation of the areola at nipple resection may be one option (Simmons, 2003). Delayed identification of nipple involvement when standard histological assessment is back may pose a dilemma on further management. The option of targeted radiotherapy may have a role and may be an alternative to the more common recommendation of secondary nipple excision.

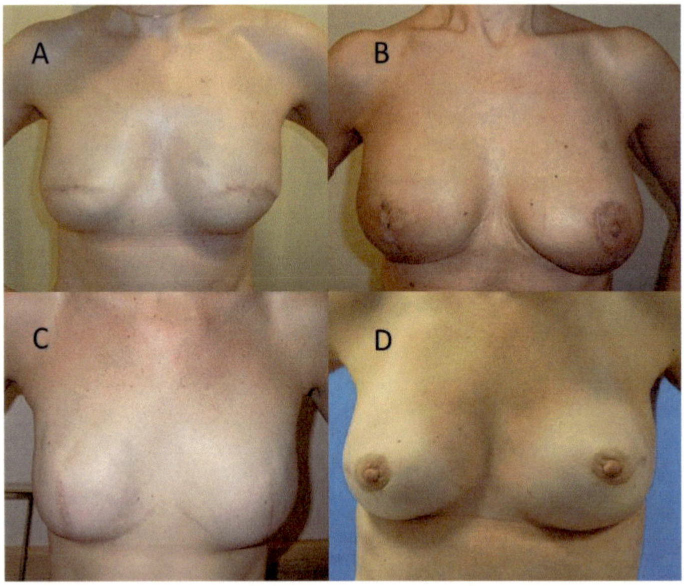

Fig. 4. Examples of skin incisions. A, transverse incisions. B, verticle incision. C, wise pattern excision without nipple preservation. D, peri-areolar incisions with lateral extension

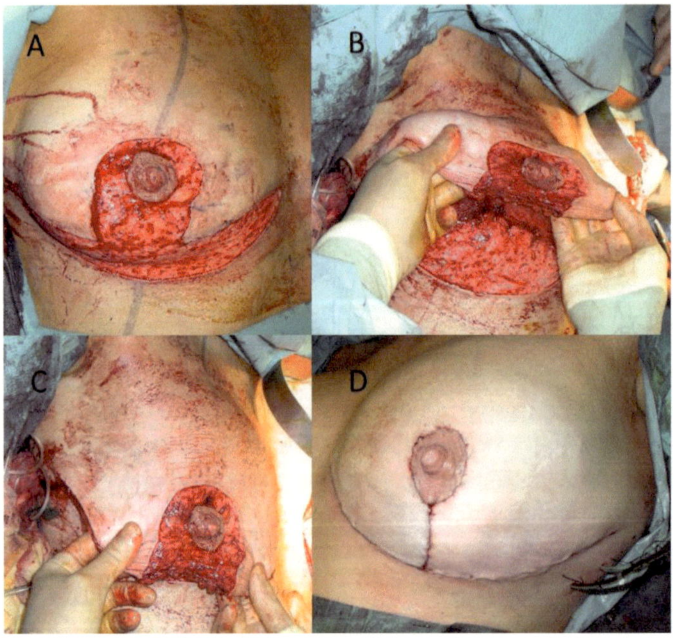

Fig. 5. Wise pattern skin excision for nipple sparing mastectomy. A, skin excision is performed and the marked areas are de-epithelialised. B, The de-epithelialised lower flap is disconnected and sutured to the inferior edge of pectoralis. C, The upper flap is drapped over the implant and the de-epithelialized lower flap. A butterfly needle has been inserted into the laterally sited injection port to allow adjustments to final inflation volume of the permanent expandable implant during pocket and skin closure. D, The incisions are closed

5.3 Creating the submuscular pocket

5.3.1 Raising pectoralis major

Following completion of the mastectomy, attention is turned to creation of a submuscular or submusculo-fascial pocket to house the implant or expander. To create a space in the submuscular plane, the fibres of pectoralis major are split 1cm lateral to the free lateral border. The inferior surface of pectoralis major is raised off the rib cage and the dissection taken medially taking care to preserve the anterior intercostal perforators as they emerge through the intercostal spaces close to the lateral sternal edge. The pectoralis major muscle should not be detached from the sternum. The upper border is taken to 1cm beyond the marked upper pole of the projected breast mound to ensure a gentle take off of the superior reconstructed breast. The inferior musculo-fascial border is created by disconnecting the attachment of pectoralis major to the ribcage from within the pocket. This takes the dissection on to a plane in continuity with the anterior rectus sheath, allowing the lower pole of the breast reconstruction to rise on the inferior implant surface. This dissection needs to be limited by the marking of the existing or new inframammary crease. Sparing the contents of the inframammary fold facilitates this dissection and avoids buttonholing of the thin fascia that can exist below the fibres of the pectoralis attachment.

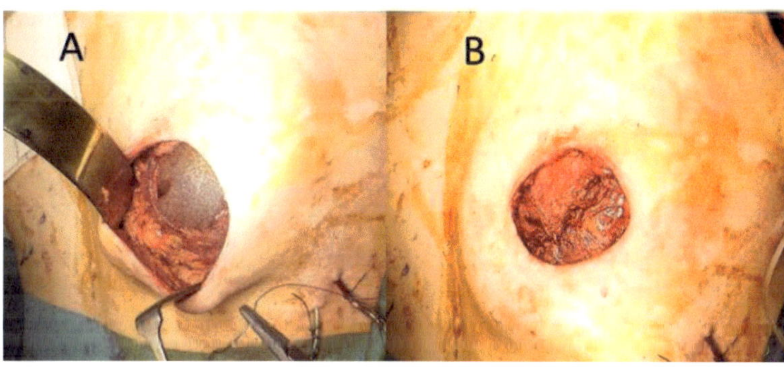

Fig. 6. Skin sparing mastectomy through a transverse incision. A, open pocket with implant visible. A butterfly needle has been inserted into the subcutaneous injection port laterally to allow adjustments to final inflation volume of the permanent expandable implant during pocket closure. B. Closed muscular pocket with the sutured edge of pectoralis major visible, the lateral border attached to serratus anterior

5.3.2 Providing cover for the inferior mammary space

When the inferior mammary musculo-fascial space does not provide adequate cover, the disconnected inferior border of pectoralis major may either be attached to the lower mastectomy flap by a series of interrupted sutures or alternatively holding sutures to the tough fascia of the inframammary crease like guide ropes, allowing the anterior surface of the muscle to adhere to the mastectomy skin flaps. In this situation, a two staged planned implant exchange is usually the preferred option enabling a return to optimise the implant pocket at a subsequent procedure. The development of acellular dermal matrices has made cover of the lower implant pole in this circumstance much simpler and interposition of a matrix sheet cut to size to interposition the required space between the free muscle border and the inframammary crease feasible as a one stage procedure.

5.3.3 The lateral pocket

The lateral musculo-fascial pocket is created by dissecting down from the lateral edge of the split pectoralis major fibres on to the lateral chest wall to find the anterior fibres of serratus anterior as they attach to the rib cage. Often this involves dividing some of the fibres at the lateral edge of pectoralis minor. The serratus anterior fibres can be freed to a varying extent to house the expander or implant. In general, in a planned two stage expansion, this dissection laterally can be limited to fit the footprint of the device, the true expansion process occurring post-surgery as an outpatient. In a planned one stage reconstruction, the dissection may need to be taken far back enough to free the anterior rib cage attachment of the serratus anterior to allow the lateral pocket to be raised fully to cover the fixed volume or expandable implant. Anatomically this extended lateral pocket consists of the lateral fibres of pectoralis major, the intervening fascia between pectoralis major and serratus anterior, and the anterior fibres of serratus anterior. The surgical dissection of the extended lateral pocket creation needs to be carefully undertaken as the fascial layer between the two muscles can be very thin.

5.3.4 Partial musculo-facial cover

Partial musculo-facial cover of the implant pocket is described, and is a simpler dissection. Advocates argue that placing the expander or implant in the subpectoral space alone allows for quicker operative time, less painful surgery, less discomfort after surgery (including during expansion) and better definition of the inframammary fold. The pectoralis major muscle is dissected free at its lateral border. The muscle is elevated and detached inferiorly at its insertion. Medially the dissection is carried to the parasternal region, but the muscle should not be detached from sternum. In particular, it is important not to detach the muscle along the sternal border superiorly, which would result in substantial dislocation of the muscle. The free inferior pectoralis major muscle should be tacked down to the lower mastectomy skin flap or to the inferior mammary crease as guide ropes as the muscle would otherwise retract resulting in poor implant cover. Spear et al. have found that placement of the implant partially under the mastectomy flap delivers predictable and cosmetically pleasing outcomes (Spear, 2004). This approach creates a breast that may be more easily placed on the chest wall and is unrestricted by the lower attachment of the pectoralis major to the rib cage. By avoiding disruption of the serratus anterior and rectus fascia, there is less postoperative pain as well as less pain during expansion. Because implant cover inferiorly is simply by the lower mastectomy flap, lower pole rippling can be more evident. It is important to minimize undermining of the inframammary fold and preserve adequate thickness of the lower mastectomy flap when possible.

5.3.5 Acellular dermal matrix

If an acellular dermal matrix sheet is to be used in the reconstruction, the dissection and creation of the submuscular pocket is simplified. The pectoralis major is freed at its lateral and inferior border, maintaining the attachment at the lower sternum. The selected acellular dermal matrix sheet is cut to size and the sheet sutured to interposition the area required to bridge the gap between the lower free muscle border and the inframammary crease. When placed in contact with viable tissue, the acellular matrix can become repopulated with circulating stem cells that differentiate into normal stromal components (endothelial cells, fibroblasts etc), resulting in the turnover of matrix components and the integration of the matrix into host beds (Buinewicz, 2003; Menon, 2003). It is available in a range of sizes and thickness (1-16cm length, 1-6cm width and 0.18 to more than 1.8mm in thickness). The matrix is fairly pliable while maintaining good tensile strength. In the short term, the matrix acts as a barrier, adding a layer of protection under compromised skin flaps.

Examples of acellular dermal matrices available include AlloDerm (Lifecell, Branchburg, NJ) and Strattice (Lifecell, Branchburg, NJ). AlloDerm is an acellular dermal matrix derived from human cadaver skin that has been processed and sterilized to remove all cells and antigenic components leaving an extracellular matrix of collagen, elastin, hyaluronic acid, fibronectin, proteoglycans and vascular channels. AlloDerm requires to be rehydrated before use for 5 minutes in sterile normal saline or Ringer's lactate. Strattice is derived from pig skin and is maintained in a rehydrated state in the packaging. The Strattice sheet needs to be washed thoroughly in sterile saline before use to minimise patient contact with the preservation fluid. The combined arc length of the IMF and lateral fold is measured to determine the length of matrix needed. A fixed volume implant can often be used to create a planned one stage breast reconstruction. Expandable implants can also be used but it is unlikely that the acellular matrix itself enables post-operative expansion. Early expansion as an outpatient, however, facilitates expansion of the pocket as a whole and has been successfully used by the authors.

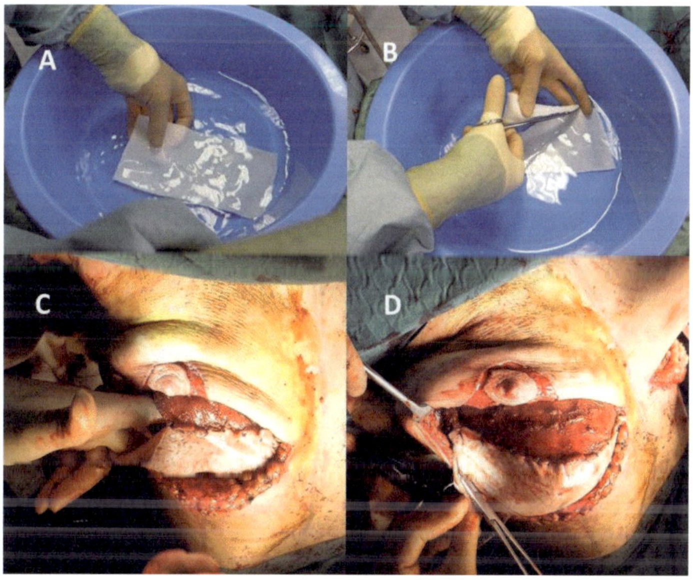

Fig. 7. (clockwise from top left): A, Strattice wash. B, Strattice cut to size. C, The superior pocket is being closed. D, Strattice sewn in with implant in pocket

5.3.6 Recreating the inframammary fold

The inframammary fold may need to be recreated by suturing the dermis or superficial fascia back down to the chest wall. A similar manoeuvre may be required to create the lateral breast fold by reattaching the advanced lateral skin flaps to the chest wall, which will prevent the tissue expander form sliding laterally or into the axilla.

5.4 Device placement and intraoperative filling

The key to successful implant reconstruction is the creation of a well-placed and adequate pocket. When a definitive fixed volume implant is planned in the immediate or delayed setting, sizers may be used intra-operatively to guide the final implant choice and position.

Expandable implants such as the Becker series (Mentor) and the Style 150 (Allergan) are designed to allow post-operative inflation. Inflation of the device creates projection on the footprint of the implant and allows correction of small volume discrepancies and projection compared with the contralateral breast. Expandable implants should not be used as tissue expanders as the tension they exert if expected to perform as expanders often are inadequate or result in implant distortion, filling at sites where expansion is easier, such as the upper pole. Expandable implants can be placed through minimal access incisions partly inflated with sterile saline and inflation completed when the device is secured in its final position within the pocket. Optimum fill is often 75% of the saline fill or more at the time of surgery and only a few post-operative inflations are generally required to achieve the desired final size (Gui, 2003). If expandable implants with remote ports are being used, the ports need to be sited and secured in an accessible subcutaneous position that does not interfere with underclothes. The lateral chest wall near the inframammary crease enables port removal with a well hidden scar, or alternatively placement adjacent to a scar that can be used for port removal such as an axillary incision avoids exposed scars when the ports are subsequently removed.

If a tissue expander is being used, accurate placement of the footprint creates the desired projection with subsequent inflation and therefore optimises the stretching of the overlying pocket tissue and skin in the expansion process. The expander is usually under filled with the intention of post-operative expansion in outpatients. The access ports can be integral or remote. Some of the integral ports with larger metallic components may not be MRI compatible or be perceived to interfere with radiotherapy planning and delivery. Choice of such expanders needs to be taken with the multidisciplinary approach to breast cancer management in mind.

Choice of sutures vary with surgeon preference. Absorbable sutures are commonly used to close the implant pocket and include PDS, Biosyn and Vicryl. Sutures to recreate the inframammary crease are more controversial as to whether a non-absorbable suture such as nylon or prolene is necessary. The important feature of recreation of the inframammary crease is well placed sutures to define the inframammary crease at the correct position on the chest wall. Even if absorbable sutures are used the healing process and the formation of a soft capsule often defines the final implant position including the inframammary crease.

5.5 Post-operative expansion

Expansion is started once pain has settled and viability of the skin flaps is assured. There are generally two schools of thought for tissue expansion. Those in favour of early expansion commence the inflation process a few days after surgery while others wait for several weeks. The quality of the overlying soft tissue and patient comfort are the primary determining factors. A 23g needle is inserted into the injection port under aseptic conditions in outpatients and 50 to 100 ml are injected once or twice weekly to reach the desired volume. Depending on the devices used, overexpansion and maintenance of this for several weeks prior to volume reduction to the desired fill may help create pseudo ptosis, remove skin folds and may decrease the incidence of capsular contracture. In women who require post-operative radiotherapy, some surgeons prefer to fully expand these patients prior to commencing radiation. A massaging protocol may be initiated and continued during the radiotherapy to minimize fibrosis.

The expander is exchanged for a permanent implant when radiotherapy changes have subsided and is often at least 6 months following the completion of radiation. In women not requiring radiotherapy, implant exchange can be performed a short interval after final expansion, commonly after one month. The inflation ports for expandable implants can be removed when the inflation process is complete and the ports are no longer required. Different implant manufacturers have their own methods described for easy and effective port removal.

5.6 Implant exchange (second stage)

The time period during which expansion occurs is a useful interval for patients to reflect on the effect the breast cancer diagnosis has had, be proactive in the reconstruction process and to be prepared for the final appearance of their breast reconstruction. Patients have the choice in decision making on breast size and position, shape and texture.

Tissue expansion is a two-stage process where the expander is exchanged for a definitive implant. The range of definitive fixed volume devices and the ability to return to optimise the implant pocket, breast form and scars at the secondary procedure has many advantages for better long term results. Other secondary procedures such as nipple reconstruction and attention to the contralateral breast for symmetry may need to be considered at the second or sometimes subsequent stages of the reconstruction process. Even when an expandable implant is placed with the intention of using it as a permanent device, secondary implant exchange may become necessary in a proportion of patients because of limitations in symmetry. This is often due to poor or differential expansion and capsule formation. One-stage surgery is a misnomer as secondary procedures are often required that are unrelated to implant exchange. In the context of expandable implants, this includes removal of the inflation port, nipple reconstruction and attention to the contralateral breast. Implant based surgery is also associated with a requirement for maintenance surgery over time.

Skin-sparing volume reducing surgery with use of the lower de-epithelialized mastectomy skin flap for lower pole implant cover has made planned one-stage surgery with reference to obviating the need to return to the implant pocket more common. The evolution of the role of acellular dermal matrices may influence the place of two stage surgery where planned implant exchange surgery has been the recommendation.

5.7 Delayed-immediate reconstruction

A two staged approach that bridges the immediate and delayed settings can be employed with the use of a temporizing implant and is suitable for a patient who desires an immediate breast reconstruction but is at a higher risk of requiring chest wall radiotherapy (Kronowitz, 2010). Following skin sparing mastectomy, a saline-filled tissue expander is inserted and serves as an adjustable scaffold to preserve the 3-dimensional shape of the skin envelope. If postmastectomy radiotherapy is not necessary, the expander is exchanged for a permanent implant, either early to avoid delaying adjuvant therapy or upon completion of chemotherapy, to preserve the ptosis in the skin envelope. If radiotherapy is required, the expander is usually maintained at a constant volume to facilitate radiotherapy planning and delivery. Some surgeons and radiation oncologists recommend deflation of the expander before radiotherapy is commenced. The resultant flat chest wall facilitates delivery of 3-beam radiotherapy. When the breast skin has recovered from the radiotherapy, a period of at least three if not six months, a skin preserving delayed reconstruction is performed by removal of the expander and transfer of an autologous tissue flap. Sometimes, the quality of the skin may have recovered adequately post-radiotherapy to consider further implant based options. The pocket may need to be optimized by fat transfer procedures prior to the implant exchange.

5.8 Delayed reconstruction

A delayed reconstruction usually requires the placement of a tissue expander to stretch the pre-existing mastectomy flaps. Delayed insertion of a tissue expander is usually a safe procedure when good quality soft tissue is available, with a reduced risk of mastectomy skin flap ischaemia, and wound healing complications. Delayed reconstruction also eliminates the uncertainty of unplanned postoperative adjuvant radiotherapy affecting a definitive reconstruction and allows more flexibility with scheduling. Delayed reconstruction however leaves patients temporarily at least without a breast mound, is usually associated with longer scars that may not be optimal and loss of skin. Tissue expansion to create a pocket must take into account whether the expansion will create sufficient skin stretch to match the contralateral side and what adjustments if necessary to both sides may become necessary to achieve symmetry.

Preoperative markings are performed with the patient in an upright position. The contralateral breast inframammary crease is outlined and the transverse base diameter and vertical base height is measured. A template may be used to transfer these measurements in the mastectomy side.

Intraoperatively, a varying length of the existing mastectomy incision is reopened for adequate access. The inferior lateral border of the pectoralis major muscle is identified and a subpectoral dissection initiated. Meticulous haemostasis is performed. Dissection beneath the pectoralis major muscle continues superiorly to the extent of the preoperative markings but not beyond to limit unwanted superior expansion and to direct expansion inferiorly. The submuscular dissection continues medially and inferiorly partially dividing the origin of the pectoralis major muscle along the parasternal border from the second rib to the fourth rib. This partial release of the muscle improves anterior projection and cleavage definition during expansion. Inferiorly the pocket dissection switches to the subcutaneous plane just above the serratus anterior, external oblique and rectus abdominis fascia. This dissection continues to the level of the marked inframammary crease. Complete release of any restricting scar or fascia extending nearly to the dermis at the desired IMF location will aid in the passive creation of a distinct fold during the expansion process. The subcutaneous positioning of the inferior portion of the expander is reliably safe in a delayed reconstruction because flap ischemia is not usually a concern. This subcutaneous placement allows easy expansion with improved projection in the inferior pole.

An appropriate expander is selected and any air within the device removed. Precise placement of the expander stretches the required soft tissue without unnecessary overexpansion. The expander is then partially filled with some saline so that the inferior border of the device rests at the level of the desired inframammary crease height. A drain is then placed in the pocket before closure of the mastectomy incision in layers. The expander may then be further filled to the maximum volume the soft tissues will allow.

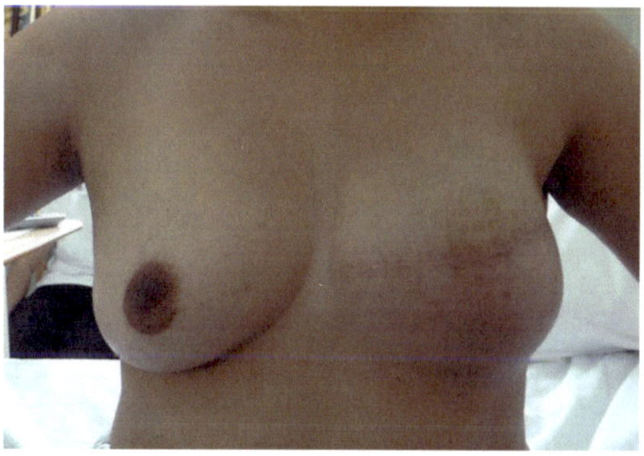

Fig. 8. Postoperative appearances followed delayed breast reconstruction following tissue expansion and implant exchange. Radiotherapy related skin changes are still visible.

Expansion can commence early, and often within a few weeks if there are no concerns with wound healing or skin flap health. Saline is added to the expander to reach the end point of moderate soft tissue tension. This should result in minimal patient discomfort if any. Expansion continues every 2 to 4 weeks until the desired maximum point of lower pole projection is obtained. The final volume within the expander should closely match the size of the opposite breast, limiting overexpansion to 10-15%. Once full expansion has been achieved, the expander should remain in place for at least one month. This allows time to achieve a mature, pliable capsule. This period of maximum expansion also prevents any recoil of the soft tissue envelop once the expander is removed. The second stage involves exchanging the expander for a permanent implant using techniques previously described for the second stage of immediate reconstructions.

6. Implant reconstruction in the irradiated breast

Radiation has significant negative effects on all types of breast reconstruction but this effect is most marked in implant based reconstructions. Irradiated tissues fibrose and contract with time, causing an apparent increasing hardness (capsular contracture) of the implant based reconstruction. Patients who present with advanced diseases or with heavily involved axillary nodes may require chest wall radiotherapy following mastectomy so are therefore less favourable candidates for implant reconstructions. Several studies have shown capsular formation rates of between 11 to 68% with varying lengths of follow-up.

Previous chest wall radiation is a relative contraindication to tissue expansion as a delayed procedure. Depending on the timing technique and quantity of radiation administered, the soft tissues can be unyielding. Expansion under these circumstances is therefore difficult with an increased risk of complications.

Study	n	n RT	% capsule formation	
			No RT	RT
Tallet 2003	77	55	0	16
Cordeiro 2004	143	68	40	68
Clough 2004	334	28		11 (2y)
				15 (5y)
Collis 2000	197	32		12
Behranwala2006	136	44	14	39

Table 3. Studies evaluating capsule formation after radiotherapy in implant IBR

A study from the Royal Marsden Hospital found capsule formation in 38.6% of reconstructed breasts using a permanent expander implant followed by radiotherapy compared to 14.1% of reconstructed breasts not needing post mastectomy radiotherapy at a median follow-up of 4 years (Behranwala, 2006). At univariate analysis, radiotherapy emerged as the only variable related to capsule formation ($p<0.001$) with significantly shorter time to capsule formation in immediate breast reconstructions that received post mastectomy radiotherapy. These results clearly demonstrate the relationship between radiotherapy post immediate implant breast reconstruction and capsular formation. However, as more than 60% of patients do not get capsules despite radiotherapy at 4 years, the use of implant assisted tissue expansion techniques still presents a viable reconstructive option in selected cases.

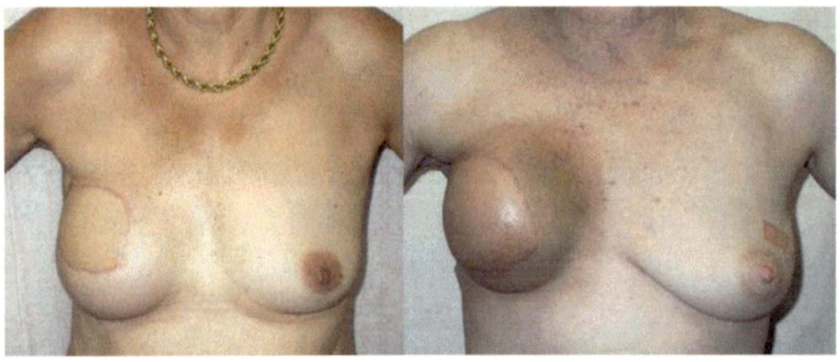

Fig. 9. Implant assisted LD reconstruction A. before post mastectomy chest wall radiotherapy. B, after post mastectomy chest wall radiotherapy.

7. Potential complications of implant based reconstructions

7.1 Rupture

Rupture of silicone filled implants presents two main areas of concern: release of silicone gel into the body and failure of the device. While there is no correlation between connective tissue disease and breast implants, a local inflammatory response to a silicone leak can result in the formation of silicone granulomas. These present as discrete breast or axillary node masses and can be mistaken for recurrence.

The rates of implant rupture range from 11 to 77% depending on the study design, generation of implant used and the age of the implant at time of study. Grouping of all devices to provide a single rupture rate is also not an accurate estimation of rupture rates which depend on type of implant where variables include shell thickness, elastomer type, surface texture and shape. True implant rupture rates are associated with time from implantation, particularly in the case of earlier generation devices which are associated with a higher rupture rate. Almost all studies have a self-selection bias of patients who present with signs consistent with implant rupture. Devices were subsequently examined for rupture and we would therefore expect a higher rate of rupture when compared to the general implant population. Most studies have used radiologic imaging to determine device integrity where overall accuracy may be limited by sensitivity or specificity. MRI imaging for instance has a high false positive rate of rupture. Allergan is conducting a 10 year Core study to assess the safety and effectiveness of their rounded implants in 715 patients. The rate of rupture is compared between patients undergoing scheduled MRIs at years 1,3,5,7 and 9 years (to screen for silent ruptures) and those not scheduled for routine MRI assessments. The 4 year results have now been reported and show an implant rupture rate of 2.7% in the MRI cohort group compared to a 0.4% rupture rate in augmented patients in the non-MRI cohort. No ruptures were reported in the 98 patients who had undergone primary implant breast reconstruction in the 4 year time period (Inamed, 2005).

Author	Infection (%)	Haematoma (%)	Seroma around implant (%)	Native skin necrosis (%)	Implant loss or extrusion (%)	Difficulty expansion (%)	Valve failure (%)	Deflation (%)
Mansel 1986	7.9 8.3			2.6	16.7 23.7			
Schuster 1990	5.4	3.6	7.1	12.5	7.1			
Hunter-Smith 1995	3.7	0	1.9	3.7	1.9		1.9	1.9
Ramon 1997	9.6	5.8		1.9	5.8	11.5	3.8	3.8
Spear 1998	3.5	1.2		5.3	10.5			4.0
Slavin 1998	2.0	0		21.6	3.9			
Peyser 2000	4.2	1.4		9.9			1.4	
Gui 2003	6.2	1.6	0	3	3.9	0	0	0

Table 4. Complications from implant reconstructions, comparison of published reports (modified from Gui, 2003)

7.2 Infection

The most serious threat to an implant based breast reconstruction is infection. The reported incidence is between 2% and 9.6%(see table 4). The first signs and symptoms may appear as early as 5 days or as late as 5 weeks after surgery. Commonly infections with staphylococcus aureus, staphylococcus epidermidis or pseudomonas appear within 5 to 7 days with dramatic symptoms suggestive of abscess formation. Diffuse redness, swelling, tenderness and systemic symptoms of fever and malaise are common. Attainment of culture material is helpful and intravenous antibiotics with hospital surveillance is recommended. If no improvement or worsening symptoms, immediate exploration is indicated in an attempt to downstage or control the process. In the presence of gross pus and inflammation at exploration, it is probably best to remove the implant, debride clearly infected tissues, thoroughly lavage the pocket, place a drain, and close the wound and cover with antibiotics. If the operative findings are favourable, it may be possible to salvage or exchange the implant after adequate cleaning of the pocket. Adequate soft tissue cover is essential with close surveillance and appropriate antibiotic cover, guided by microbiology culture and sensitivity. If salvage strategies fail, the device needs to be removed and further reconstructive attempts delayed for a reasonable period for tissue to recover, usually at least 6 months. Mycobacterium infection may present differently and may be suspected following repeated negative cultures. Signs and symptoms may be delayed for 3-5 weeks after surgery and are mostly local and minor, often consisting of a clear discharge from the incision with no systemic symptoms.

7.3 Capsular contracture

Symptomatic capsular contracture occurs in 3 to 5% of patients (Mandrekas 1995). Retaining the filling port permanently allows some surgeons to treat early signs by over inflation of the implant at the onset of symptoms and maintaining the over expanded state for 2 to 3 months, followed by a return to the recommended fill range. As capsular contracture progresses, pocket revision may become necessary. Modest capsule formation may be treated by capsulotomy but often the implant capsule is thick and may need to be excised by capsulectomy. If soft tissue coverage is inadequate, consideration needs to be made as to whether this could be improved by increasing the subcutaneous adiposity by fat transfer, implant cover by incorporation of an acellular dermal matrix or autologous tissue such as using a latissimus flap. In cases of recurrent capsule formation, especially early or after radiotherapy, an autologous component for implant cover may become necessary or an elective strategic change to autologous reconstruction without implant would avoid further capsule related complications.

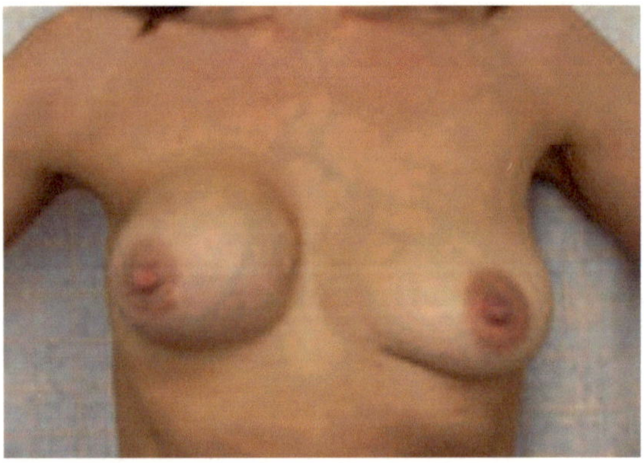

Fig. 10. Grade 4 capsule contracture

7.4 Scalloping and rippling

Over or under filling of the device may cause visible and palpable wrinkling of the outer envelope. This becomes even more obvious when thin, loose or irradiated soft tissue fail to provide adequate padding. Irregular visible or palpable implant edges mostly in the upper inner quadrant of the reconstructed breast may be avoided by conforming to the saline fill range recommended by the manufacturer. Another site at which rippling may be more prominent is the inferior pole of the reconstructed breast in a dual plane approach where the pectoralis major covers the upper pole of the implant while the lower pole lies in the subcutaneous plane.

Textured surfaces that provide tissue ingrowth also result in tissue adhesion to the anterior implant pocket. The resultant tethering may contribute to visible and palpable wrinkling of the tissue overlying the implant. A loose pocket or a smooth surface on the other hand does not eliminate this problem as elasticity of the overlying skin may similarly result in a wrinkled appearance. Other solutions that could be considered include skin tightening, fat transfer, internal capsulorrhapy, incorporation of an acellular dermal matrix or the addition of a latissimus dorsi muscle flap.

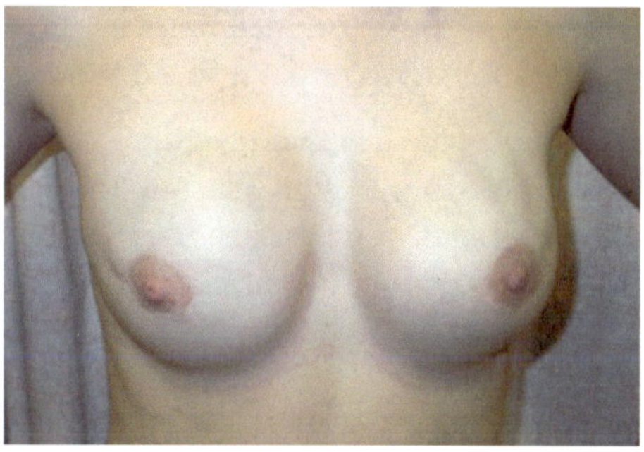

Fig. 11. Left upper pole rippling following nipple sparing mastectomy

7.5 Skin and nipple ischaemia and necrosis

Compromise to the blood supply of the mastectomy skin flaps or to a preserved nipple can result in tissue ischaemia and necrosis. The risk of skin and nipple ischaemia is elevated when skin sparing techniques have been used because of the increased length of the mastectomy flaps from the perforating blood vessels supplying the skin. Care must be taken to ensure that the flaps are not compromised. Supportive measures in the immediate post-operative period such as warming (with a warming blanket and warmed intravenous fluids), nursing in a supine position, correction of profound anaemia and avoidance of hypotension may reduce the incidence of skin and nipple ischaemia. Superficial necrosis may be managed conservatively with supportive measures in the first instance and then with appropriate dressing and wound care. Infection, inflammation and skin necrosis should be aggressively treated either with antibiotics or excision of the necrotic skin with primary closure. It is particularly important to excise and repair any necrotic skin early as if necrotic tissue is left for longer, the risk of a wound infection increases significantly.

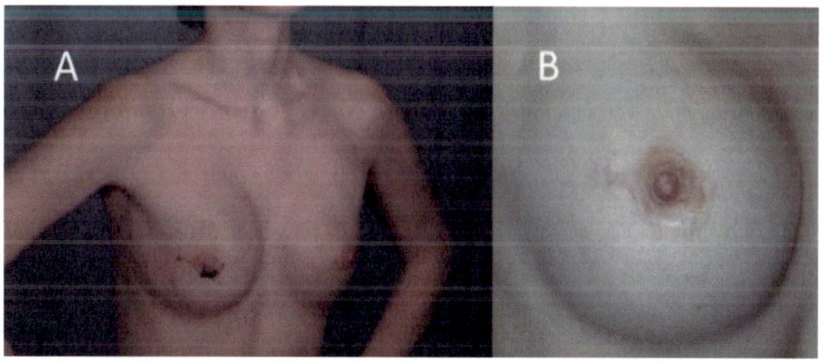

Fig. 12. A,partial nipple necrosis following nipple sparing mastectomy. B, Close-up view of nipple-areolar complex showing recovery of necrotic areas

8. Conclusion

Implant based breast reconstruction remains the most common method utilized to reconstruct a breast after mastectomy for cancer. Implant reconstruction has advanced through the years with better devices and improved surgical techniques. Skin-sparing volume reducing procedures that utilize de-epithelialized skin for implant cover have broadened the scope of patients suitable for implant based breast reconstruction beyond the traditional concept of slim to moderately built women with modest breast size and minimal ptosis. The further development of acellular dermal matrices and fat transfer techniques will see further evolution of patients suitable for implant based techniques.

Autologous breast reconstruction is an option for many women. The choice of breast reconstruction depends on multiple factors when selecting the best reconstruction option for a patient. One consideration is the level of patient motivation and the patient's willingness to undergo complex or extensive procedures, including the risk of failure or comorbidities associated with those procedures. The magnitude of surgery, the length of recovery, potential complications, resultant extensive scarring, and potential functional loss associated with some forms of autologous breast reconstruction may be a valid reason why patients opt for implant based surgery, recognising that maintenance surgery is more likely. Breast reconstruction using expanders and implants offers an excellent opportunity to achieve high quality results in breast reconstruction.

Breast reconstruction should be tailored to meet the individual needs of patients. The options available and the decision making process should be fully discussed and a balance of benefits and risks used in the final analysis of patient choice. Units that offer breast reconstruction should have access to the range of options in current practice to meet these needs.

9. References

American Society of Plastic Surgeons. (2010). Report of the 2010 Plastic Surgery Statistics, In: ASPS website, Accessed 24th July 2011: http://www.plasticsurgery.org/Documents/news-resources/statistics/2010-statisticss/Top-Level/2010-US-cosmetic-reconstructive-plastic-surgery-minimally-invasive-statistics2.pdf

Beasley, M.E. & Ballard, A.R. (1990). Immediate breast reconstruction: a comparison of techniques utilizing the pedicled TRAM and tissue expanders. *Proceedings of the annual meeting of the American Association of Plastic Surgeons*, Hot Springs, Va, May,1990

Behranwala, K.A., Dua, R.S., Ross, G.M., et al. (2006). The influence of radiotherapy on capsule formation and aesthetic outcome after immediate breast reconstruction using biodimensional anatomical expander implants. *British Journal Plast Surg*, 59, pp. 1043-51

Buinewicz, B. & Rosen, B. (2004). Acellular cadaveric dermis (AlloDerm): a new alternative for abdominal hernia repair. *Ann Plas Surg*, 52, pp.188

Carlson, G.W., Bostwick, J.B., Toncred, M.S., et al. (1997). Skin-Sparing Mastectomy Oncologic and Reconstructive Considerations. *Annals of Surgery*, 225, pp.570-578

Clough K.B., Thomas S.S., Fitoussi A.D., et al. (2004). Reconstruction after conservative treatment for breast cancer: cosmetic sequelae classification revisited. *Plast Reconstr Surg*, 114, pp.1743-53.

Collis N. & Sharpe D.T. (2000). Breast reconstruction by tissue expansion. A retrospective technical review of 197 two-stage delayed reconstructions following mastectomy for malignant breast disease in 189 patients. *Br J Plast Surg*, 53, pp. 37-41

Cordeiro P.G., Pusic A.L., Disa J.J., et al. (2004). Radiation after immediate tissue expander/implant breast reconstruction: outcomes, complications, aesthetic results, and satisfaction among 156 patients. *Plast Reconstr Surg*,113, pp 877-81

Gui, G.P.H., Tan, S-M., Faliakou, E.C., et al. (2003). Immediate breast reconstruction using biodimensional anatomical permanent expander implants: a prospective analysis of outcome and patient satisfaction. *Plast Reconstr Surg*, 111, pp.125-138

Hunter-Smith D.J. & Laurie S.W. (1995). Breast reconstruction using permanent tissue expanders. *Aust N Z J Surg*. 65, pp. 492-5

Inamed (2005) Summary of safety and effectiveness data, silicone gel filled breast implants, FDA website, accessed on 24th July 2011, available http://www.accessdata.fda.gov/cdrh_docs/pdf2/P020056b.pdf

Kronowitz, S.J. (2010). Delayed-immediate breast reconstruction: technical and timing considerations. *Plast Reconstr Surg*, 125, pp 463-74

Mandrekas, A.D., Zambacos, G.J. & Katsantoni, P.N. (1995). Immediate and delayed reconstruction with permanent expanders. *Br J Plast Surg*, 48, 572

Mansel R.E., Horgan K., Webster D.J., et al. (1986). Cosmetic results of immediate breast reconstruction post-mastectomy: a follow-up study. *Br J Surg*., 73, pp. 813-6.

Menon, N.G., Rodriguez, E.D., Byrnes, C.K., et al. (2003). Revascularization of human acellular dermis in full-thickness abdominal wall reconstruction in the rabbit model. *Ann Plast Surg*, 50, pp. 523

Peyser P.M., Abel J.A., Straker V.F., et al. (2000). Ultra-conservative skin-sparing 'keyhole' mastectomy and immediate breast and areola reconstruction. *Ann R Coll Surg Engl*. 82, pp. 227-35

Ramon Y., Ullmann Y., Moscona R., et al. (1997). Aesthetic results and patient satisfaction with immediate breast reconstruction using tissue expansion: a follow-up study. *Plast Reconstr Surg*. 99, pp. 686-91

Rosen, P.B, Jabs, A.D., Kister, S.J., et al. (1990). Clinical experience with immediate breast reconstruction using tissue expansion or transverse rectus adbominis musculocutaneous flaps. Ann Plast Surg, 25, pp. 249

Schuster RH, Rotter S, Boonn W., et al. (1990). The use of tissue expanders in immediate breast reconstruction following mastectomy for cancer. *Br J Plast Surg*., 43, pp. 413-8.

Simmons, R..M., Hollenbeck, S.T. & Latrenta, G.S. (2003). Areola-sparing mastectomy with immediate breast reconstruction. *Ann Plast Surg*, 51, pp 547-51

Slavin S.A., Schnitt S.J., Duda R.B.,et al. (1998). Skin-sparing mastectomy and immediate reconstruction: oncologic risks and aesthetic results in patients with early-stage breast cancer. *Plast Reconstr Surg*.102, pp. 49-62

Spear S.L. & Majidian A. (1998). Immediate breast reconstruction in two stages using textured, integrated-valve tissue expanders and breast implants: a retrospective review of 171 consecutive breast reconstructions from 1989 to 1996. *Plast Reconstr Surg*. 101, pp. 53-63

Spear, S.L. & Pelletiere, C.V. (2004). Immediate breast reconstruction in two stages using textured, integrated-valve tissue expanders and breast implants. *Plast Recons Surg*, 113, pp. 2098

Tallet A.V., Salem N., Moutardier V., et al. (2003) Radiotherapy and immediate two-stage breast reconstruction with a tissue expander and implant: complications and esthetic results. *Int J Radiat Oncol Biol Phys*, 57, pp. 136-142

One-Stage Immediate Breast Reconstruction with Implants in Conservative Mastectomies

Marzia Salgarello, Giuseppe Visconti and Liliana Barone-Adesi
University Hospital "Agostino Gemelli", Catholic University of "Sacro Cuore", Rome, Italy

1. Introduction

The evolution of breast cancer surgery is focused on optimization of the balance between the oncologic radicality and the maximization the cosmetic outcomes. The final goal of reconstructive breast surgery is to achieve a pleasant and attractive breast that matches as much as possible what is considered a "normal breast."To do that, it is important first to understand which features define the normal female breast identity. Followings the works of Blondeel et al., the breast identity can be defined by a balanced combination of all the followings four elements:

- *Breast Footprint*: the foundantion of the overlying breast, including the inframammary fold (IMF).
- *Breast Conus*: shape along with ptosis, volume and projection. These mean the "contents" of the breast.
- *Breast Skin Envelope*: the "container", what hold the breast "contents" on the footprint.
- *Nipple-Areola Complex*: unique structure, normally located on the point of maximal antero-posterior projection.

The absence of even only one of these elements prejudices the breast identity.

It is on these concepts that we can better understand and explain the advances of breast cancer surgery from radical modified mastectomy to conservative mastectomies such as skin-sparing mastectomies and nipple-sparing mastectomy.

So far, what is and what is not "conservated" by mastectomies? The breast conus is the only element that is always removed, being the parenchymal tissue its main component. The radical modified mastectomy violates all the other three elements. The skin-sparing mastectomies violate the conus and nipple-areola complex while preserve the skin envelope and an important breast structure such as the IMF (part of the breast footprint). The nipple-sparing mastectomy preserves everything except the conus.

More is violated, more has to be replaced, more demanding is the reconstruction, more difficult is the achievement of an an "attractive" breast. Since we are talking about the aesthetic appearance of the breast, it is also quite intuitive that more the "missed" element is visible more the mastectomy is recognized as "mutilative" and more the aesthetic outcome is less favorable. So far, the absence of breast conus only that can be replaced by an implant or autologous tissue (being both not readily noticeble) is less of concern if compared to a replaced skin envelope or reconstructed NAC.

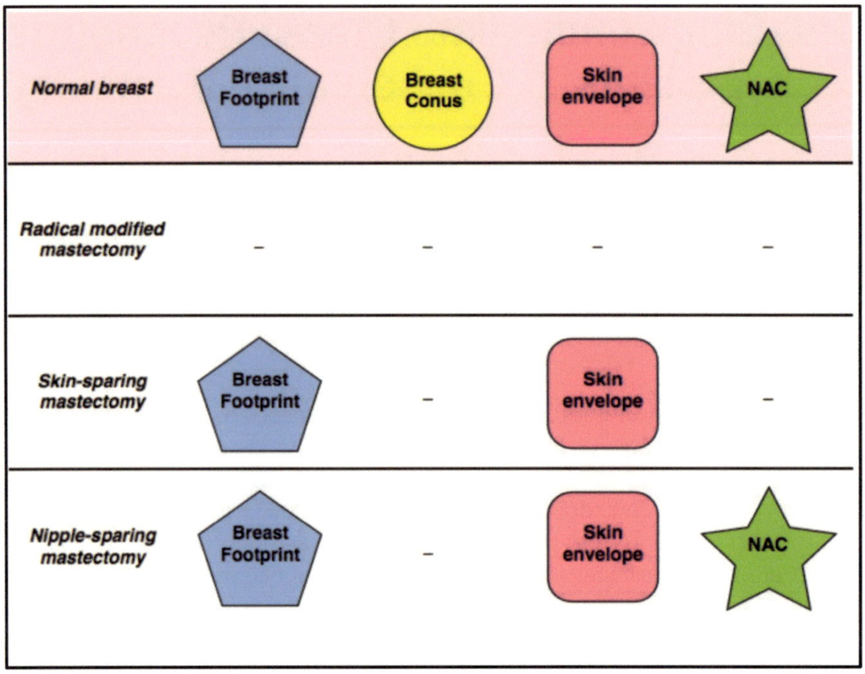

Since it was introduced by Toth and Lappert, skin-sparing mastectomy (SSM) has gained wide popularity over the last twenty-years. It is now considered a safe oncologic procedure, being its indications limited to the treatment of early breast cancer.

As for the concepts outlined above, the absence of the NAC leads patients to still identify SSM as a "mutilative procedure", even if the breast mound is immediately reconstructed with implant or autologous tissues.

NAC reconstruction is usually performed 2-3 months later in outpatient setting. The aesthetic outcomes of different NAC reconstruction techniques are variable and no-one really matches the original features of the removed NAC.

For these reason and because of the successful application of skin-sparing mastectomy in breast surgery, surgeons worldwide have started to reconsider the feasibility of preserving the NAC during the mastectomy to maximize the cosmetic outcome in breast cancer surgery. Nipple-sparing mastectomy (NSM) represents, in fact, a further evolution of the "conservative" mastectomy concept, because by also preserving the NAC, reduces the mutilation consciousness to the breast conus only.

2. Indications

In this section we broadly summarize the oncologic indications for conservative mastectomies as this argument goes beyond the goal of this chapter.

- *Risk reduction/prophylactic mastectomy.*
- *Therapeutic mastectomy.*

In high-risk patients, risk reduction/prophylactic NSM is widely accepted because it has been demonstrated that it dramatically reduces the incidence of breast cancer, allowing at the same time a very satisfying reconstruction.

In breast cancer patients, SSMs has been demonstrated by large series to have no significant increase in local recurrence rates when compared to conventional mastectomies in patients with early breast cancer, except the ones with the skin tethering by tumour. In our centre, SSM is indicated in extensive ductal carcinomas in situ (DCIS), in multicentric tumors, in tumors that do not infiltrate the skin, with T1 and T2 tumors and an unfavorable breast-to-tumor ratio, and in patients who did not respond to chemotherapy. SSM is not indicated in inflammatory tumors or in locally advanced tumors.

NSM is indicated in carefully selected patients as the main concerns are related to both the risk of local recurrence of the cancer and development of a de-novo tumor in the NAC. This is justified by studies from 70s and 80s that have demonstrated an incidence of NAC tumor involvement ranging from 12 to 58%. However, these findings date from an era of later diagnosis and more advanced diseases. In fact, more recent reports have shown that NSM could carry an acceptable level of risk in selected patients with small (< 3cm), peripheral breast cancer with a negative axillary node. Nevertheless, there is no uniform consensus worlwide on the strict inclusion criteria of NSM as different technique are being used worldwide in NSM. In fact, some Authors use to excise the nipple core, others leave a thin button of tissue beneath the NAC with the aim to improve its viability, whereas others use the intraoperative radiotherapy with electrons (ELIOT) to further diminish the oncologic risk of the procedure. However, all these approaches, even with different inclusion criteria, are promising in the treatment of of some type of early breast cancer. In our centre, Nipple-sparing mastectomy is restricted to oncologic patients within the following inclusion criteria: tumor size of less than 5 cm, tumor at least 2 cm from the nipple-areola complex, no skin involvement or inflammatory breast cancer, clinically negative axillae or negative frozen-section of the sentinel node, negative intraoperative frozen section of the tissue immediately beneath the nipple, and patients' choice between breast conservative surgery and nipple-sparing mastectomy.

In addition to the oncologic considerations, the reconstructive concerns are equally determinant in NSM as this procedure is being performed to maximize the cosmetic outcomes after mastectomy. An unsatisfying reconstructive result would not justify the NSM to SSMs.

In this chapter we will analyze the one-stage immediate implant breast reconstruction using the submuscular subfascial pocket following conservative mastectomies, focusing on the aesthetic outcomes and reconstructive issues.

3. Relevant applied anatomy

The comprehension of anatomy of the musculo-fascial structures of the thorax is essential for understanding and performing the submusculo-subfascial pocket dissection in breast reconstruction.

The Thorax muscles are anatomically divided by their depth in three layers:

- the first (more superficial) layer is defined by Pectoralis Major muscle (PM);
- the second (intermediate) layer is defined by Pectoralis Minor and Subclavian muscle;
- the third (deeper) layer is defined by the Serratus Anterior muscle (SA).

The submuscular-subfascial pocket is mainly defined by structure belonging to the first layer, as follow:

- superiorly by the released pectoralis major muscle (PM) with its fascias - deep pectoralis major fascia (DPF) and superficial pectoralis fascia (SPF).
- Inferiorly by the SPF.
- Laterally by the lateral pectoralis fascia (LPF) and axillary fascia (AF) with or without the serratus anterior muscle (SA).

3.1 Pectoralis major muscle

PM is a large, fan-shaped muscle. It originates from the medial clavicle, the sternum, the anterior second to sixth/seventh ribs and inserts onto the upper humerus about 10 cm from the humeral head on the anterior margin of the bicipital sulcus. On the median line of the sternum, it approaches the contralateral PM. It borders on rectus abdominis muscle inferiorly, the external oblique muscle infero-laterally, the serratus anterior muscle laterally and the deltoid muscle superiorly. The PM is superficial to rectus abdominis, serratus anterior and external oblique muscles.

The lateral margin of the PM forms the anterior axillary fold.
The main function of the PM is adduction and medial rotation of the arm.

3.2 Deep pectoralis fascia (DPF) and superficial pectoralis fascia (SPF)

The PM is wrapped by the pectoralis major fascia that anatomically represents a downward continuation of the superficial cervical fascia.

From anatomy books, the relationship of this fascia with the surrounding anatomical structures is usually not described in depth. That's why, we believe it is important to focus on some key-point of the anatomical relationship of these structures as they play a fundamental role in defining the submuscular-subfascial pocket.

The pectoralis major fascia wraps the PM by splitting itself in the deep pectoralis fascia and the superficial pectoralis fascia.

The DPF is located on the inner side of PM. Inferiorly it ends where PM ends and laterally it fuses itself with the SPF to define the pectoralis fascia laterally, or lateral pectoralis fascia (LPF).

The SPF is located on the outer side of PM, just below the deep layer of the superficial fascia (i.e breast capsule). Many fibrous connections exist between the SPF and the deep layer of the superficial fascia, making a bluntly dissection very difficult. These are:

- numerous thin, fibrous bundles in the upper third of PM;
- the presence of the Wuringer septum at the level of the fourth and fifth intercostal spaces;

- a tight connective tissue connecting the inframammary fold (IMF) with SPF.

The SPF thickness varies with different site of fascia. According to Jindle et al., SPF average thickness is 0.49, 0.60, 0.52 and 0.68 mm in the upper, lower, medial and lateral side. In our cadaver dissection experience, we found the SPF a thin and fragile but well defined fascia with strict anatomical relationship with PM epimysium (Fig. 1), confirming Jindle findings.

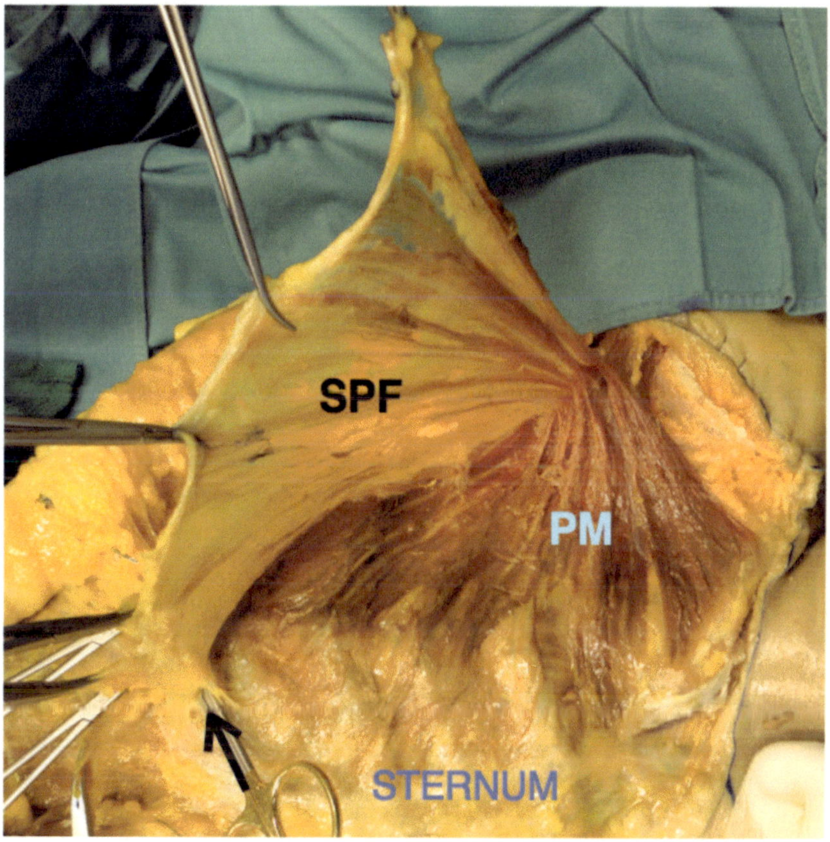

Fig. 1. SPF, cadaver dissection.

Cadaver dissection of right superficial pectoralis fascia. The deep layer of superficial breast fascia (breast capsule) has been dissected from SPF and PM. SPF has been dissected from the underlying PM starting from the superomedial to the inferolateral direction. The SPF continuation upward in the superficial cervical fascia as well as its adhesions to the sternum have been interrupted at the clavicle and at the sternum to allow the dissection. The cleavage between SPF and PM is anatomically not well distinct because of the strict relationship between SPF and PM epymisium. For this reason, few PM fibers have to be included in the fascia dissection. The black arrow points where the SPF anatomically have a fan shape behaviour. (see also figure 2, right)

The SPF cover the outer side of the PM. Laterally, it fuses with the DPF (figure 2, left) defining the pectoralis fascia laterally or lateral pectoralis fascia. Inferiorly, it pass over the inferior border on PM for few centimeters to end on the rectus sheath.

We found a peculiar behaviour of the SPF at the level of the IMF. At this point the SPF has a fan-shaped structure with two main divergent directions: one, that goes superficially ending on the skin at the level of the IMF and the other one goes inferiorly, vanishing on the rectus sheath. This structure plays a fondamental role in defining the IMF as, through this aproneurotic structure, the IMF is firmly attached to the chest wall. (figure 2, right)

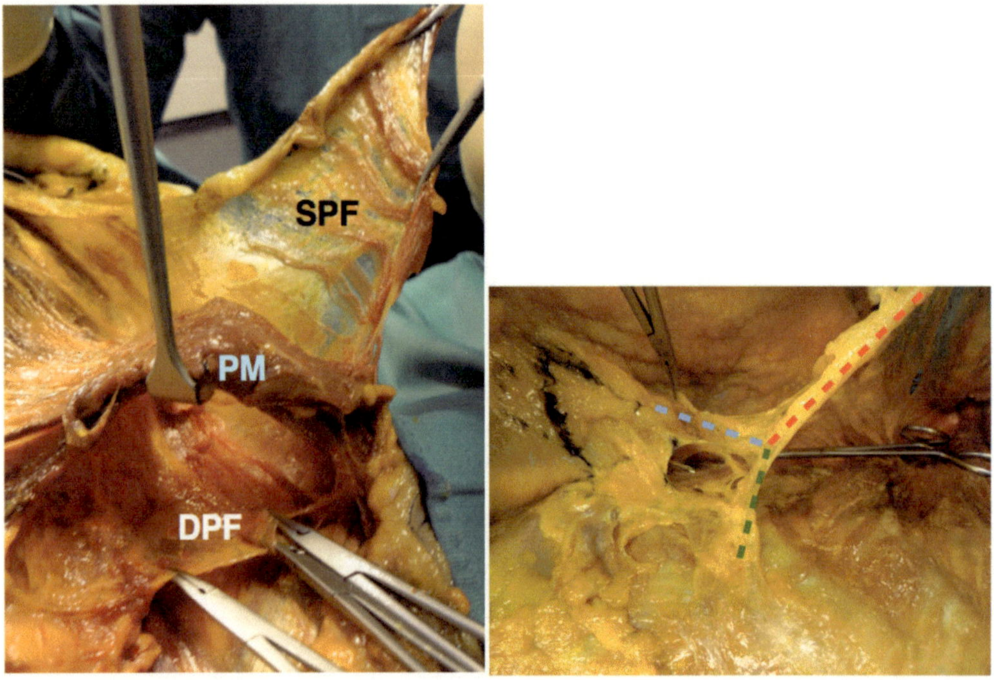

Fig. 2. (Left). SPF and DPF, cadaver dissection of right SPF. Close up at the lateral part of the PM defining the anterior axillary pillar. The SPF and DPF has been dissected off the muscle. Both fascias fuses themselves laterally defining an unique fascial layer, the lateral pectoralis fascia that continues laterally over the serratus anterior muscle as axillary fascia. (Right) Close up of SPF cadaver dissection at the IMF. At the IMF level, a needle has been inserted percutaneously. The SPF is a flat and thin structure over the PM (red dotted line). SPF shows a fan-shaped structure once at the IMF level with fibers showing two main directions: superficial fibers insert themselves at the level of the IMF (blue dotted line) while deep fibers point the abdominal wall by vanishing on the rectus sheat (green dotted line). The fan-shaped structure has been entered (where the needle emerges) to clarify the behaviour of the SPF at the IMF.

The structural features of the SPF makes it not useful in breast implant surgery if the SPF is completely dissected by the surrounding structures. In fact, it is a very fragile and thin fascia that can be easily smashed, thus having any supportive role alone. However, if used in combination with the surrounding structures, it can add valuable benefits in breast implant surgery.

In sub-fascial breast augmentation, the implant is placed beneath the SPF and above the PM. However, the SPF is only dissected by the PM being firmly attached to the breast capsule and breast itself.

In our submuscular-subfascial breast placement, the implant is placed beneath the PM being the fascia attached to the PM itself. The SPF relationships with PM epymisium are not violated, thus not weakening the fascia itself. In the submuscular-subfascial pocket, the SPF is only dissected beyond PM border, where the SPF is thicker. Inferiorly it is dissected by the rectus sheath and laterally by the SA.

3.3 Lateral pectoralis fascia (LPF) and axillary fascia (AF)

The LPF is defined by the fusion of the SPF and DPF lateral to PM border. The LPF continues with AF.

The AF extends between the lateral border of the PM anteriorly and the lateral border of Latissimus Dorsi muscle posteriorly, forming the floor of the axilla. It is suspended from the clavi-coraco-pectoral fascia, a triangular shaped aponeurotic system that envelopes the second layer of the thoracic muscles (i.e. Pectoralis minor, subclavian), being the downward continuation of the deep cervical fascia.

Lateral to PM, the AF is superficial to the SA and its fascia (third layer).

In the submuscular-subfascial pocket dissection, the AF is dissected in continuity with the LPF over the SA almost reaching the median axillary line. When this fascial layer is disrupted during the mastectomy or it is found very thin, we prefer to continue the plane of dissection beneath SA muscle and its fascia to assure lateral coverage.

3.4 Serratus anterior muscle (SA)

The SA is a large, fan-shaped muscle and the deepest extrinsic thoracic muscle. It origins with digitations from the upper eight ribs, intedigitating with origins of the external oblique muscle. The function of the SA is to stabilize the scapula against the chest wall. The SA is covered by its fascia, deeper to the AF and clavi-coraco-pectoral fascia.

In the submuscular-subfascial pocket dissection, the SA with its fascia is sometimes raised in continuity with the AF. This, when the LPF has been disrupted during the mastectomy or it is very thin.

4. Clinical decision-making in SSMs and NSM - How to maximize the results

4.1 SSMs and breast reconstruction: Why, when and how

We routinely offer SSMs in early stage breast cancer patients within our oncologic inclusion criteria. SSMs differ from radical modified mastectomy as the native breast skin is being preserved, allowing a more pleasant breast reconstruction. The type of skin incisions and the amount of skin removed define the type of SSM according to Carlson et al. Type I to III are reserved to patients with small to medium size breasts and the mastectomy carried out through a periareolar approach. A challenge arises in patients with macromastia. Whether reconstructed with implant or with the autologous tissues, a discrepancy between the spared skin envelope and the reconstructed breast mound tend to be. Because a contralateral reduction is usually required for symmetry, the Type IV and V SSM are offered to these patients, also known as skin-reducing mastectomies (SRM) as the oncologic procedure is carried out using a reduction pattern.

4.2 NSM and breast reconstruction: Why, when and how

Nipple-sparing mastectomy is offered to selected patients with the aim of maximizing the cosmetic outcome in high-risk and breast-cancer patients. Hence, the teamwork between plastic and breast surgeons is paramount. In our series of risk-reduction and oncologic nipple-sparing mastectomies, we did not register any subsequent nipple-areola complex cancer involvement. The final pathology of the retro-areolar tissue confirmed the negative intraoperative frozen section. Our nipple-areola complex cancer involvement rate is found to be within the range reported in the literature. Patients whose tumors are within 5 cm, at least 2 cm from the nipple-areola complex, without skin involvement or inflammatory breast cancer may be candidates when the intraoperative frozen section of the tissue immediately beneath the nipple-areola complex is negative.

4.3 The patient selection process in SSMs and NSM

4.3.1 SSMs

Patients with breast cup from A to C are better served with a type I to III SSM. The SRM patterns have been designed for patients with macromastia undergoing SSM as these patients would typically present a mismatch between skin redundancy and implant volume if type I to III SSM are performed. The SRM allows excess skin envelope removal and at the same time a pleasant shape and symmetry with the contralateral breast that usually needs a reduction, using the same reduction pattern as the SRM breast. The resulting final scars are similar to those from cosmetic surgery. The type IV SSM identifies a SSM with a reduction pattern embracing both the inverted-T reduction as well as the vertical reduction patterns. If the vertical reduction pattern is feasible in patients with medium to large breast, the inverted T approach is best suited for patients with very large and ptotic breasts. The type V SSM has been described to overcome the limitations of the type IV SSM in patients with superficial tumors located above the proposed reduction pattern.

Compared to SSMs, inverted-T SRM are characterized by a higher rate of skin ischemic complications as the mastectomy flaps are more devascularized by the pattern itself. For this reason, the selection criteria for SRM patients should be more strict than SSM patients. Risk factors such as smoking, diabetes and neoadjuvant chemotherapy has to be considered prior surgery.

4.3.2 NSM

Patients with breast cup A/B/C with a Regnault ptosis grade within 2 and hemiperiareolar scars/lateral scars with nipple-areola complex lateralization/ scars in the medial quadrants and from breast reduction/mastopexy should be informed that a higher rate of nipple-areola complex-related minor complications could occur. We discourage nipple-sparing mastectomy with implant reconstruction in very large and ptotic (cup D and over with Regnault ptosis grade 3) breasts, large breasts with scars, and in patients radiated or planned for radiation therapy.

Besides the type of incision and the NSM technique used, other factors may concur to the development of nipple-areola complex ischemic complications. Among these, heavy smoking, diabetes, and large-size and very ptotic breasts have been generally recognized as risk factors.

Evaluation of candidates for Implant-based Reconstruction in SSMs

Excellent candidates

- Thin patients undergoing bilateral SSM.
- Monolateral SSM with normal, small-medium size, no/minimally ptotic contralateral breast.

Good candidates

- Monolateral SSM with medium-big size, ptotic contralateral breast.

Poor candidates

- Radiated patients.
- Obese and smoking patients.
- Some neo-adjuvant chemotherapy protocol in SRM (still under investigation)

Evaluation of candidates for Implant-based Reconstruction in NSM

Excellent candidates

- Thin patiens with breast cup A to B and ptosis grade 1 without breast scars.
- Bilateral NSM.
- Monolateral NSM with normal, small-medium size, no/minimally ptotic contralateral breast.

Good candidates

- Thin patiens with breast cup C and ptosis grade 1 without breast scars.
- Thin patients with breast cup A to C and ptosis grade 1 to 3 with previous scars: external radial without NAC lateralisation and supero-lateral quadrant.
- Monolateral NSM with normal, small-medium size, ptotic contralateral breast.

Poor candidates

- Patients with breast cup D or major.
- Previous breast scars: lateral scars with NAC lateralization, medial quadrant scars, scars in the mammary fold and from previous breast reduction/mastopexy.
- Radiated patients.
- Obese and smoking patients.

4.4 Planning the skin incision

Besides the well-defined type I to III SSMs, planning the incision plays a key role in both SRM and NSM.

4.4.1 SSMs (type I to III)

Following Toth and Lappert paper on skin-sparing mastectomy, Carlson GW el al. classified the procedure in four types based on the type of incision made and the amount of skin removed.

- *Type I.* In SSM type I, the skin incision is periareolar only with, sometimes, a lateral radial extension to enhance the exposure. (i.e patients with small nipple-areola complex). SSM type I is normally offered to patients with breast cancer diagnosis made by needle biopsy, thus without other breast scars. Only the NAC is removed. (figure 3, left)
- *Type II.* The skin incision is periareolar in continuity with previous breast scars or skin overlying superficial tumors. It is intuituve that SSM type II is normally offered to patients with previous breast scar or superificial tumour tethering the skin in proximity to the NAC itself. When these are distant from the NAC, the SSM type III is applied to these patients. The NAC along with the previous scars/tumours are removed including the intervening skin.(figure 3, center)
- *Type III.* The mastectomy is developed through a periareolar incision. Distant excision of a previous breast scar or skin overlying superficial tumours is added. In this case, the intervening skin can be preserved. (figure 3, right)

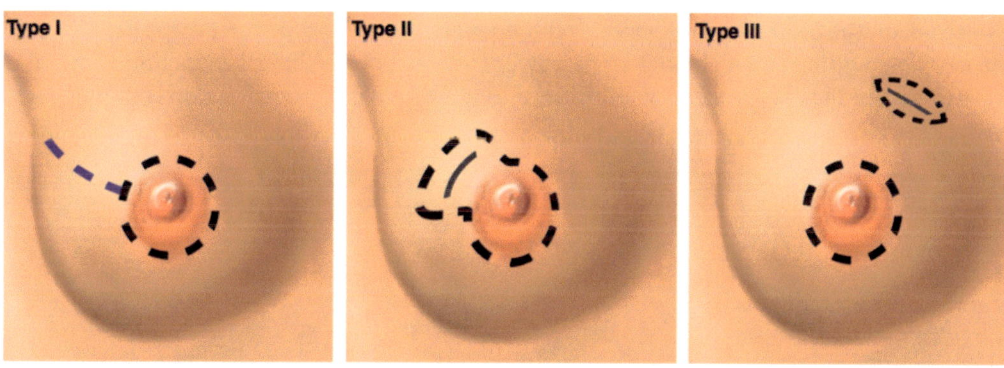

Fig. 3. (Left) Type I SSM. The lateral radial incision is made only for better exposure (dotted violet line). (center) Type II SSM. The intervening skin between the breast scar and the periareloar incision in included in the pattern. (right) Type III SSM. The intervening skin between the breast scar and periareolar incision in not included in the pattern.

4.4.2 SSM type IV or SRM

The SSM type IV or SRM are normally offered to patient with macromastia and/or ptotic breasts. The skin incisions resemble the inverted-T or the vertical reduction pattern, even if an important concept should be underlined for the incision planning. When a inverted-T SRM is planned, the mastectomy is developed through the inverted-T pattern, thus removing en-bloc the breast cancer with the skin pattern. In our series, when a vertical skin excess is present, the mastectomy is performed through a circumareolar approach (type I SSM) and a vertical dog-ear is removed at the end of the reconstruction to better shape the skin envelope on the implant. So far, the ending scar is vertical along with a central purse-string suture.

The SRM pattern follows the contralateral breast reduction pattern being the latter defined as follows. IMF and breast meridian are marked. The location of the IMF is transposed onto the anterior surface of the breast, using the Pitanguy maneuver and marked on the breast meridian. One cm above this point, point A is marked on the breast meridian. This will be the new nipple site. With the aid of a compass set on 7-8 cm, with one tip held on point A, a line with an upward concavity is drawn. (figure 4 – black dotted line) Seven-eight centimeter is the sum of one-half the diameter of the areola and the length of the vertical limbs of the inverted T. Along the IMF, three points are marked: the medial (E) and lateral (F) extremities, and the place where the breast meridian crosses the IMF (D). Using point E as pivot, a compass set on the length as long as segment DE is rotated upward until it reaches the curved line drawn before. (figure 4 – red dotted line) Point B is marked there. In the same way, using point F as pivot and a compass set on the length as long as the segment DF (figure 4- green dotted line), point C is marked laterally on the same curved line. The inverted-T breast reduction pattern can now be easily completed connecting F to C, E to B and B and C to A. The drawing is checked twice by the surgeon. By using the fingers, point B and point C are pinched and transposed to point D to check the tension.

Once the breast reduction markings are completed, the SRM pattern is then drawn. The SRM pattern is marked similarly to the breast reduction one with few main differences. With the aid of a compass pointing the sternal notch and point A, point A′ is marked on the SRM side one centimetre below than the contralateral side. The vertical limbs of the inverted-T on the SRM side are marked with a length 1-2 cm longer than the reduction side. The key-hole width is kept about 2cm narrower than that on the breast reduction side. All in order to reduce the skin tension on the scars and to foresee the extensive skin retraction after mastectomy.

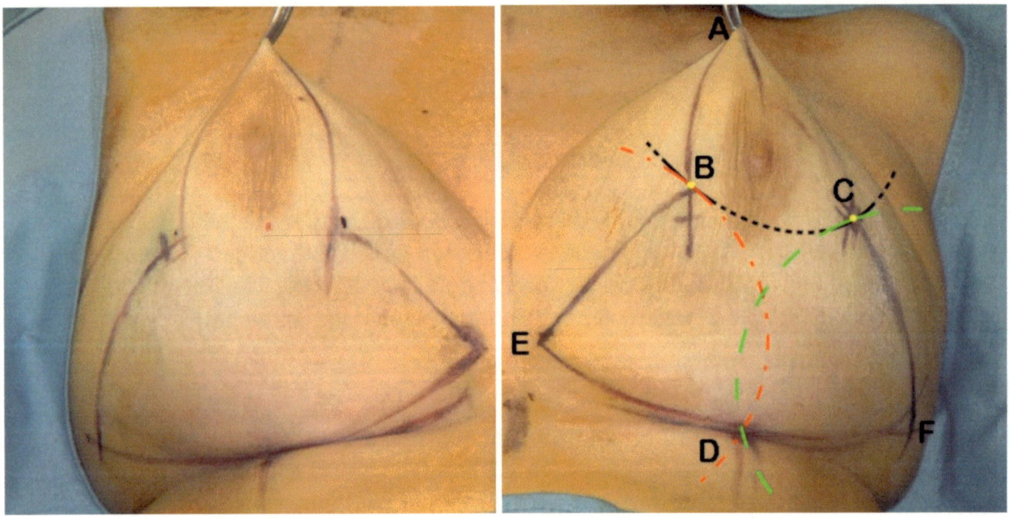

Fig. 4. The left inverted-T breast reduction pattern is showed along with the right SRM pattern. Note that the reduction pattern is wider than the SRM pattern.

The SRM pattern is checked twice. Point B′ and point C′ are pinched and transposed to point D′ to be sure that the vertical limbs are tension-free. Otherwise, the SRM pattern is corrected to gain the target of a tension-free skin closure. In every case the skin area encircled by the markings is wider on the breast reduction side compared with the SRM one.

When a bilateral SRM has to be performed, the SRM pattern is transposed on the contralateral breast for symmetry. If breast asymmetry is present, the skin areas encircled by the markings will be different, wider on the bigger breast.

When using the inverted-T SRM pattern, the major concerns are related to the viability of the skin flaps, especially at the T-junction where the breakdown rate has been reported to be up to 30 percent because of the skin flaps ischemia due to their length and thinness. To reduce the incidence of skin flap necrosis, the reduction skin pattern needs to be more "conservative" than the conventional one used for cosmetic reason, as also showed in our series. This results in longer vertical skin flaps with a more acute angle. The target is to close the skin flaps over the reconstructed breast in a tension-free fashion.

4.4.3 NSM

The incision must be suitable for an appropriate mastectomy, for easy access to the retro-areolar tissue without impairing the nipple-areola complex viability, and for reconstructive pocket dissection.

Initially, we used the inferior hemiperiareolar incision in the breast with a normal to large areola diameter to better hide the scar. When the areola diameter was small, we extended the inferior periareolar incision in a short lateral radial fashion. After experiencing major and minor nipple-areola complex complications with the periareolar approaches, we opted for radial incisions.

The radial approaches consisted of lateral radial and vertical radial incisions. The lateral radial incision (3 and 9 hours for left and right breast, respectively) began from just outside the areola and extended laterally for a variable distance, depending on the breast size/ptosis and the needs of the breast surgeon. The vertical radial 6 hours approach is preferred for big and ptotic breasts (ptotic C cup and D and DD cups) when a slight skin excision is required. In young patients that exhibits a good skin quality, the skin redraping over the implant makes this excision useless. The vertical radial 6 hour approach consists of a vertical lozenge along the breast meridian, starting from 1 to 2 cm above the inframammary fold and ending at the nipple, inferiorly. The lozenge may include a little triangle of the areola. The incision is then extended lateral periareolarly for a maximum of one-half of the nipple-areola complex circumference. The vertical approach allows some shaping of the skin after the insertion of the implant, as some redundant skin is removed along the vertical incision to match the implant size. This explains the need of smaller implants in these patients when compared with C cup- sized ones.

Breasts with scars from reduction mammaplasty/mastopexy have been accessed using a part of the existing scars. In the presence of other scars, the breasts were accessed using the existing scars.

Radial approaches and incisions using existing scars located in the superolateral quadrant are related to lower rate of minor complications, no major complications, and high patients' and surgeons' satisfaction.

The periareolar incisions have been found to be related to the higher rate of nipple-areola complex complications. Our findings are in agreement with those observed by other authors. In our opinion, radial lateral incisions allow the best exposure of breast parenchyma and nipple-areola complex tissue, and easy access to perform reconstruction.

4.4 The selection of the reconstructive option.

The reconstructive options after SSM and NSM are one-stage or two-stage alloplastic reconstruction and an autologous one, alone or combined with the implant. In a study comparing the cosmetic outcome of three different reconstruction techniques following nipple-sparing mastectomy (implant only, pedicled latissimus dorsi flap with implant, and deep inferior epigastric perforator flap), Mosahebi et al. reported no significant differences in those who did not undergo postoperative radiotherapy.

In our series, we found good to excellent results in 83 % of cases of NSM and in 90 % of cases of SSMs and SRM. Thus, we favor one-stage immediate implant reconstruction for many reasons. When compared with the autologous one, the one-stage implant reconstruction presents less morbidity, more technical simplicity, and absence of the need for donor-side recovery. We routinely perform autologous reconstruction in case of implant reconstruction failure and in patients previously irradiated or planned for radiation therapy.

In high selected radiated patient, nowadays, we can offer an alternative reconstructive procedure called "Lipobed", consisting of 1 to 3 sessions of breast fat grafting followed by implant-placement.

When compared with the two-stage implant reconstruction, the one-stage approach allows immediate definitive reconstruction and contralateral symmetrization procedures when needed. We found that by using the submuscular-subfascial pocket technique, a gentle expansion of lower-pole tissue coverage can be obtained. This, combined with the skin redundancy, leads us to consider tissue expansion as unnecessary in most of the case. Moreover, in SSM and SRM, the placement of a tissue expander would allow undesirable skin retraction of the mastectomy flaps. This phenomenon, in NSM cases, would promote nipple-areola complex lateralization. Some authors have expressed their concern in using definitive prostheses in the immediate set, because the skin stretching owing to the definitive implant could increase the risk of nipple-areola complex ischemia and skin-flap sufferance. This never happened in our cases.

Regarding inverted-T SRM, the implant-based reconstruction is often preferred as these patients are often obese making the autologous tissue reconstruction more challenging. In these patients, the major concerns are related to the viability of the skin flaps, especially at the T-junction where the breakdown rate has been reported to be up to 30 percent because of the skin flaps ischemia due to their length and thinness. To overcome this drawback, complete implant coverage with viable tissues beneath the skin flaps has been advocated. This allows to minimize complications over implants by giving a lifeboat for the skin healing process. This can be easily managed in an outpatient setting. The submuscular-subfascial pocket, being made only of autologous tissue, will favor the healing process by second intention in case of breakdown.

Thus, the technical advantages of the immediate implant reconstruction are as follows:

1. One-stage immediate reconstruction and contralateral symmetrization procedure when needed.
2. A natural breast shape for the significant lower-pole projection and no need of further coverage at the lower pole (i.e., acellular human dermis).
3. Reduction of the rate of implant reconstruction failure in SRM patients which experience T-junction breakdown as complete autologous tissue coverage is gained.

4. Preservation of the quantity and quality of the breast skin envelope, reducing the rate of skin retraction experienced with tissue expander placement.
5. Control of the nipple-areola complex tendency to migrate laterally. (NSM cases)
6. Reduction in the patient's physical and psychological impact from breast mutilation.
7. Reduction in healthcare costs.

On the other hand, this surgery is discouraged when the adipofascial layer is impaired during nipple-sparing mastectomy.

By ending this paragraph, we have to underline that there are some cases where the one-stage immediate implant reconstruction is not feasible because it would lead to unpleasant results. This normally happens for brachitype patients with short PM and little extensible SPF for whom it is not possible to obtain a good pocket space at the lower pole. It is in these cases, where the implant does not fullfill correctly the lower pole and is displaced in the upper pole, that we place a tissue-expander to better expand the lower pole thus creating the condition for a pleasant implant reconstruction.

4.5 The choice of the breast implant

Nowadays, both gel- and saline-filled implants with smooth, textured and polyurethane-foam covered are available on the market.

Currently, we found that anatomical cohesive silicone-gel textured implants with high projection were the most suitable for breast reconstruction; in fact, with the slightly filled upper pole as well as the full roundness and overprojected lower pole, they resembled the contour of a natural breast.

The determination of implant size depends on many factors. In literature, there are many mathematical-based algorithm for the choice of breast implant that can be helpful moreover for the young surgeons. However, we think that experience cannot be replaced by any mathematical algorithm, even the more dynamic and complete one.

Preoperatively, we estimated a range of implant sizes based on the following factors:

- contralateral breast mound, base and height.
- the actual breast mound, base and height of the mastectomy side as well as the expected breast volume to be replaced.
- Clinical evaluation of any chest-wall asymmetry.
- Patients' request. There are patients that are asking for bigger breast and other ones that prefers the same or even smaller volume.

It is mandatory for us that the range of implant sizes estimated preoperatively are available in the OR along with implant sizers. Nowadays, the advances in breast implant surgery offers the surgeons a large available choice on breast implant sizes, even within the same brand, that an almost "customized" reconstruction can be performed.

This advantages cannot be under-estimated if an excellent result is searched.

Intraoperatively, the final decision on the breast implant size and type is determined by evaluating the volume of the mastectomy specimen and either with the help of transverse width and vertical height of the contralateral breast and implant sizers.

In our experience on more than 350 patients, we did use Silimed Nuance silicon-gel filled implants with textured surfaces in 75 % of the cases and in the remainder Allergan Natrelle Style 410 silicon-gel filled implant with textured surfaces. Both the implant types share the anatomic shape and a high to extra projection in the lower pole.

4.6 The contralateral breast

When the conservative mastectomy is not bilateral, the final result in breast reconstruction cannot be limited to the reconstructed breast because it is a matter of symmetry between the reconstructed and contralateral breast. During preoperative patient consult, the plastic surgeon must assess also the contralateral breast along with patient desire, to correctly plan the reconstruction as well as the need of contralateral breast surgery. Patient has to be informed at the same time about the reconstruction along with the timing and plan, if any, for contralateral breast.

The contralateral breast can be left untouched only when facing with a normal, small-medium size breast with no ptosis when a conservative mastectomy with immediate one-stage implant reconstruction is performed.

Patient with breast hypoplasia are better managed with a breast augmentation. Patient with small-medium and ptotic breasts, from pseudo to real ptosis, are better managed with mastopexy with ot without implant.

Patients with medium to big and ptotic breast that underwent a SSM type I to III or a NSM can be managed with breast reduction with vertical or J-scar with or without implant.

Patient undergoing SRM are normally planned for immediate contralateral inverted-T breast reduction.

5. Surgical technique

Conservative mastectomies were carried out by the breast surgeon using different incisions, as explained above. These were planned preoperatively by the plastic surgeon in consultation with the breast surgeon.

The breast parenchyma was removed by sparing the superficial layer of the superficial fascia, leaving standard-thickness skin flaps and by deeply sparing the pectoralis major fascia. (Fig. 5,left) Following the mastectomy, the definitive implant was placed in a submuscular-subfascial pocket. The lateral pectoralis fascia is opened by blunt dissection in its upper part (at the level of the 1st and 2nd rib) and the subpectoral plane (beneath PM) entered at this level. (Fig. 5,right)

A fiber-optic retractor with incorporated suction is then inserted. Under direct vision, the subpectoral plane is dissected as the muscular fibres to the chest wall are divided with the cautery till the lower part of the pectoralis major. (fig. 6)

The PM has been detached from its costal insertion. Two fingers are introduced in the submuscular-subfascial pocket to show the dissection. Note that the musculo-fascial integrity are completely preserved inferiorly and laterally.

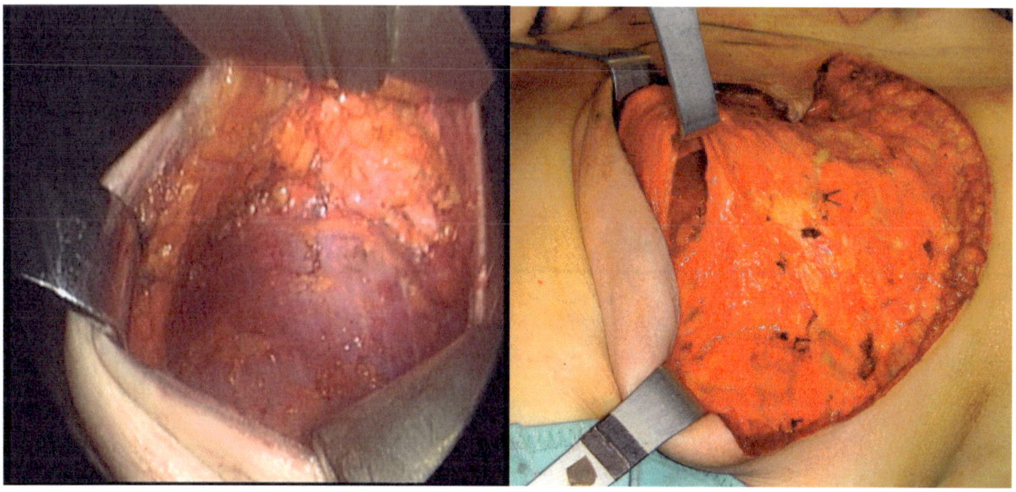

Fig. 5. (Left) SSM, picture made with endoscopic camera. Three retractors are lifting the mastectomy skin flaps. On the bottom, the PM with its overlying fascia. (right) Introperative picture of right SRM. Beginning of submuscular-subfascial pocket dissection. The submuscular space is bluntly entered laterally to PM at the level of the second rib. A retractor is lifting the PM at its upper part.

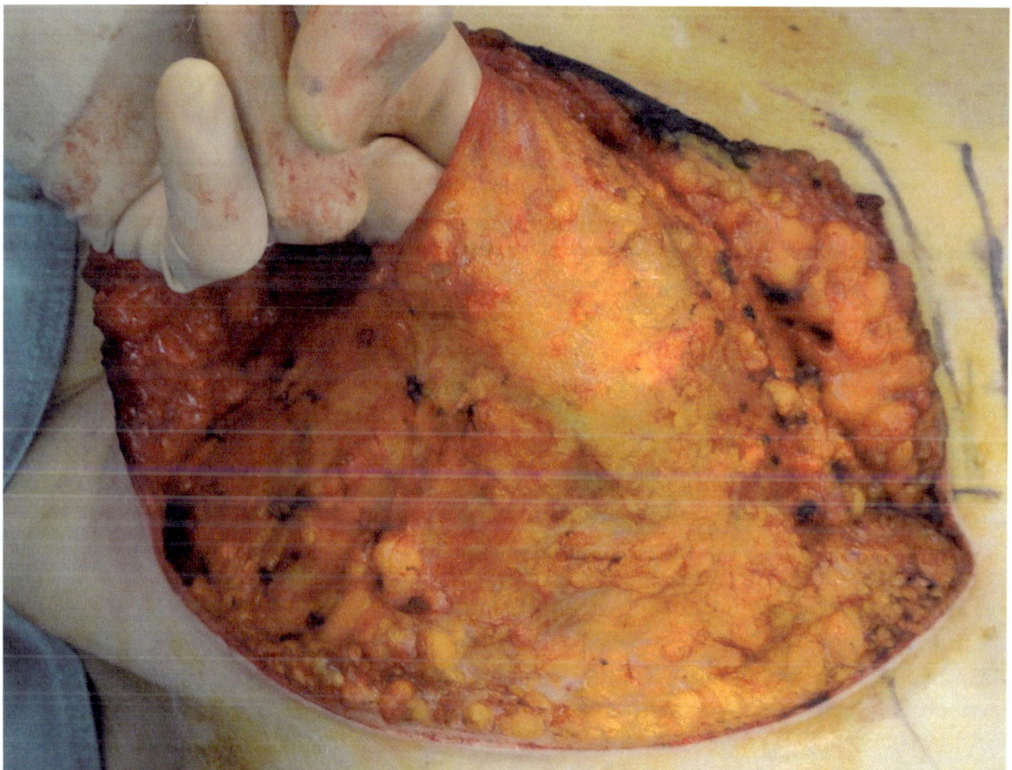

Fig. 6. SRM, sumuscular-subfascial pocket dissection.

At this level, the dissection is continued downward with cautery under the adipofascial layer (i.e. superficial pectoralis fascia (SPF) and overlying subcutis)(16,17), up to the inframammary fold (IMF). Then, the SPF is incised at the level of the IMF, exposing the overlying subcutaneous tissue. (Fig. 7)

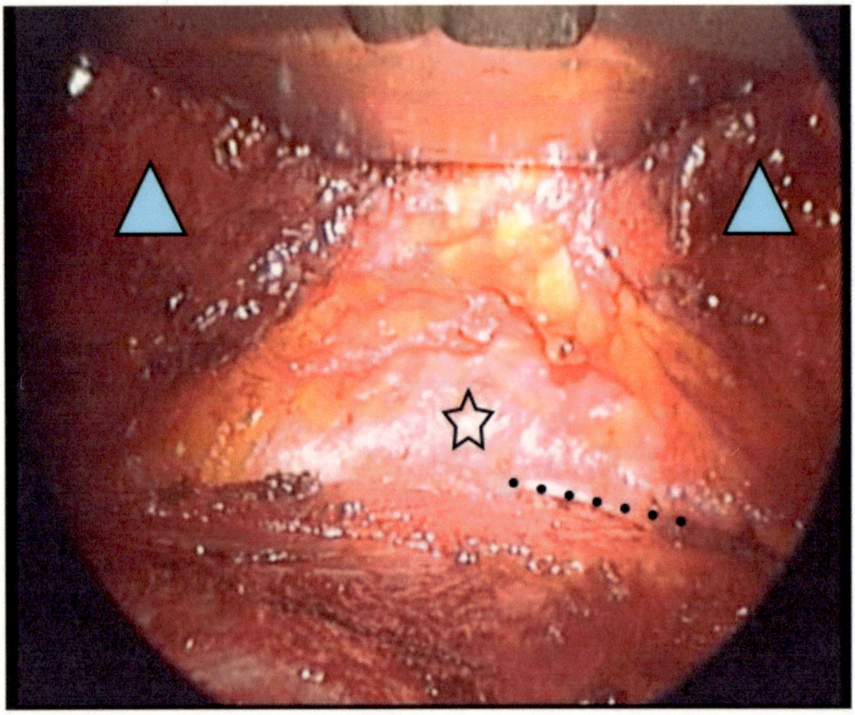

Fig. 7. SPF the PM, picture made with endoscopic camera. From *Salgarello M, Visconti G, Barone-Adesi L. (2010) Nipple-sparing mastectomy with immediate implant reconstruction: cosmetic outcomes and technical refinements. Plast Reconstr Surg.* 2010 Nov;126(5):1460-71.

PM costal insertion has been completely detached and PM freed (blue triangles). The retractor is pointing the inferior border of PM. SPF came into view as opalescent white structure with overlying subcutaneous tissue (star). The beginning of the rectus sheath is seen as a white, thick structure (dotted line).

This manoeuvre allows a re-definition of the IMF and a slight expansion of the lower pocket that may host even an implant with bigger volume than the excised gland.

Size choice of the implant was made with the help of implant sizer for Silimed prostheses and with the help of transverse breast width and vertical breast height for Mentor and McGhan implants. Nowadays, for the latter we use Allergan Natrelle 410 series ® FX and MX restrilizable implant sizer. After implant insertion, the upper part of the lateral pectoralis fascia was closed with absorbable stitches. Then the patient was semi-sitting positioned to check out the result.

The mobility of skin flaps, the larger quantity of tissue on the breast lateral pole and skin retraction would tend to attract the NAC laterally. The definitive implant filled the skin envelope (i.e. the mastectomy flaps) thus allowing the repositioning of the breast skin and preventing the NAC lateralisation. However, when needed, the NAC position was assured with 1 or 2 absorbable stitches from the retroareolar tissue to the pectoralis fascia.

Thence, the implant was covered by the pectoralis major superiorly and by SPF and the overlying subcutis inferiorly. The submusculo-subfascial pocket was closed over the implant as this was completely separated from the subcutaneous tissue of the mastectomy flap. (Fig.8)

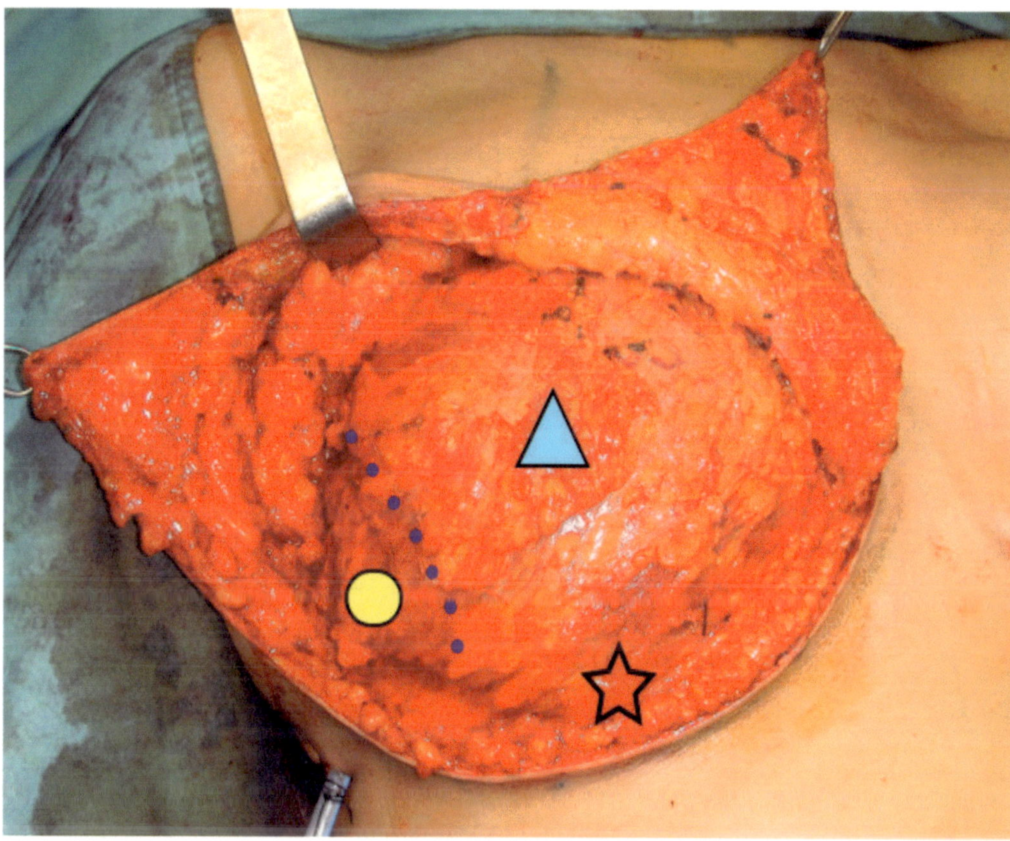

Fig. 8. SRM with definitive implant in the submuscular-subfascial pocket.

The submuscular-subfascial pocket seen from the mastectomy space in a SRM reconstruction. The dotted line shows the lateral margin of PM (blue triangle). The SPF has been lifted from rectus sheath inferiorly (star) and from serratus anterior laterally (yellow circle). The biomechanical features of these freed musculo-fascial structure allow the placement of big implant (in this case a 400 cc definitive implant) with good compliance of the musculo-fascial structure to the implant shape. Note the lower pole fullness along with a pleasant shape.

6. Results

6.1 SSM

We did perform more than 350 SSM with immediate one-stage breast reconstruction in our centre, being bilateral in 15% of the cases. Almost all monolateral cases (95%) had contralateral breast surgery to achieve simmetry. All these patients had not received radiotherapy and were not planned to undergo postoperative radiotherapy.

Neverthless, 3% of the patients underwent postoperative radiotherapy because of the following reasons after the final histology: extended multicentric tumour; peritumoral lymphatic invasion; more than 4 positive nodes. The final aesthetic outcome was judged as excellent to good in 78.6% (figure 9), fair in 14%, and poor in 7.3%.

Patients' satisfaction was from high to very high in 90% of the results.

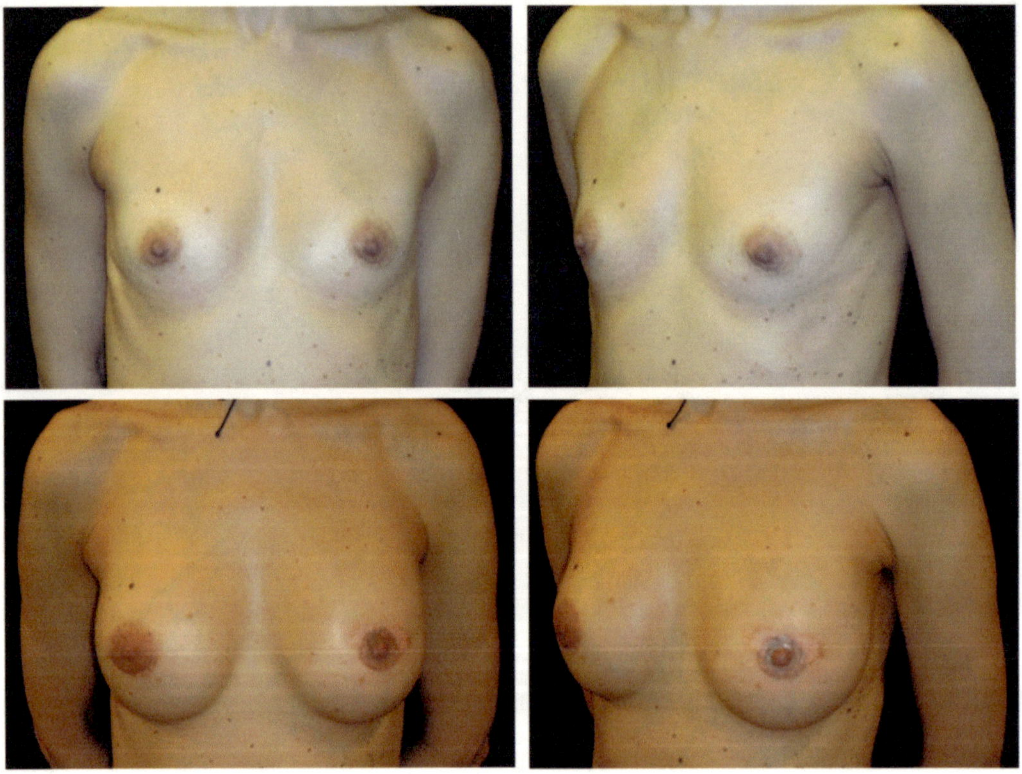

Fig. 9. (Above; left, right). Preoperative picture. The patient underwent left SSM type I with immediate implant reconstruction (McGhan 410 FX 280cc) plus right breast augmentation using McGhan 410 FM 205 cc. (Below; left, right) Thirteen month postoperative picture. NAC reconstruction has been performed 2 months later.

6.2 SRM

The average implant volume used was 416.5cc (range 300 to 500cc). The reconstructive outcomes were graded as excellent in 45 % of the patients (figure 10), very good in 40%, good 7%, fair and bad in 8 % of the cases which experienced full thickness necrosis of the vertical mastectomy limbs and at the T-junction. Patients' satisfaction was high to very high, except the case with "major" skin flap necrosis.

Major complications (i.e. extensive mastectomy skin flap necrosis) were noticed in 1 breasts that underwent debridement, implant removal and tissue-expander placement 2 days postoperatively. The only one minor skin necrosis have been experienced and managed by debridement and STSG in local anaesthesia 20 days postoperatively.

We did not experience any pathologic capsule contracture as well as any other early/late complications. Contour deformities have been found in 12.5%, which were all successfully treated with fat graft. (table 1)

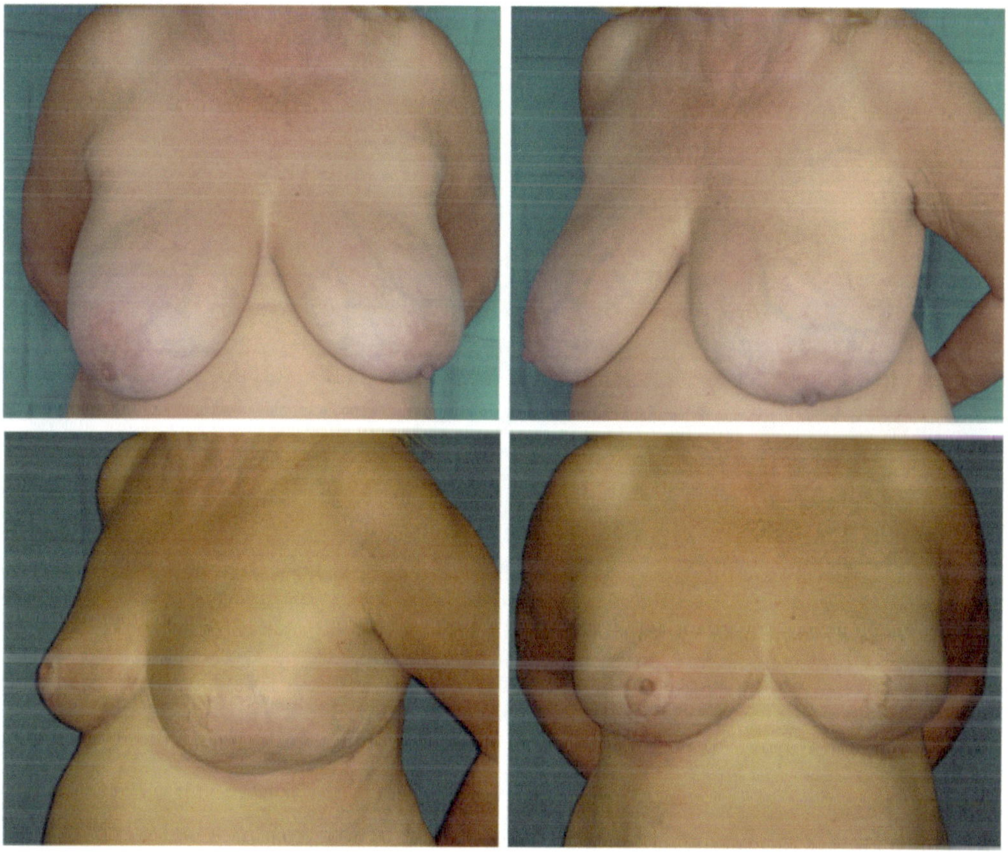

Fig. 10. (Above; left, right). Preoperative picture. The patient underwent left inverted-T SRM (mastectomy specimen weight:800gr) with immediate implant reconstruction (Silimed Nuance 300cc) plus right inverted-T breast reduction (reduction specimen weight 550gr). (Below; left, right) Eleven month postoperative picture. The patients refused the NAC reconstruction.

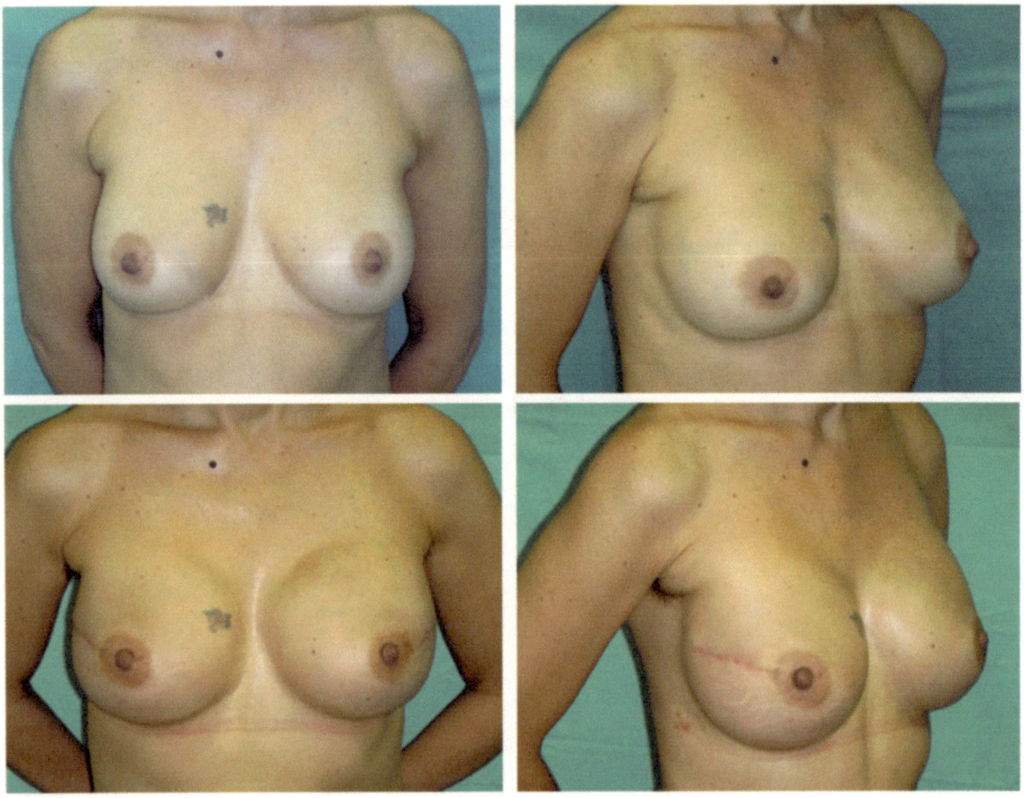

Fig. 11. (Above; left, right). Preoperative picture. The patient underwent bilateral NSM through radial lateral incisions plus immediate implant reconstruction (McGhan 410 MX 455cc). (Below; left, right) Three month postoperative picture.

6.3 NSM

On more than 60 cases with NSM, 40% were bilateral and 60% monolateral. All the monolateral cases underwent contralateral breast surgery simultaneously with nipple-sparing mastectomy for cancer (skin-sparing mastectomies and immediate implant reconstruction) and symmetry. The average implant volume use was 340 (range 200 to 485 cc).

The reconstructive outcomes were graded as excellent in 37.8% of the cases (figure 11), very good in 16%, good in 29.5%, fair in 10%, poor in 5% and bad in 1.7% in which total nipple-areola complex loss was experienced. Patients' satisfaction was high to very high, except the case with total nipple-areola complex loss.

6.4 Complications peculiar to each type of conservative mastectomy

6.4.1 SSM and SRM

Complications that may be experienced after SRM mastectomy and immediate implant reconstruction can be grouped in "early" and "late" complications. Among "early" complication, we identify mastectomy skin flap necrosis requiring revision surgery as "major skin necrosis". Skin flap necrosis susceptible to conservative treatment/minor surgery has been named "minor skin necrosis". Hematoma, seroma, infections represent other "early complications".

Thinning of skin with visible implant, implant rupture and capsule contracture represent the "late complications".

6.4.1.1 Major skin necrosis

The risk of mastectomy skin flap necrosis can be dramatically reduced if an appropriate patient selection is made preoperatively.

As outlined before, smoking, obesity, hypertension, diabetes, microvascular disease must be ruled out during preoperative patient consult as they have been recognized as risk factors. Even if literature evidence is lacking on the matter, some chemotherapy protocols seems to interfere with mastectomy skin flap viability.

Intraoperatively, it is never overstressed that mastectomy skin flap must be gentle manipulated during the oncologic surgery and a meticulous mastectomy with preservation of the subdermal plexus is mandatory.

Large mastectomy skin flap necrosis that extends over the T-junction means the failure of the conservative approach as a surgical revision consisting of debridement is needed. The debridement further reduces the skin envelope usually meaning removal of the breast implant. We did experience major skin flap necrosis in the only one case which underwent neo-adjuvant chemotherapy. (fig. 12)

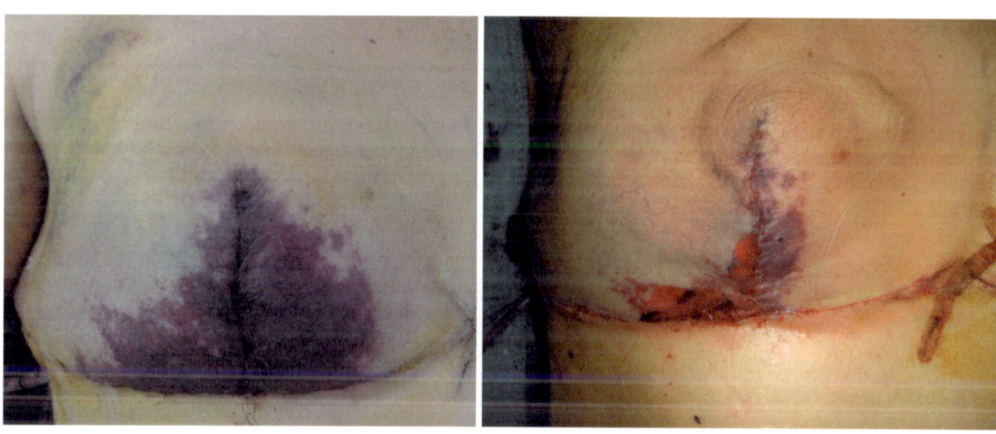

Fig. 12. Major skin necrosis after SRM. (Left) Postoperative day 2 of right SRM and immediate implant reconstruction with a Silimed Nuance 350 XH. Ischemic sufferance is visible at the T junction and at both the vertical mastectomy flaps. This patient underwent neoadjuvant chemotherapy and showed a preoperative chemotherapy related anemia. (right) Patient in the OR after debridement, implant removal and tissue-expander insertion.

6.4.1.2 Minor skin necrosis

The most experienced drawback in inverted-T SRM is the breakdown at the T-junction, reported up to 30 % in literature.(figure 13) When an implant reconstruction is performed, complete implant coverage with viable tissues is desirable to protect the areas at risk of breakdown. In case of skin necrosis, the presence of a viable tissue beneath the skin flaps would allow wound healing by second intention or by STSG. This would minimize implant reconstruction failure due to implant extrusion/infection, being this complication reported close to 15 percent in literature.

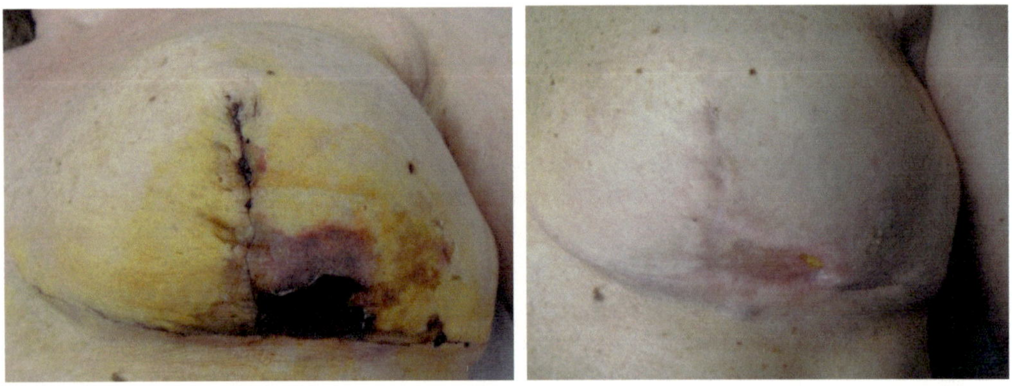

Fig. 13. Mastectomy skin necrosis at the T-junction after left SRM. (Left) Postoperative day 15 picture with a 3x2 cm frank eschar at the T junction. (right) Ten days after debridement and STSG taken from the bottom. There is a residual millimetric area in healing process.

6.4.2 NSM

Peculiar complication in NSM and immediate implant reconstruction can be divided in "early" and "late" complications. We grouped total nipple-areola complex loss and nipple-areola complex cancer involvement as "major complications." In fact, these cases represent a total failure of the NAC preservation both from an oncologic and cosmetic point of view.

Partial nipple-areola complex loss, skin flap-edge necrosis, impaired wound healing, were termed "early minor complications." Nipple-areola complex distortion and/or lateralization were termed "late minor complications."(table 1)

6.4.2.1 NAC cancer involvement

No nipple-areola complex cancer involvement was registered in our series.

The risk of NAC cancer involvment represents the main concern in breast cancer surgery when performing NSM. Inconsistent data from studies of 70s and 80s reported a risk of NAC cancer involvment from 12 to 58 %. However, these data came from an era of later diagnosis and more advanced disease. To reduce the likelihood of NAC cancer involvment, breast cancer patients have to be within stricts inclusion criteria. Even if there is still no general consensus on the inclusion criteria for NSM and on the predictor factors of NAC cancer involvment, the results from different centers outlined that NSM represents a safe oncological procedure in patients with tumour inferior to 3cm in size, at least 2cm from the NAC and with negative nodes. In fact, recent NSM series reports a NAC cancer involvment being from 0 to 16%.

We will not focus on the oncological aspect of NSM because it goes beyond the goal of this chapter, but it is important to underline that it is still a matter of debate, especially regarding the inclusion criteria and the predictor factors of NAC cancer involvment.

	Complications*		Major		Early minor**		Late minor				
		Breasts	**NAC total loss**	**NAC cancer involvement**	**NAC partial loss**	**Skin flap-edge necrosis**	**NAC lateralisation**	**NAC distortion**	**NAC lateralisation and distortion**	**Capsule contracture**	**Contour deformities**
PERIAREOLAR APPROACHES	***Hemiperiareolar*** 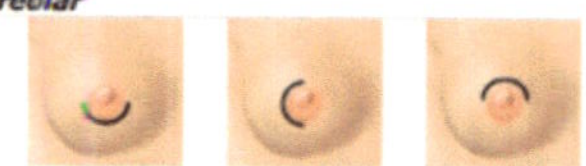 Inferior (13) Lateral (1) Superior (1) *The lateral and superior ones were used in breast with these existing scars.*	15	1 (B/1)	0	2	0	0	0	0	0	0
	Periareolar with lateral or vertical radial extensions 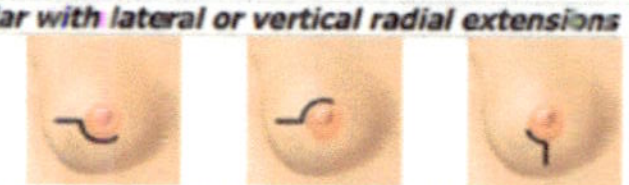 *(left, center)* Inferior (3) and superior (1) periareolar with radial lateral extension (hours 3 and 9 for left and right breasts respectively). 2 breasts showed existing lateral radial scar (post-lumpectomy) near the NAC	4	0	0	1 (A/0)	1	0 (in 1 case already displaced from BCS) (A/0)	1 (A/1)	0	0	2
	(right) Lateral periareolar with vertical radial hours 6 extension (3 cases) *(breasts with existing scars from reduction mastoplasty/mastopexy)*	3	0	0	2 (B/3) (C/3)	0	0	1 (C/3)	0	0	2
RADIAL APPROACHES	***Breast without existing radial scars*** 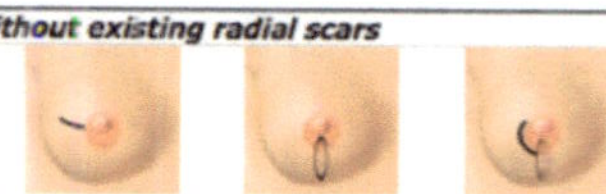 *(left)* Lateral radial incision (at hours 3 and 9 for left and right breasts, respectively) *For not very large and ptotic breast* (22 cases) *(center, right)* Vertical radial lozenge., with lateral periareolar extension when the access to the subpectoralis plane is limited. *For large and ptotic breasts* (4 cases)	26	0	0	0	0	0	1 (DD/3)	0	0	0
	Breast with existing radial scars from BCS 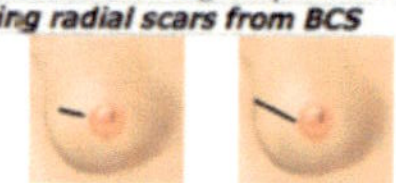 Lateral radial existing scars from BCS.	4	0	0	0	0	0 (in 4 cases already displaced from BCS) (A/1,C/3,B/0,?)	0	1 (Xrt) (C/1)	1 (Xrt) (C/1)	0
OTHER INCISIONS USING EXISTING SCARS	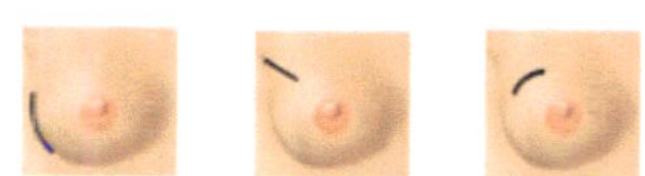 Lateral mammary Fold (LMF) (2) Between axilla and supero-lateral quadant (1) Supero-laterral Langer's line (6)	9	0	0	0	0	0 (in 1 case approached through LMF, already displaced from BCS) (C/3)	0	0	0	5
	TOTAL	61	1 (1.6%)	0 (0%)	5 (8.2%)	1 (1.6%)	0 but 6 cases already displaced from BCS	3 (4.9%)	1 (1.6%)	1 (1.6%)	9 (14.7%)

*: under each complication it is showed the breast cup size/ptosis grade according to Regnault.
** : other "early minor complications" such as infection, hematoma, seroma, skin flap sufferance has not been reported in the table because not experienced (0%).
BCS : breast-conserving surgery. Xrt : radiation therapy.

Table 1. Overview of our experience in NSM and immediate implant reconstruciton. The complications experienced are related to the skin incisions. From *Salgarello M, Visconti G, Barone-Adesi L. (2010) Nipple-sparing mastectomy with immediate implant reconstruction: cosmetic outcomes and technical refinements. Plast Reconstr Surg. 2010 Nov;126(5):1460-71.*

6.4.2.2 NAC total loss

After excluding the risk of NAC cancer involvment, all the surgical efforts should be spent in preserving the NAC viability when performing a NSM. This mainly means a gentle manipulation of the NAC during the mastectomy and the reconstruction time and preservation of subdermal plexus. These facts have to be always emphasized by the plastic surgeon, moreover when not working with the same breast surgeon. In our opinion, this complication itself would not justify NSM .

The risk of total NAC loss should be better assessed preoperatively or at most intraoperatively. When the surgeon is high suspicious about NAC viability he can opt to harvest the NAC in order to graft it at the end of the surgery. Alternatively, the NSM can be converted in SSM by removing the entire NAC.

In our series total nipple-areola complex loss was found in one breast. This patient was managed with early nipple-areola complex excision and purse-string closure, and did not require implant removal. (figure 14)

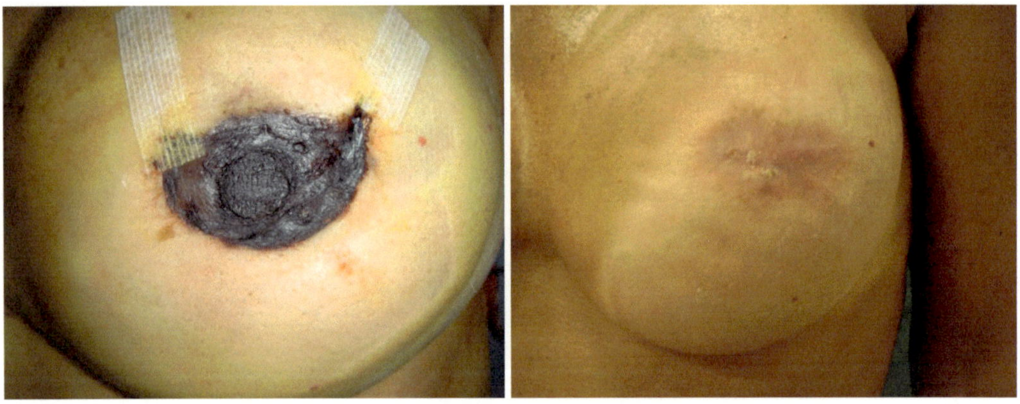

Fig. 14. NAC total loss (Left) Postoperative day 15 after left NSM and right SSM type II with immediate implant reconstruction. (Right) NAC total loss has been managed by debridement and purse-string closure in local anaesthesia; three-month later, it looks the patient underwent SSM.

6.4.2.3 NAC partial loss

Among early minor complications, partial loss involving less than 50 percent of the nipple-areola complex was found in 8% (Fig. 15). These were treated with dressing changes and healed uneventfully within 8 weeks.

6.4.2.4 NAC hypopigmentation

NAC hypopigmentation has been recognized as a sequelae of tissue ischemic sufferance without developing necrosis.

In our series, we did find one case of NAC hypopigmentation. (fig.16)

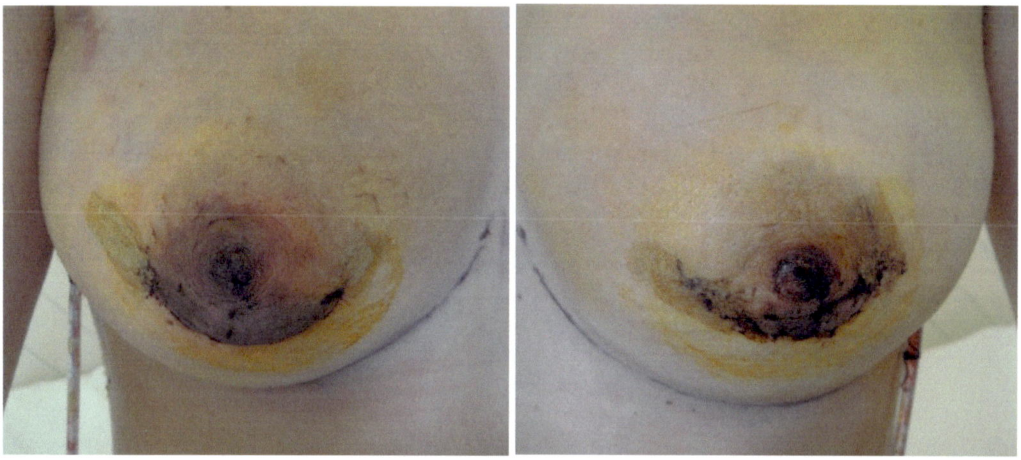

Fig. 15. Bilateral Partial NAC loss. Postoperative day 7 after bilateral NSM using inferior hemiperiareolar skin incision. (left, right)

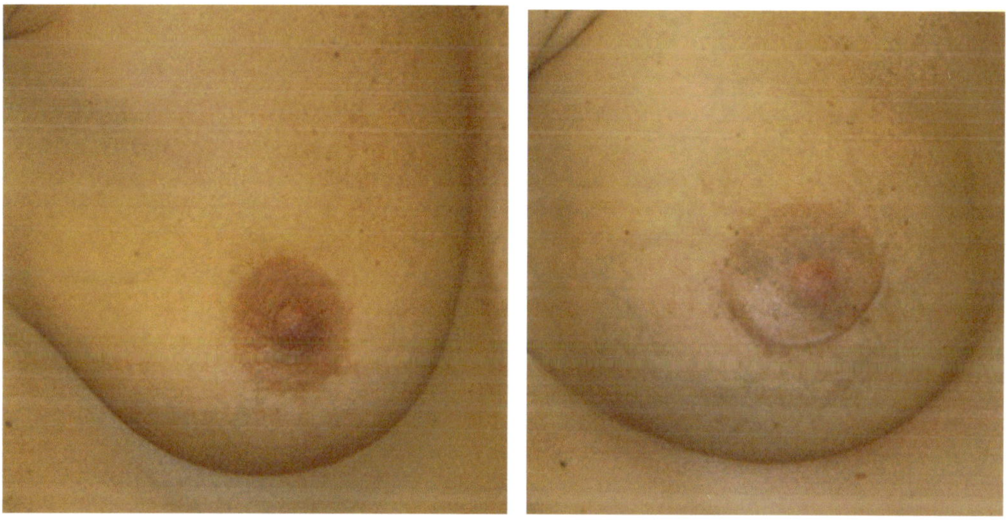

Fig. 16. NAC hypopigmentation. (left) Preoperative picture of NSM planned with inferior hemiperiareolar skin incision. (right) Two-month postoperative appearance. The NAC hypopigmentation in the inferolateral NAC quadrant is evident.

6.4.2.5 NAC lateralization / asymmetry / distortion

NAC lateralization defines a lateral malposition of the NAC when compared to preoperative location. For the breast aesthetic principles, the NAC should be located on the breast meridian. Some authors advocate that nipple-areola complex lateralization is related to either implant reconstruction or breast size/ptosis because of the likely dissociation between nipple-sparing mastectomy skin envelope, pectoralis nipple-areola complex major muscle, and implant. A recent 8-year survey on patient satisfaction after nipple-sparing mastectomy reconstruction(mainly with skin expander or autologous methods) by Mosahebi et al. demonstrates that nipple-areola complex malposition is a common complication and represents the most frequent aspect that patients would change, after lack of sensation. If sensation loss is not avoidable, our series demonstrates that nipple-areola complex malposition can be prevented. In our opinion, we did not experience nipple-areola complex lateralization because we directly inserted a definitive implant that completely filled the skin envelope and opposed skin retraction that would lateralize the nipple-areola complex position. In our series, we did not found any case of NAC lateralization even when using a radial lateral incision, except the cases which already showed this condition preoperatively, as sequela of previous breast-conserving surgery through radial lateral scars. (fig. 17)

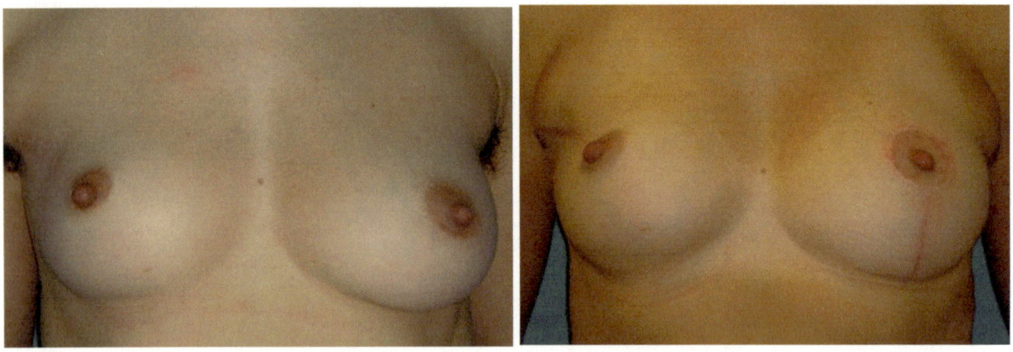

Fig. 17. NAC lateralization (Left) Preoperative picture of right NSM and left mastopexy. Patient underwent superolateral lumpectomy 1 year before on the right breast. The lumpectomy scar on the right breast is evident. It goes from the anterior axillary pillar to the areola and it brings to NAC lateralization. (right) One month postoperative after right NSM and immediate implant reconstruction and left vertical mastopexy. The NAC lateralization persists and it is more pronunciated as right breast volume is increased after NSM and immediate implant reconstruction.

NAC asymmetry is experienced when NAC position is not symmetryc with the contralateral one. This can be a consequence of monolateral NAC lateralization.

However, a symmetric bilatetal lateralization is a sign of symmetry. The likelihood of NAC asymmetry is expected to be higher in monolateral NSM than bilateral procedures.

NAC distortion is defined by an altered NAC shape. This minor complication can be due to a pull-effect of the NSM scar on the NAC or a impaired wound healing.

We did experienced this complication in 5% of the cases. (fig. 18)

6.5 Complications common to all conservative mastectomies

6.5.1 Hematoma, seroma, infection

None of these complications has been experienced in any case of NSM and SRM.

However, we did experience infection in 6% of SSMs, seroma in 1,5% and haematoma in 3%.

90 % of implant infection were solved with e.v. antibiotics. One patient developed a seroma that became infected, and subsequently, it required the explantation of the implant. Furthermore, one patient experienced an infection 50 days after the surgery during the first

cycle of adjuvant chemotherapy and required implant explantation. Regarding the patients who developed an infection and retained their implant, 15% showed severe capsular contractures at 6 month follow-up.

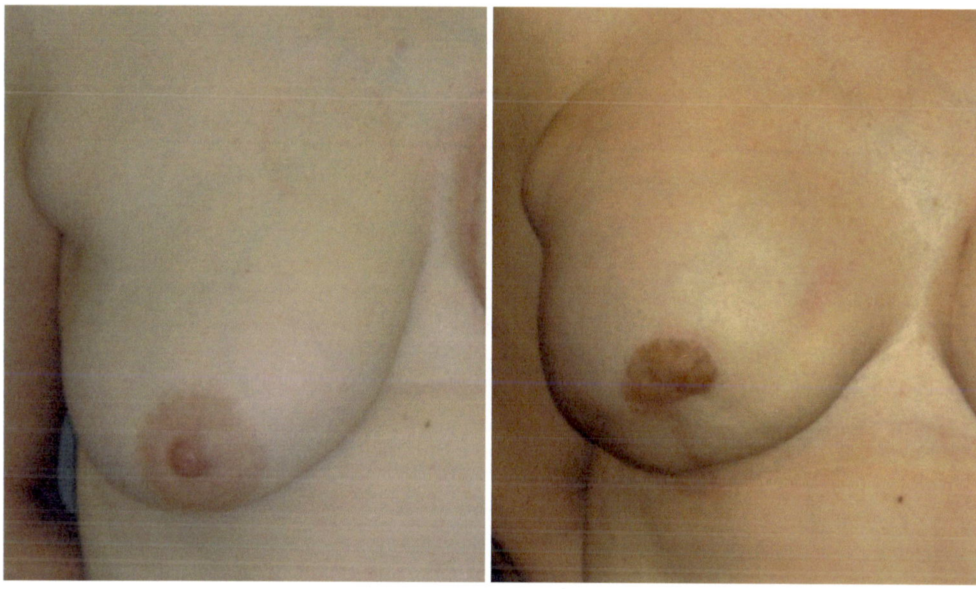

Fig. 18. NAC distortion along with nipple loss. (Left) Preoperative view of right NSM using a complete periareolar incision with vertical radial h 6 estension. Nine-month postoperative view. Note the NAC distortion and nipple loss after ischemic sufferance.

6.5.2 Rippling, implant rupture, implant malposition/rotation

We experienced 2% of rippling. We did not experience any case of implant rupture. Implant rotation has been experienced in only 2 SSM cases which underwent revision surgery.

6.5.3 Contour deformities

With the advances in modern breast reconstruction, the expectations from surgeons and patients for a great aesthetic result of a reconstructed breast are very high. The main goals are to recreate a harmonic breast mound in terms of size, projection, ptosis, providing natural contour in both the superior and inferior poles, so far matching the contralateral breast. According to Kanchwala et al., the contour deformities of the reconstructed breast and chest wall can be categorized in three groups:

- *Type 1.* The so-called "step-off" deformity occurring at the interface between the native chest wall and the reconstructed mound. It can be related to an "out-of-border" mastectomy that usually interests the superior pole, to an inappropriate implant or both. (fig. 19)
- *Type 2.* Intrinsic defect, secondary to irregularities from autologous tissue, fat necrosis or implant rippling.
- *Type 3.* Resulting from extrinsic factors, such as radiation therapy, scarring and post-lumpectomy defects. (fig 20)

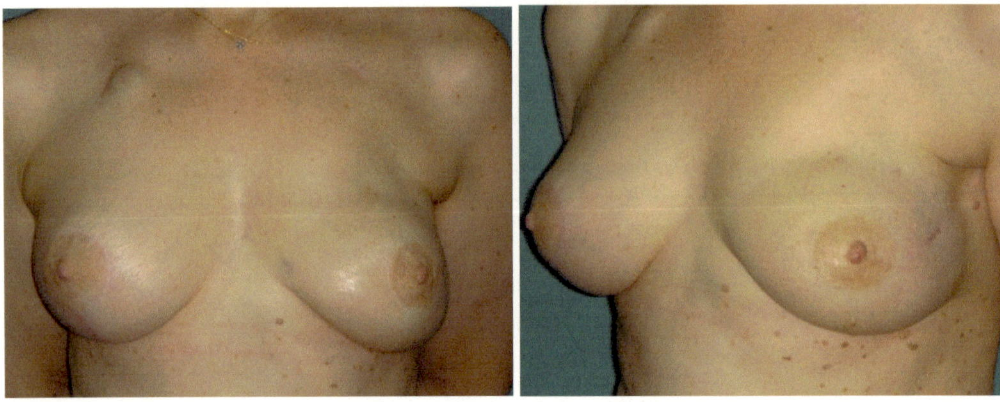

Fig. 19. (left, right) One-year postoperative view of left NSM thought previous lateral biopsy with immediate implant reconstruction using a Allergan Natrelle 410 LF 205cc scar and right J-scar mastopexy. The step-off deformity on the left breast is evident.

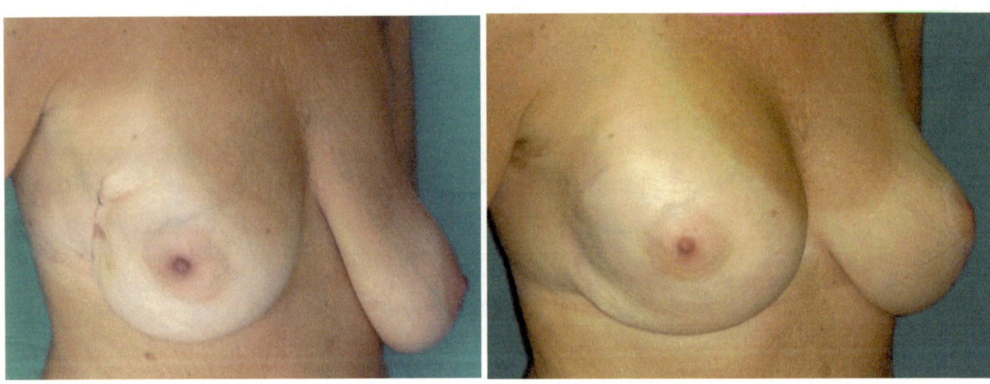

Fig. 20. (Left) Preoperative picture of right NSM and left J-scar mastopexy. Note the breast scar in the lateral mammary fold as sequelae of previous full lateral quadrantectomies. (right) Ten month postoperative view of NSM through previous lateral mammary fold scar and immediate reconstruction with Silimed Nuance 370cc. The lateral contour deformity due to previous extensive lumpectomy and scarring is evident.

The most experienced contour deformity in SSM patients is the type 1 deformity, where in NSM is the type 3. All these patients underwent from 1 to 3 sessions of fat grafting, experiencing different degrees of improvement. (fig. 21).

Autologous fat graft represents, nowadays, the best filler to correct soft tissue contour deformities as well as the ones experienced in the reconstructed breast. In fact it replaces "like-to-like", adipose tissue missed with the same tissue, providing excellent results in terms of contour, softness and camouflage. Depending on the extent of the defects, more than 1 session may be needed to achieve a satisfactory result. It is a low invasive operation, with few scarring and well-tolerated by patients.

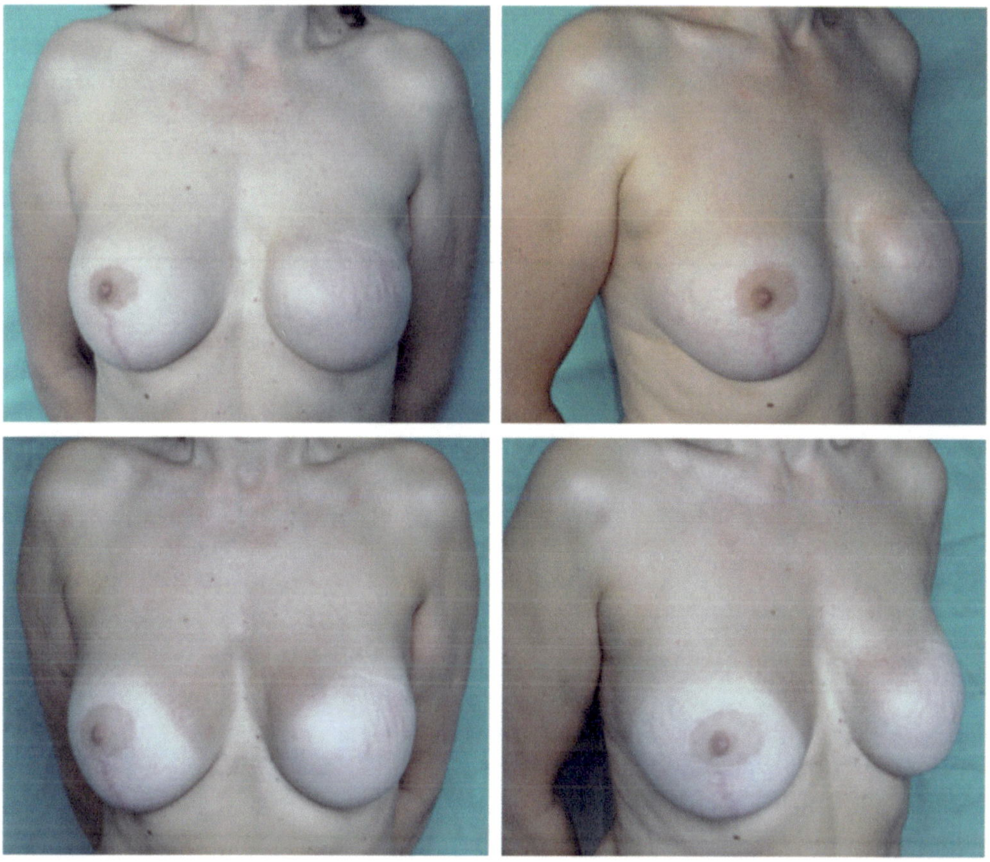

Fig. 21. (above; left, right) Fifteen month postoperative result after left SSM and immediate reconstruction with Silimed Nuance 480 cc and right breast mastopexy with implant (Silimed Natural 120cc). The "step-off" deformity in the upper quadrant of the left breast is evident as well as the implant contour in evident in the medial quadrant. (Below; left, right) Three month postoperative picture after 1 session of fat graft (32cc of grafted fat in the upper quadrant and 30cc grafted in the medial quadrant). The patient is waiting for the NAC reconstruction.

6.5.4 Capsule contracture

In breast implant surgery, capsule contracture represents an important issue. The human body response to the presence of a foreign body is the development of fibrous capsules, as it normally happens around breast implant. However, when this response leads to change of breast shape, induration and even pain it is recognized as capsule contracture. It represents one of the most significant complication in breast implant surgery.

Even if four decades has passed since the introduction of breast implants, the exact physio-pathogenesis of capsular contracture remains unknown. From more recent trends, capsular contracture is attributed to subclinical infection in breast pocket, presence of foreign bodies (i.e. Surgical gloves talc), suture line fibers, silicone particles coming from breast implant surface and last but not the least, especially in breast cancer patients, radiation therapy.

In our SSM series, we did experience 5% of capsular contracture of which 80% developed a Baker IV grade all sharing postoperative radiation therapy and 20% a Baker IV capsular contracture sharing history of infection and retained implants. No capsular contracture has been experienced in SRM cases. In our NSM series, we experience capsular contracture in the only one patient with a history of breast radiation therapy.

In case of capsular contracture in a radiated field, we normally pone indication to implant removal and autologous tissue reconstruction with DIEAP flap. If the patient has contraindication to the autologous tissue reconstruction or refused it, we perform 3 sessions of lipofilling all around the implant capsule followed by total capsulectomy and implant changing.

7. Conclusion

The immediate one-stage submuscular-subfascial implant reconstruction with hyperprojected silicone-gel filled anatomical implant represents a versatile and valid option in patients undergoing conservative mastectomies if not radiated or planned for radiation therapy. By using this surgical technique, very good aesthetic results, low complication rates, and high patient satisfaction are experienced. The clinical-decision making process in these patients is paramount to maximize the results.

8. Acknowledgment

Thanks to Prof. Dr. P.M.N. Werker, Mr. Hepke Gjaltema and Mr. Sip Zwerver for the opportunity, kindness and hospitality for the cadaver dissections at Weckenbach Institute - Skillslab, Universitair Medisch Centrum Groningen, Groningen, The Netherlands.

9. References

Blondeel PN, Hijjawi J, Depypere H, Roche N, Van Landuyt K. (2009) Shaping the breast in aesthetic and reconstructive breast surgery: an easy three-step principle. *Plast Reconstr Surg*. 2009 Feb;123(2):455-62.

Carlson GW, Bostwick J 3rd, Styblo TM, Moore B, Bried JT, Murray DR, Wood WC. (1997) Skin-sparing mastectomy. Oncologic and reconstructive considerations. *Ann Surg* 1997 May;225(5):570-5.

Caruso F, Ferrara M, Castiglione G, Trombetta G, De Meo L, Catanuto G, Carillio G. (2006) Nipple sparing subcutaneous mastectomy: sixty-six months follow-up. *Eur J Surg Oncol.* 2006 Nov;32(9):937-40.

Chen CM, Disa JJ, Sacchini V, Pusic AL, Mehrara BJ, Garcia-Etienne CA, Cordeiro PG. (2009) Nipple-sparing mastectomy and immediate tissue expander/implant breast reconstruction. *Plast Reconstr Surg.* 2009 Dec;124(6):1772-80.

Crowe JP, Patrick RJ, Yetman RJ, Djohan R. (2008) Nipple-sparing mastectomy update: one hundred forty-nine procedures and clinical outcomes. *Arch Surg.* 2008 Nov;143(11):1106-10.

Garcia-Etienne CA, Cody Iii HS 3rd, Disa JJ, Cordeiro P, Sacchini V. (2009) Nipple-sparing mastectomy: initial experience at the Memorial Sloan-Kettering Cancer Center and a comprehensive review of literature. *Breast J.* 2009 Jul-Aug;15(4):440-9. Epub 2009 May 22.

Gasperoni C, Salgarello M. Preoperative breast marking in reduction mammaplasty. (1987) *Ann Plast Surg.* 1987 Oct;19(4):306-11.

Gerber B, Krause A, Reimer T, Müller H, Küchenmeister I, Makovitzky J, Kundt G, Friese K. (2003) Skin-sparing mastectomy with conservation of the nipple-areola complex and autologous reconstruction is an oncologically safe procedure. *Ann Surg.* 2003 Jul;238(1):120-7.

Hartmann LC, Schaid DJ, Woods JE, Crotty TP, Myers JL, Arnold PG, Petty PM, Sellers TA, Johnson JL, McDonnell SK, Frost MH, Jenkins RB. (1999) Efficacy of bilateral prophylactic mastectomy in women with a family history of breast cancer. *N Engl J Med.* 1999 Jan 14;340(2):77-84.

Hartmann LC, Sellers TA, Schaid DJ, Frank TS, Soderberg CL, Sitta DL, Frost MH, Grant CS, Donohue JH, Woods JE, McDonnell SK, Vockley CW, Deffenbaugh A, Couch FJ, Jenkins RB. (2001) Efficacy of bilateral prophylactic mastectomy in BRCA1 and BRCA2 gene mutation carriers. *J Natl Cancer Inst.* 2001 Nov 7;93(21):1633-7.

Hunter JE, Malata CM. (2007) Refinements of the LeJour vertical mammaplasty skin pattern for skin-sparing mastectomy and immediate breast reconstruction. *J Plast Reconst Aesthet Surg* 2007;60(5):471-81.

Hwang K, Kim DJ. (2005) Anatomy of pectoral fascia in relation to subfascial mammary augmentation. *Ann Plast Surg.* 2005 Dec;55(6):576-9.

Jinde L, Jianliang S, Xiaoping C, Xiaoyan T, Jiaqing L, Qun M, Bo L. (2006)Anatomy and clinical significance of pectoral fascia. *Plast Reconstr Surg.* 2006 Dec;118(7):1557-60.

Kanchwala SK, Glatt BS, Conant EF, Bucky LP.(2009) Autologous fat grafting to the reconstructed breast: the management of acquired contour deformities. Plast Reconstr Surg. 2009 Aug;124(2):409-18. Review.

Kroll, S. S., Khoo, A., Singletary, S. E., et al. Local recurrence risk after skin-sparing and conventional mastectomy: A 6-year follow-up. *Plast. Reconstr. Surg.* 104: 421, 1999.

Laronga C, Kemp B, Johnston D, Robb GL, Singletary SE. The incidence of occult nipple-areola complex involvement in breast cancer patients receiving a skin-sparing mastectomy. *Ann Surg Oncol.* 1999 Sep;6(6):609-13.

McDonnell SK, Schaid DJ, Myers JL, Grant CS, Donohue JH, Woods JE, Frost MH, Johnson JL, Sitta DL, Slezak JM, Crotty TB, Jenkins RB, Sellers TA, Hartmann LC. Efficacy of contralateral prophylactic mastectomy in women with a personal and family history of breast cancer. *J Clin Oncol.* 2001 Oct 1;19(19):3938-43.

Menon RS, van Geel AN. Cancer of the breast with nipple involvement. *Br J Cancer.* 1989 Jan;59(1):81-4.

Mosahebi A, Ramakrishnan V, Gittos M, Collier J. (2007) Aesthetic outcome of different techniques of reconstruction following nipple-areola-preserving envelope mastectomy with immediate reconstruction. *Plast Reconstr Surg.* 2007 Mar;119(3):796-803.

Nahabedian MY, Tsangaris TN.(2006) Breast reconstruction following subcutaneous mastectomy for cancer: a critical appraisal of the nipple-areola complex. *Plast Reconstr Surg.* 2006 Apr;117(4):1083-90.

Nava MB, Catanuto G, Pennati A, Garganese G, Spano A. Conservative mastectomies. (2009)*Aesthetic Plast Surg.* 2009 Sep;33(5):681-6.

Nava MB, Cortinovis U, Ottolenghi J, Riggio E, Pennati A, Catanuto G, Greco M, Rovere GQ. (2006) Skin-reducing mastectomy. *Plast Reconstr Surg* 2006 Sep;118(3):603-10.

NCCN, National Comprehensive Cancer Network. (2011) Clinical practice guidelines in oncology: breast cancer - version V.2.2011. NCCN, 2011. (last access 30th of August, 2011)

Petit JY, Veronesi U, Orecchia R, Rey P, Martella S, Didier F, Viale G, Veronesi P, Luini A, Galimberti V, Bedolis R, Rietjens M, Garusi C, De Lorenzi F, Bosco R, Manconi A, Ivaldi GB, Youssef O. (2009) Nipple sparing mastectomy with nipple areola intraoperative radiotherapy: one thousand and one cases of a five years experience at the European institute of oncology of Milan (EIO). *Breast Cancer Res Treat.* 2009 Sep;117(2):333-8.

Regolo L, Ballardini B, Gallarotti E, Scoccia E, Zanini V. (2008) Nipple sparing mastectomy: an innovative skin incision for an alternative approach. *Breast.* 2008 Feb;17(1):8-11.

Rivadeneira, D. E., Simmons, R. M., Osborne, M. P., et al. Skin-sparing mastectomy with immediate breast reconstruction: A critical analysis of local recurrence. *Cancer J.* 6: 331, 2000.

Sacchini V, Pinotti JA, Barros AC, Luini A, Pluchinotta A, Pinotti M, Boratto MG, Ricci MD, Ruiz CA, Nisida AC, Veronesi P, Petit J, Arnone P, Bassi F, Disa JJ, Garcia-Etienne CA, Borgen PI. Nipple-sparing mastectomy for breast cancer and risk reduction: oncologic or technical problem? *J Am Coll Surg.* 2006 Nov;203(5):704-14.

Salgarello M, Farallo E.(2005) Immediate breast reconstruction with definitive anatomical implants after skin sparing mastectomy. *Br J Plast Surg* 2005; 58: 216-222

Salgarello M, Visconti G, Barone-Adesi L. (2010) Nipple-sparing mastectomy with immediate implant reconstruction: cosmetic outcomes and technical refinements. *Plast Reconstr Surg.* 2010 Nov;126(5):1460-71.

Salgarello M, Visconti G, Barone-Adesi L.(2011) Fat grafting and breast reconstruction with implant: another option for the irradiated breast cancer patients. *Plast Reconstr Surg.* 2011 Oct 18. [Epub ahead of print]

Santanelli F, Paolini G, Campanale A, Longo B, Amanti C. (2010) The "Type V" skin-sparing mastectomy for upper quadrant skin resections. *Ann Plast Surg* 2010 Aug;65(2):135-9.

Santini D, Taffurelli M, Gelli MC, Grassigli A, Giosa F, Marrano D, Martinelli G. (1989) Neoplastic involvement of nipple-areolar complex in invasive breast cancer. *Am J Surg.* 1989 Nov;158(5):399-403.

Spear SL., Willey SC, Feldman ED, Cocilovo C, Sidawy M, Al-Attar A, Hannan C, Seiboth L, Nahabedian MY. Nipple-sparing mastectomy for prophylactic and therapeutic indications. *Plastic & Reconstructive Surgery.*, POST ACCEPTANCE, 5 July 2011

Stolier AJ, Sullivan SK, Dellacroce FJ. (2008) Technical considerations in nipple-sparing mastectomy: 82 consecutive cases without necrosis. *Ann Surg Oncol.* 2008 May;15(5):1341-7. Epub 2008 Feb 7.

Toth BA, Lappert P. (1991) Modified skin incisions for mastectomy: the need for plastic surgical input in preoperative planning. *Plast Reconst Surg* 1991 Jun;87(6):1048-53.

Vlajcic Z, Zic R, Stanec S. (2005) Nipple-areola complex preservation: predictive factors of neoplastic nipple areola complex invasion. *Ann Plast Surg* 2005; Vol 55(3): 240-244.

Warren Peled A, Itakura K, Foster RD, Hamolsky D, Tanaka J, Ewing C, Alvarado M, Esserman LJ, Hwang ES. (2010) Impact of chemotherapy on postoperative complications after mastectomy and immediate breast reconstruction. *Arch Surg.* 2010 Sep;145(9):880-5.

4

The Effect of Breast Reconstruction on Maintaining a Proper Body Posture in Patients After Mastectomy

Sławomir Cieśla[1] and Małgorzata Bąk[2]
[1]*Oncoplastic Division of General Surgery Department Hospital Leszno,*
[2]*Institute of Phisical Education, Higher Vocational State School Leszno,*
Poland

1. Introduction

Breast cancer remains the most common malignant neoplasm in women. Surgical treatment options include radical mastectomy (RM), breast conservative treatment (BCT), radical mastectomy and immediate (IBR) or delayed breast reconstruction (DBR). Treatment of breast malignancies is currently focused on reducing surgical intervention while still eradicating the neoplasms.

Sentinel lymph node biopsy (SLNB) has been explored as a method to determine the need for axillary lymph node dissection (ALND) in breast cancer patients. In theory, a properly performed negative SLNB should accurately identify those patients without axillary node involvement, thereby obviating the need for a more morbid ALND. The risk of arm morbidity, particularly lymphedema, chronic pain, shoulder-arm dysfunctions and other complications is significantly lower after SLNB than ALND.

Despite an increasing proportion of indications to surgical intervention with breast conservation in early breast cancer stages, as many as 10% of stage I and 30% of stage II patients do not qualify for BCT (Morrow M et al., 2001). In addition to difficulties in offering each patient a 5-week course of radiotherapy, the number of unwilling patients, and the difficulties in staging the disease before surgery, there are many women who still undergo RM in early stages of the disease (Parker PA et al., 2007).

A strong family history of breast or ovarian carcinoma indicates a genetic predisposition to the disease and should prompt investigation of mutations in the BRCA gene. Women with identified BRCA1 or BRCA2 mutation have a high risk of breast cancer and are prime candidates for prophylactic bilateral total mastectomy. Still currently in Europe 40% to 60% of women diagnosed with breast cancer undergo amputation (Ferlay et al., 2007). In such cases, breast reconstruction minimalises scarring. Most women, who have had a mastectomy and are in otherwise good health, are candidates for breast reconstruction that can be done immediately (IBR - immediate breast reconstruction) or in delayed fashion (DBR - delayed breast reconstruction). Nowadays the rate of breast reconstruction after mastectomy ranges between 8% to 42%. This wide variation is attributed to geographic locations, ethnicity, patient's age, education & social status as well as cancer stage. The goal of breast reconstruction is to create a breast mound that matches the opposite breast and to achieve symmetry (Rietman et al., 2003; Elder et al., 2005). Breast reconstruction attempts to restore a patient's breast(s) as closely as possible to pre-mastectomy size, shape and appearance.

There are several surgical methods used to perform breast reconstruction and they include:

- patient's own tissues only (TRAM, LD, DIEP, free flaps)
- tissue expanders or sillicon prosthesis
- connecting both procedures -using autologous tissue and implants for breast reconstruction.

To date, the benefits of breast reconstruction have been mainly associated with the improvement of quality of life and breast appearance, both factors leading to better self-esteem and emotional well-being in women after mastectomy.

There have been almost no attempts to determine the effect of mastectomy and breast reconstruction on maintaining the proper body posture after the surgery. A huge number of women after mastectomy complain of increased back pain a few months to years after surgery even when they use external breast prosthesis in a professionally fitted bra or self-adhesive directly stack to the chest wall. Moreover recent investigations show that only 75% of mastectomised women wear the external breast prosthesis every day and only a few percent during the night (Bąk et al., 2000). In addition the full weight of the external prosthesis is carried by the bra, which causes higher pressure from the straps to the shoulder, pulling the shoulder down at the operated side.

2. Proper body posture

The proper body posture is vital to human health. It is closely linked to balance and fundamentally affects the key functions of a human being: the correct movement, correct breathing and efficient cardiovascular system.

Disturbances in proper body posture can lead to many health issues like scoliosis, headaches, dizziness, lower back problems, stuck energy feeling, functional impairment of respiratory and circulatory systems.

Posture is the position in which human body holds upright against force of gravity while standing, sitting, moving or lying down. Good posture requires the least amount of muscle activity to maintain an upright position and people have to train their bodies to place the least strain on supporting muscles and ligaments during movement or weight-bearing activities. Proper posture keeps bones and joints in the correct alignment so that muscles are being used properly, helps to decrease the abnormal wearing of joint surfaces that could result in arthritis, decreases the stress on the ligaments holding the joints of the spine together, prevents the spine from becoming fixed in abnormal positions and reduces fatigue because muscles are being used more efficiently, allowing the body to use less energy, avoiding strain, backache and muscular pain. The posture constantly changes depending on the human activity; the musculosceletal system is constantly working to maintain alignment whether sitting or standing for long periods of time or dancing.

In maintaining a good posture, two groups of factors are important:

- related to the anatomy: bones of the spine, joints, intervertebral discs, nerves and soft tissues - ligaments, fascia and muscles
- associated with managing the above structures: central and peripheral nervous system that keeps changing and adjusting the tension of individual muscle groups, both in motion and at rest (while standing, sitting and lying).

The spine allows the agile movement of the human body. It not only supports the body and all its organs, it also protects the sensitive and delicate spinal cord and spinal nerves exiting it. It is composed of 24 freely movable segments and is taxed by activities of daily living. Every activity, even breathing, demands a movement of the spine, ribs, and all attachments. The spine gives the human structure both strength and agility. A humans "biped" position gives the advantage of agility, leverage and mobility, while also creating certain structural stresses. The human body must adapt to the continual stress of gravity in order to maintain its balance.

Posture affects and moderates every physiologic function from efficient breathing to hormonal production. It allows musclo-skeletal system to hold the body parts in place, provides space for vital organs to function at optimal efficiency and promotes efficient functioning of the nervous system. Spinal pain, headache, mood, blood pressure, pulse and lung capacity are among the functions most easily influenced by posture. The most obvious benefits of good posture are efficiency and comfort.

Yet, because of the interrelationship of the structural (bone) and functional (organ) systems of the body, posture is also a factor that can impact health. For example, poor posture compromises the movements of the rib cage and does not allow the lungs to function at maximum capacity in order to bring much needed oxygen to the tissue and eliminate carbon dioxide wastes. Other vital organs of the body are also restricted when body posture is improper, creating structural stress. By reducing these postural imbalances we can start to improve all functions of the body and improve our health as well as quality of life.

3. 3D measurement techniques for human body surface scanning

3.1 Photogrammetry

Photogrammetry is one of the many fields of three dimensional measurement associated with surveying. The theoretical basis of the measurements was Moire conturography, described in 1880s in optics. (Takasaki H., 1970)

A ray of white light hitting an uneven surface leads to this light reflecting at various degrees. Photogrammetry has been used for medical applications since midway through the nineteenth century, and is now beginning to regain its past popularity due to recent developments in real time instrumentation. Medical photogrammetry is now part of the broader field known as biostereometrics.The major shift in the analytical approach to photogrammetry came about by considering each image as representing a bundle of rays from the center of the lens system through points on the image to the object photographed. These individual rays could be corrected for distortion in the lens system, the focal length of the lens and the geometry of the film or digital chip. With several images from different stand-points, the bundles of rays would then intersect in space where they would have struck the real object. (Meadows DM et al., 1970) The reflected image was registered by a camera, digitally configured and analysed by a special computer program.

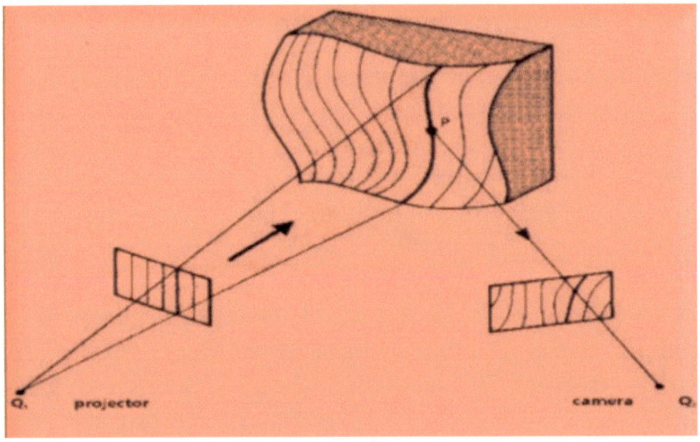

Picture 1. The principle of photogrammetry

Structured light projection and laser scanning represent the optical measurement technologies mostly employed for the three-dimensional digitalisation of the surface of the human body. They are both based on the same rule, namely triangulation, in the way that light structures are projected onto the human body, whereas light sensors acquire the scene; by known geometry of the set-up, 3D information can then be drawn from the imaged data. Digital imaging has greatly improved and changed photogrammetry because the "metric" parameters that were originally engineered into the cameras are now solved, and compensated for, by software. It is a great advantage to use such systems in combination with analysis and measurement performed by computer software for the comparison between pre- and post-operative shape of human body. These systems allowed for real-time registration and comparison of the resultant changes in body posture of the examined women. Two positive aspects of Moire conturography are the non invasive nature of the test and the possibility to perform repeated examinations over time. (Wong HK et al., 1997)

3.2 Use of moire conturography

The first results of investigations that compared the changes in proper body posture in two groups of women (after radical mastectomy (RM) and women who underwent immediate breast reconstruction (IBR)) were published in 2004 and then 2006 and 2010 (Cieśla & Bąk, 2004, 2006; Cieśla & Połom, 2010).

All women before and after surgery were examined to determine their body posture using three-dimensional (3D) analysis of the body surface with photogrammetry. This method involves objective anthropometric measurements based on the computer analysis of the 3D image constructed of the spine of each examined woman. This non-invasive and non-burdening manner of obtaining measurements allowed for multiple measurements in each woman pre and post-operatively. Before taking a measurement, characteristic bony structures were marked on the patient's back: the C7 to S1 spinous processes, the lower borders of the scapulae, and the superior posterior iliac spines.

The measurements were taken in specific, reproducible conditions, accounting for the same parameters of the visual apparatus, at a constant distance between the camera and the patient. This examination allowed for the measurement of 54 parameters in the coronal, sagittal, and transverse planes, which made it possible to evaluate the body posture of the patients objectively.

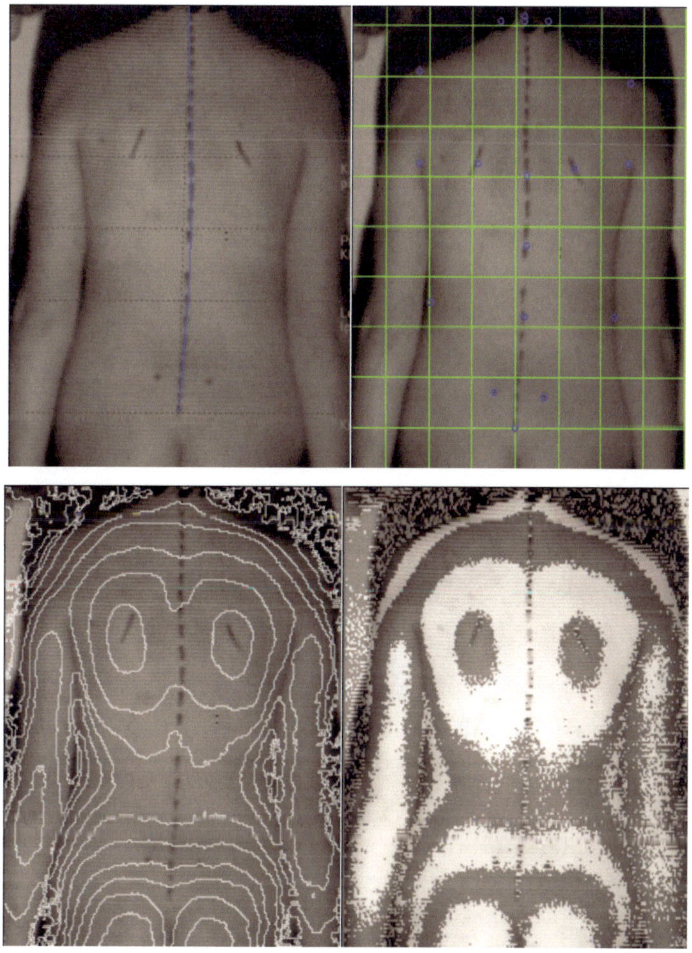

Picture 2. Patients' images obtained from studies using computerised photogrammetry

3.3 Asymmetry of body posture after mastectomy

Every human body is unique and from the moment we are born various factors (gravity and the activities we engage in) alter our posture therefore muscle imbalance and misalignment will affect all of us to a greater or lesser extent. It also has to be taken into account that the posture and health change during our lifetime under the influence of internal (degree of overall fitness, training, illness) and external factors (trauma). Radical surgical treatment of patients with breast cancer may contribute to a locomotor dysfunction. Damaged muscle weakness, pain associated with extensive postoperative wound, reflexive attempt to compensate for the absence of the breast - "a complex of half woman" as well as soft tissue fibrosis as a result of radiotherapy are the direct causes of adverse changes in the posture of women after mastectomy (Al Ghazar et al., 2000; Janni et al., 2001). Research conducted on a large group of patients showed the presence of posture defects in 82.3% of women after breast amputation compared with only 35.1% in healthy group women. (Bąk & Cieśla 2009) The research confirmed clearly abnormal posture in women after radical mastectomy that appeared in all three planes: sagittal, coronal and transverse. Women after mastectomy have an increased tendency to exhibit kyphotic posture, tilt the trunk forward and extend kyphosis in the thoracic spine. Even with properly conducted intensive postoperative rehabilitation, it is observed that patients demonstrate a constant tendency to tilt forward while the shoulder on the operated side is lifted, ejected forward and medially. In the frontal plane, the symmetry disturbances of bony points are clearly visible especially of the shoulder heights on both sides, the position of the blades, twist of the pelvis and the deviation of vertebrae spinous from the vertical line.

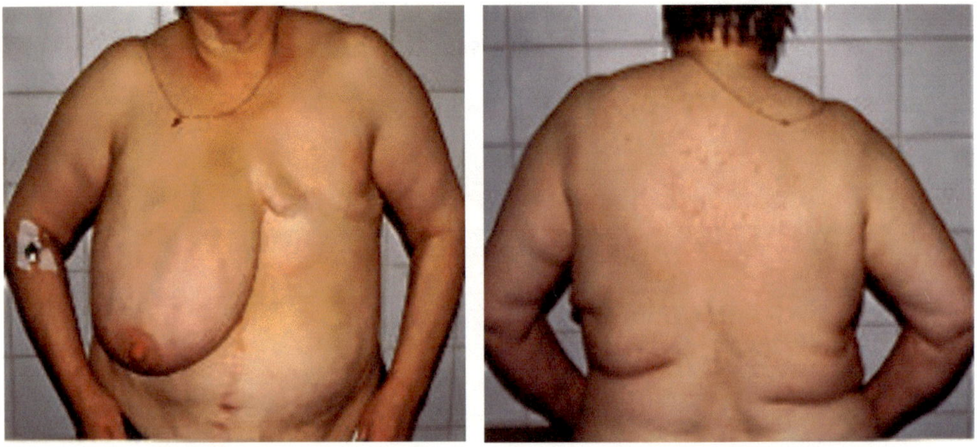

Picture 3-4. Photographs showing the typical abnormalities of posture in women after radical breast amputation. Fifty two years old woman shown two years after radical mastectomy for cancer.

The asymmetry of the buttocks in women after RM was studied before. The results of these studies indicated that the asymmetry was related to the position of the shoulders and scapulae. In cases of radical mastectomy (RM) without breast reconstruction, external prosthesis worn as a special bra was a significant factor in the degree of buttock asymmetry. Women who wore such prosthesis regularly, both during day and night, demonstrated a lesser degree of body posture disturbances. It is also necessary for the patient to undergo rehabilitation to minimise the changes in body posture (Kopanski et al., 2003, Rostkowska et al., 2006).

In our study it was shown that body posture disturbances significantly affect the vertebral column in patients after RM. The scapula on the operated side was higher than the scapula on the un-operated side. Women who were older at the time of surgery more frequently have a right rotation to their buttocks and their pelvis was located more posterior on the right side. The spinous process with the greatest deviation from a vertical line perpendicular to the ground was expressed to a greater degree in women after mastectomy. This deviation was most significant in the lower thoracic spine (Th 7-12) of older women, while in younger women it was at a higher part of the thoracic spine (Th 1-6). Another interesting clinical observation is the change in body posture depending on time passed after the surgery. In the early postoperative time, there is a tendency to thrust the buttocks forward, and as more time passes after the surgery the buttocks are thrust posteriorly. This is due to the fact that thrusting the buttocks forward in the early postoperative period has an aesthetic and psychological effect, which passes over time (Bąk & Rostkowska, 2000).

The recent studies have shown a statistically significant disturbance of proper body posture in women after mastectomy. These disturbances have even been demonstrated in women who underwent intensive rehabilitation. It has also been noted that these disturbances in body posture are decreased in women who used an external prosthesis not only during the day but also at night, while sleeping (Bąk & Rostkowska, 2000).

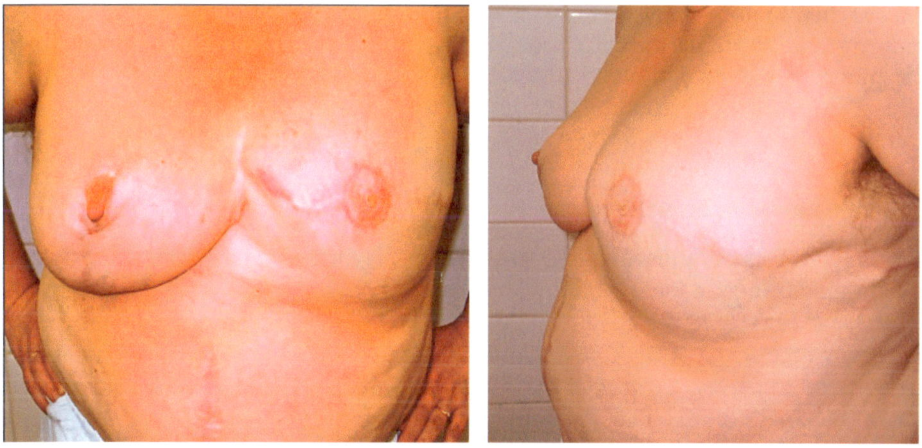

Picture 5-6. Photographs showing women from picture 1-2 four years after radical mastectomy for cancer and two years after delayed left breast reconstruction with Becker-25 (800cc) expandero-prosthesis and Mc Kissock reduction of the right breast.

This leads to the assumption that breast reconstruction may have a positive effect in maintaining the proper body posture in women after mastectomy.

4. The influence of breast reconstruction on correct body posture

4.1 Reconstruction with prosthesis and expander-mammary prosthesis

A common method of breast reconstruction after breast surgery is the use of silicon prostheses, expanders or expander-prostheses. They are placed under pectoralis major muscle in a special muscle pocket including a part of serratus anterior muscle and even the upper part of rectus abdominis muscle. A great advantage of this kind of reconstruction is the use of the breast's shape, its weight and a high flexibility of silicone prosthesis. This solution limits the surgery to the wall of the chest of the breast after mastectomy. The most important elements of implant breast reconstruction are the inframammary fold, the inferior pole, the superior slope, and the projection (Cordeiro & McCarthy, 2006). However, in this type of breast reconstruction it is necessary to incorporate the above mentioned chest muscles in the process of shaping the new breast.

4.1.1 Pectoralis major muscle

Pectoralis major muscle (musculus thoracic major) is a large, wide and triangular muscle that belongs to a group of superficial muscles of the chest. It is innervated by the medial pectoral nerve and lateral pectoral nerve. A superficial lamina of thoracic fascia covers its front surface and separates the muscle from the subcutaneous layer of adipose tissue and, in women, from the mammary gland. The rear surface of the pectoralis major muscle is covered through chest deep fascia. Medial part of pectoralis major has three trailers. The upper part - clavicles (pars clavicularis) is attached to the medial portion of clavicle. It is separated from the sterno-rib part by inter-rib furrow (sulcus interpectoralis).The central part - sterno-rib (pars sternocostalis) attaches on the front surface of the sternum and to rib cartilage from I to VI. Lower part - abdominal (pars abdominalis) attaches to the blade anterior abdominal rectus sheath. Part of the lateral muscle tendon passes into a common tendon attached to the greater tubercle crest of the humerus. The lower part of the pectoralis major forms axillary folds forward (plica axillaris anterior). The contraction of the whole muscle moves the shoulder blade forward, drops and draws an arm moving it slightly forward and making its rotation inside. Pectoralis major muscle is also an auxiliary respiratory muscle.

4.1.2 Serratus anterior muscle

Serratus anterior muscle (musculus serratus anterior) is located on the lateral chest wall. This flat, quadrangular muscle innervated by long thoracic nerve $C_{5\text{-}8}$ is one of the largest muscles in humans and belongs to the group of superficial muscles of the chest. From the front it has wide trailers in the shape of ten saw blades originating on the outer surface of the upper nine ribs. It is placed to the rear surface of the chest, and inserts along the entire anterior length of the medial border of the scapula. Anatomically, there are three parts of the serratus anterior muscles. The thickest and shortest superior part spans between the first and second rib and rib side of the superior angle of scapula. The thinnest intermediate part spreads out between the second and third rib and the medial border of the scapula. The inferior part stretches between the fourth and the ninth rib and the rib side of the inferior angle. The superior part is an antagonist of the middle trapezius muscle pulling the shoulder joint forward. The inferior part pulls scapula downward and the lower angle of the shoulder forward and laterally toward the armpit while setting the acetabulum articular shoulder upwards, which allows raising the upper limb above the level. In addition, serratus muscle pushes the shoulder blade against the chest wall. It is an auxiliary inspiratory muscle.

4.1.3 Abdominal rectus muscle

Abdominal rectus muscle (musculus rectus abdominis) is a muscle interoperating with a flat abdominal muscles, diaphragm and perineal muscles in the formation of the abdominal prelum. His initial trailers are the rib cartilage V-VII, appendix of the sternum and rib-gladioli ligament, and the end - pubic symphysis and pubic crest of the pelvic bone. It is prolonged in men in the suspensory ligament of penis (ligamentum suspensorium penis) and the suspensory ligament of clitoridis in women. It is covered by a sheath of the rectus abdominis muscle (vagina musculi recti abdominis*)*. It has so called tendinous *intersections* (intersectiones tendineae). The blood supply is from inferior epigastric artery a terminal branch of the internal thoracic artery. It is innervated by intercostal nerves (Th6-Th12) and is often the first lumbar nerve (L1). Lower and upper abdominal arteries are responsible for vascularisation. Abdominal rectus muscle participates in bending the body, strengthens the abdominal prelum, raises pelvis and lowers the chest and ribs which supports the exhaust function.

BREAST RECONSTRUCTION	Musculus pectoralis major	Musculus serratus anterior	Musculus rectus abdominis	Musculus latissimus dorsi
Implant	+ + +	+	+	-
Implant+AlloDerm	+ +	-	-	-
TRAM	-	-	+ + +	-
Free TRAM	-	-	+ +	-
DIEP	-	-	+	-
LD	-	-	-	+ + +
Ms-LD	-	-	-	+
SIEA	-	-	-	-
SGAP	-	-	-	-
IGAP	-	-	-	-

+++ large
++ average
+ small
- no importance
TRAM – transverse abdominis muscle flap , Free TRAM - free transverse abdominis muscle flap,
DIEP- deepinferior epigastric perforator flap,
LD - latissimus dorsi flap,
Ms-LD - muscle sparing latissimus dorsi flap,
SIEA- superficial inferior epigastric artery flap,
SGAP - superior gluteal artery perforator flap,
IGAP - inferior gluteal artery perforator flap.

Table 1. The degree of trunk and abdominis wall muscle exploitation in different type of breast reconstruction.

4.1.4 Implantable biomaterials supporting implant coverage

Recent methods of using implantable biomaterials, or patient's own abdominal rectus fascia or skin flap during simultaneous breast reduction preclude the need for using of the serratus anterior muscle and the rectus abdominis. In this way, not only there is a much greater opportunity to create a natural ptosis even with larger breasts, the possibility of obtaining the symmetry with the natural breast of the opposite side, but also the damage to the muscles of the chest to completely cover the implant is limited to the minimum.

4.1.4.1 Acellular dermal matrix (ADM)

Acellular dermal matrix (ADM) has been used in surgery as soft tissue replacement since 1994. The first report about the use of human acellular dermis in prosthetic breast reconstruction was in 2005 (Breuing & Warren, 2005). Alloderm, Neoform or Flex HD are dermal grafts obtained from deceased human donors, which can be used for immediate breast reconstruction as a "sling" to cover the lower outer quadrant of the reconstructed breast, thereby redefining the base and outer limits of the breast. It fuses with the mastectomy flap and serves to put the chest wall muscle on stretch, so that the entire expander or implant is more fully covered. This technique creates a subpectoral and sub-AlloDerm pocket only that completely encloses the breast implant. By tailoring the width of the AlloDerm, it is possible to precisely control the degree of lower-pole fullness. This technique shortens or eliminates the need for tissue expansion.

4.1.4.2 Inframammary fold reconstruction (IFR)

A new approach for inframammary fold reconstruction (IFR) that focuses on the breast and muscles fascial system establishes next very important point in implant breast reconstruction. The inframammary fold is an important landmark that frequently is disrupted or destroyed by modified radical mastectomy.

4.1.4.3 Skin-reducing mastectomy (SRM)

Skin-reducing mastectomy (SRM) is a technique that creates a dermomuscular pouch with adequate volume in the lower-medial quadrant and, at the same time, provides satisfactory coverage of the silicone implant. Much of the surgical scarring lies in relatively concealed areas of the breast. (Nava et al., 2011)

It also has a beneficial influence on keeping the right body posture among women after surgery.

4.1.5 The results of the photogrammetric measurements in women after breast reconstruction with Becker prosthesis

The photogrammetric results obtained from women after surgery for breast cancer demonstrate a significant difference in body posture between the patients who underwent immediate breast reconstruction (IBR) and those with radical mastectomy (RM) who never had reconstruction. Prospective studies were performed in a group of women with stage I and II breast cancer operated in 2000-2005 at the Oncoplastic Division General Surgery of the State Regional Hospital Leszno. There were three groups of examined women: A (n=38) - women underwent radical Madden mastectomy, B (n=38) - women underwent skin sparing mastectomy with single stage immediate breast reconstruction (ssm+IBR) , C (n=38) healthy women who have not had any surgery before (control group). Groups A and B were comparable in terms of age, body mass index, height, the degree of cancer advancement and comorbidities. All the women qualified for ssm+IBR agreed to this kind of surgery and declared their intention to actively participate in postoperative breast modeling and rehabilitation. This examination allowed for the measurement of 54 parameters in the coronal, sagittal and transverse planes, which made it possible to objectively evaluate the body posture of the patients.

The measurements taken preoperatively, but after clinical diagnosis and qualification to surgical treatment, did not differ significantly in group A (ssm+IBR) and B (RM), either between each other or in comparison to the control group. (Cieśla & Bąk, 2004, 2006; Bąk & Cieśla, 2009)

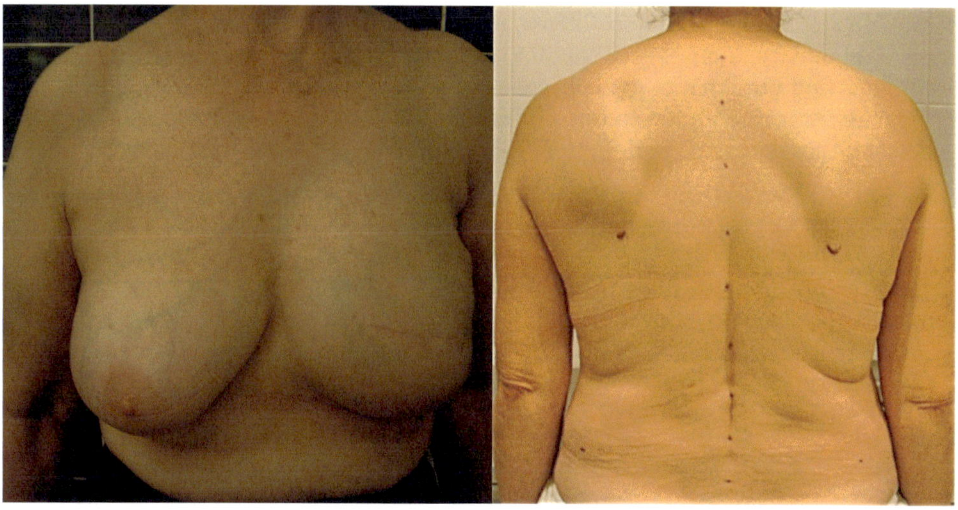

Picture 7. Photographs showing a fifty six years old woman with breast cancer 2 years after amputation with sparing the skin and simultaneous breast reconstruction using prosthesis ekspander-Becker-35 (565 cc). Visible correct positioning of the shoulders, shoulder blades, pelvis and no deviation from the vertical of vertebral processes of the spine.

Examination of those patients 6 months postoperatively demonstrated a considerable increase in body posture divergence in the patients who had RM without breast reconstruction. Twelve months postoperatively, this body posture divergence was even more obvious and was significantly different from the results obtained from the ssm+IBR and control (healthy women) groups. In the eighteenth postoperative month, the difference between the RM and ssm+IBR groups reached its peak, with the RM group showing even more divergence in body posture. Two years after surgery, there was no further increase in divergence demonstrated by the parameters of body posture in the coronal, sagittal and transverse planes in the patients with RM. It can be therefore assumed that adaptation of the body stabilises approximately 18 months after surgery and does not progress any further. There were no statistical differences between ssm+IBR patients and healthy controls in all five terms of measurements before and after surgery. (Cieśla & Połom, 2010)

There are visible, statistically significant, abnormal postures in the RM group appearing after 6 months with the upward trend until 18 months after surgery. In the group ssm+IBR the abnormal body postures after the surgery were small and did not differ statistically from the control group.

4.2 Autologous breast reconstruction

4.2.1 Pedicle flaps

4.2.1.1 Transverse rectus abdominis musculocutaneous flap reconstruction

TRAM is still a standard procedure in autologous reconstruction with the use of soft tissues from abdomen in the form of rectus abdominis muscle pedicle skin-muscle flap. As a result, the reconstructed breast is flexible, soft and its shape is similar to the healthy one. However, the use of one or both rectus abdominis muscles for transferring tissues weakens the abdomen muscle wall and may influence the incorrect static position and therefore body posture. Preliminary unpublished photometric studies seem to confirm this. It will be interesting to find out what is the influence of the TRAM reconstruction on the changes in body posture. A good solution to this problem seems to be the free transfer of own tissues with deep inferior epigastric perforator (DIEP) flap.

Michigan Breast Reconstruction Outcome Study made some interesting findings analising the impact of TRAM reconstruction on the abdominal wall function. Two-year prospective study was conducted in 12 surgical centers. A feedback from 460 patients treated by 23 surgeons was analysed. Studies using isometric dynamometer showed the deficit of the abdominal wall functions both in methods of free and pedicle TRAM flap over two years. This deficit ranged with different authors between 6 to 19% while in women with pedicle TRAM was always larger (Alderman AK et al. 2006).

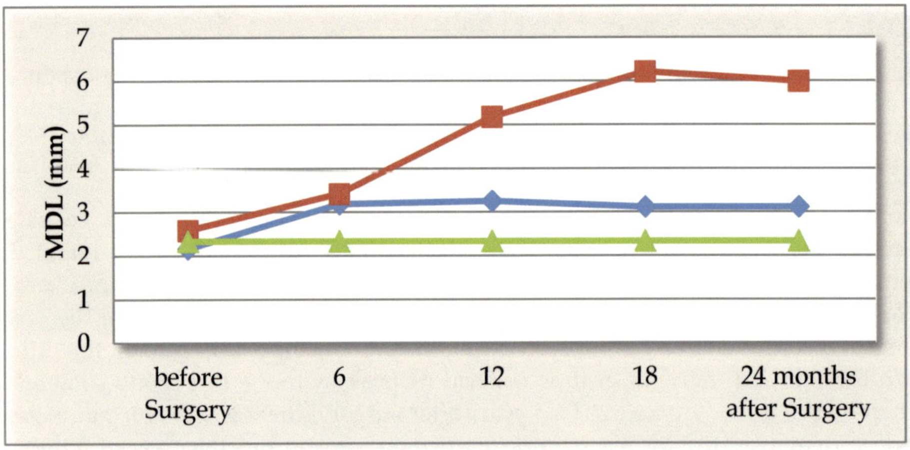

MDL - the maximal deviation of the line of the superior-posterior iliac spines from C7-S1.

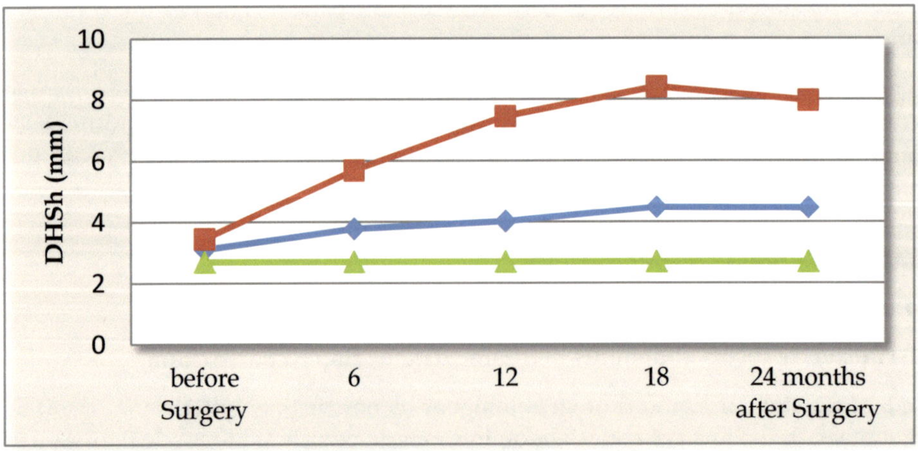

DHSh -the difference in height of the shoulders

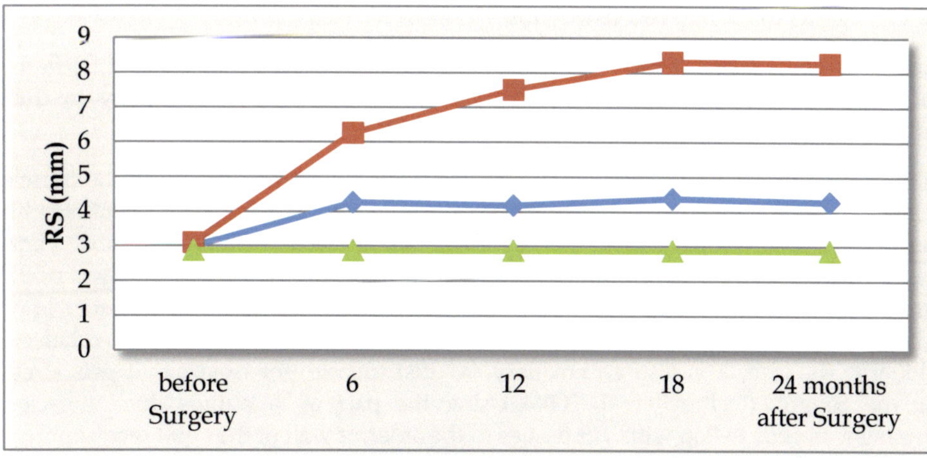

RS – the difference in depth of the lower border of the scapulae (rotation)

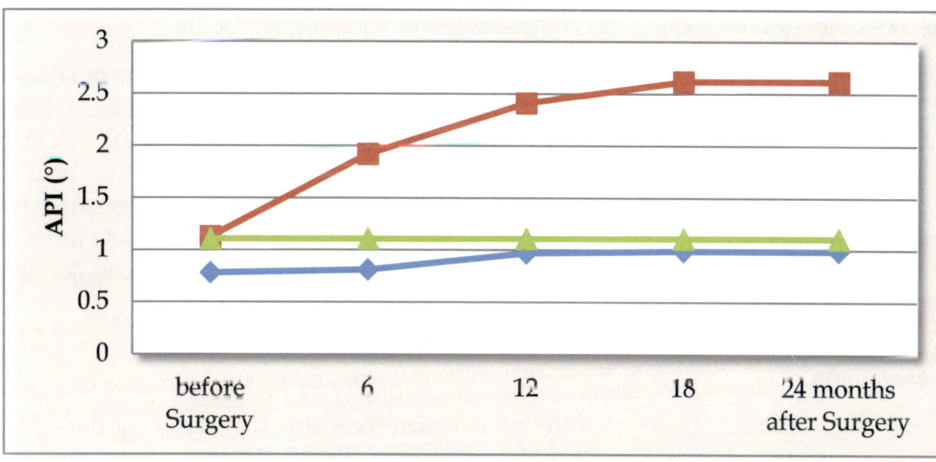

API – the angle of pelvis inclination (°)

Picture 8. Graphs showing the results of measurements of various parameters of body posture in planes: frontal, sagittal and transverse in three groups of women: after radical breast amputation (RM), after amputation of the sparing of skin and simultaneous breast reconstruction (IBR ssm +) and a group of healthy women, not operated (Control).

It was also found that up to 53% of the reconstructions using pedicle TRAM flap showed deficits in both rectus abdominal muscle and the oblique muscles.

In women with bilateral breast reconstruction using pedicle TRAM, the trunk flexion deficit reaches 40% and trunk extension deficit is 9%. This group of patients also experienced a subjective muscle dysfunction of the abdominal wall.

In varying degrees, this influenced the overall assessment of quality of life of patients after breast reconstruction with abdominal flaps.

4.2.1.2 Latissimus dorsi flap reconstruction

Another problem is a breast reconstruction with the use of latissimus dorsi (LD) flap. It is still a very common and useful method of breast reconstruction especially in difficult conditions or corrective surgeries.

Latissimus dorsi muscle (musculus latissimus dorsi) has the largest area of all the muscles in the human body. It is innervated by the thoracodorsal nerve. The initial points of attachment of this muscle are: vertebral processes of lower six thoracic vertebrae, lumbal vertebral processes, median sacral crest, the outer lip of the iliac crest (in the back of the third part) and the outer surface of the 9th and 10-12 ribs. The final trailer is a crest of lesser tubercle of the humerus (crista tuberculi minoris humeri). In addition to adduction, inward rotation and straightening the arm, it is also an auxiliary exhaust muscle (for example, it gets stretched during the cough). (Daltrey et al. 2006) Using the part of latissimus dorsi muscle and transferring it as pedicle flap with soft tissues to the anterior wall of the chest may significantly influence torso symmetry, which has been confirmed in photogrammetric studies. However, the extent of torso statics disturbances after LD reconstruction is still unknown. To some extent, the operational movement and function change of the latissimus dorsi muscles also affects the chest expiratory action and compromises the shoulder morbidity.

An interesting solution was proposed based on detailed studies of the anatomy of latissimus dorsi muscle vascularization - the muscle latissimus dorsi flap sparing (MS-LD) breast reconstruction (Mojallal et al. 2010). A tiny lateral part of muscle containing the descending branch of the thoracodorsal artery with its perforators (TDAPs) can be used as a pedicle to carry a large skin-fascial flap. This way, the donor site morbidity in this manner is much less than classical or extended adipomuscular technique and latissimus dorsi muscle function is spared (Brackley PT et al. 2010). It results in no or minimal functional deficit of donor site, low rate of flap complications, absence of seroma and acceptable scarring.

4.2.2 Free flaps

Perforator flaps represent the state of the art in breast reconstruction replacing the skin and soft tissue removed at mastectomy with soft, warm, living tissue is accomplished by borrowing skin and fatty tissue from the abdomen or hip. This is made without sacrificing muscles and strength as compared to less sophisticated techniques.

The most important reason to use free flaps for breast reconstruction is the improved blood supply and reduced donor site morbidity. Moreover the use of free flaps with vascular microanastomosis transferred from remote regions of the body may offer a favourable solution in terms of maintaining a proper posture, minimising muscle morbidity. Accurate isolation of the vascular pedicle while sparing the muscle prevents the damage.

4.2.2.1 The free transverse rectus abdominis musculocutaneus flap reconstruction (free TRAM)

The free transverse rectus abdominis musculocutaneus flap reconstruction (free TRAM) is vascularised from the inferior epigastric artery. With this method a small amount of the rectus abdominis muscle containing blood vessels supplying the skin and fat are used. The inevitable weakness in the abdominal wall does increase the risk of a bulge or hernia. In the free TRAM reconstruction group only a slight deficit of rectus abdominal muscle was identified. Of course, even more abnormalities of the correct abdominal wall function were noticed in the bipedicle TRAM flap reconstruction and bilateral breast reconstruction using both pedicle and free TRAM.

4.2.2.2 The deep inferior epigastric perforator flap reconstruction (DIEP)

The deep inferior epigastric perforator flap reconstruction (DIEP) is an evolution of the free TRAM flap, developed in Germany in the early 1990s. The flap - fat and overlying skin survives on a blood supply via one or two perforators or side branches from the inferior epigastric artery. Perforators are generally smaller in diameter than the main vessel, and vary in size between different people. If the perforators are too small, this type of reconstruction cannot proceed as there is the risk of flap failure due to inadequate blood supply. An interesting comparison of the results of dysfunction of the abdominal wall in two groups of patients after breast reconstruction: using free TRAM and DIEP reconstruction was conducted. The DIEP flap group had significantly higher trunk flexion torque compared with free TRAM flap group. This could suggest a better function of the abdominal wall reconstruction in patients with DIEP (Blondeel et al. 1997).

A publication of a systematic review of reports of dysfunction of the abdominal wall function after different abdominal flaps breast reconstructions appeared in 2009 (Atisha D & Alderman AK, 2009). Conclusions are based on the analysis of 20 documented reports. It confirmed the largest deficit of trunk flexion in patients with pedicle TRAM flap reconstruction (up to a 23%), lower in patients with free TRAM flap reconstruction (up to a 18%) and lowest in the DIEP flap reconstruction group. There was no statistically significant difference between the pedicle and free TRAM groups. However, a statistically significant difference between the free TRAM and DIEP methods was confirmed, in favour of the latter method of reconstruction. The analysis of the ability of trunk extension showed 14% deficit in the group of pedicle TRAM, and only a slight deficit in the free TRAM flaps and DIEP groups.

4.2.2.3 The superficial inferior epigastric artery flap (SIEA)

This flap is vascularised from the superficial epigastric artery arises from the front of the femoral artery about 1 cm below the inquinal ligament. This vessel supplies the skin and the fat of the lower abdomen. In this case there is no need to make incisions within the abdominal wall, thus hypothetically the problem of hernias and functional disorders of the abdominal wall muscle is eliminated. Unfortunately, only about 50% of patients have this vessel present

4.2.2.4 The superior gluteal artery perforator flap (SGAP)

This flap is vascularised from the superior gluteal artery. Because of very short vascular pedicle it is difficult to perform this technic without additional vein graft. It is mainly used as second-line treatment option for patients ineligible for TRAM, and having breasts without or with minimal ptosis.

4.2.2.5 The inferior gluteal artery perforator flap (IGAP)

This flap is vascularised from the inferior gluteal artery. Due to the improved donor site contour and scar, the IGAP can be a flap of choice when a tissue from the buttock is required. There are several advantages to use this flap: a predictable consistent vascular pedicle, an adequate cutaneous paddle and well concealed donor site.

4.2.2.6 The Rubens fat pad free flap

This flap consist of redundant fatty tissue vascularised by the deep circumflex iliac vessels. The main benefit of this method is the aesthetics of the donorsite contour and scar.

The use of SGAP and IGAP as well as the Rubens flaps in a well-planned bilateral breast reconstruction may be important in maintaining normal body symmetry.

However all above mentioned metods of breast reconstruction with the use of free flaps are very promising, the wide feasibility for breast surgeons can be difficult to perform because of need of hight quality microvascular expertise and financial constrains.

4.3 Immediate or delayed breast reconstruction?

Breast reconstruction carried out during one surgery as a second stage after the oncological treatment is finished has many advantages. The woman wakes up with a new breast after surgery. In this way many negative consequences resulting from not undertaking immediate reconstruction or delaying it are avoided. Immediate reconstruction is the only way to save own skin of the operated breast and significantly improve aesthetical results (SSM- skin sparing mastectomy or ASM - areola sparing mastectomy). The benefits of choosing immediate breast reshaping during mastectomy allow for the best aesthetic results according to many plastic surgeons. The breast tissue, skin and nipple are more easily preserved. The breast cancer patient also benefits from the close collaboration of both oncologic and plastic surgeon at the same theatre to obtain satisfactory results. Photometric studies of body posture explicitly indicate correct body posture parameters among this group of women. Moreover, it has been shown that adverse changes in correct body posture among women after mastectomy without reconstruction occur after 6 months after surgery and they get worse in time reaching a peak after 18 months (Cieśla & Bąk 2006; Cieśla & Połom 2010). Therefore, delaying reconstruction may have a negative effect on body posture among women after mastectomy. Still, the extent of the negative effects of delaying breast reconstruction needs to be looked into.

4.4 The role of rehabilitation

It is very important for women after radical mastectomy and mastectomy with immediate or delayed breast reconstruction to attend regularly physical rehabilitation in a gym. The programme of essential therapeutic rehabilitation included:

- increasing or maintaining mobility of shoulder joint on the operated side,
- increasing or maintaining muscle strength of the upper limb on the operated side,
- correcting the faulty posture which arose as a result of amputation,
- balancing the strength of postural muscles and developing postural endurance,
- increasing the efficiency of respiratory system,
- preventing the lymph stasis in the limb and in the area of operation,
- improving the physical efficiency and body fitness,
- changing the mindset in order to adapt to new living conditions

In the rehabilitation of women after mastectomy the exercises are based on isotonic contraction and short isometric tension. Apart from active exercises proper also active exercises without pressure (in suspension) were applied, as long as functional abilities of the women allowed it. In individual cases (with weakened muscles, significant limitations of mobility, soreness in the shoulder girdle or other complications) passive exercises were introduced. Low exercise positions were mainly used, since physical exercises in high position (standing) are the greatest burden to the circulatory system, in particular its venous part. Low isolated positions force the subjects to perform proper movements, and do not allow compensating for a limited mobility of shoulder girdle with movement of neighbouring joints (for example using the spine).

Since in women after mastectomy the static and body symmetry are disturbed, scoliosis arises, kypholordosis is changed it is important to locate the place where effects on the spine are exerted according to the steering rule. Control from above (of upper limbs) and from below (lower limbs) is used. In breathing exercises special attention is paid to breathing route – upper-costal (diaphragmatic and mixed) and to teaching correct breathing rhythm. The aim of breathing exercises is to improve pulmonary ventilation after the operation, gradual stretching of the scar and pressure on the cistern of chyle and abdominal part of thoracic duct (squeezing the lymph out of them towards the head).

During therapeutic rehabilitation educational effects were considered relating to the patient's behaviour at home, using anti-oedematous prophylaxis and making women realise the significance of physical activity in the prevention of secondary malignant disease. Future research on the motional rehabilitation of women after mastectomy should head in two directions. First, the alterations in body posture should be monitored during regular physical exercises. There is an urgent need to work out an exact program of those exercises that improve particularly difficult features in the body posture. Patients should also be protected against compensatory changes. Another research topic is based on observation of alterations in body posture and their prevention in women after different kind of breast reconstruction.

5. Conclusions

It should be strongly noted that breast reconstruction surgery has a significant effect on the patient's postoperative body posture. Although the changes in body posture are not completely eliminated, breast reconstruction considerably decreases the amount of divergence from normal body posture, as compared to patients who do not have reconstruction after mastectomy. This may be the basis for justifying immediate breast reconstruction not only from multiple psychological and physical perspectives - self-image, ease of dressing, interpersonal relationships, quality of life, but also improved posture as a positive outcome of breast reconstruction.

Future studies should aim at determining the effects of breast surgery on the body posture, as such procedures can also impact the patient's quality of life. It seems that the immediate, one or two-stage breast reconstruction using tissue expanders, implants or expander-prostheses should be a very important and integral part of treatment of patients with breast cancer who need mastectomy.

The advantage of the immediate breast reconstruction is that it protects a woman from traumatic loss of breast(s), make it possible to perform a radical oncological amputation while preserving natural own breast skin (ssm) or even nipple-areola complex (asm). The wider use of this procedure is possible in breast surgery centers and does not require complicated methods for own tissue transfer from other parts of the patient's body. However, this does not relieve the surgeon from mastering other techniques of breast reconstruction. The need for reconstruction using patient's own tissue is particularly useful in case of a failure of primary reconstruction with the use of implants or in case of severe postoperative complications. Freedom and skills of using techniques for reduction, mastopexy or augmentation of a healthy breast is necessary to achieve the proper symmetry of both breasts.

6. References

Alderman AK, Kuzon WM, Wilkins EG. A two-year prospective analysis of trunk function in TRAM breast reconstructions. Plast Reconstr Surg 2006; 117(7):2131-2138.

Al-Ghazal SK, Fallowfield L, Blamey RW. Comparison of psychological aspects and patient satisfaction following breast conserving surgery, simple mastectomy and breast reconstruction. Eur J Cancer 2000;36:1938–43.

Atisha D, Alderman AK. A systematic review of abdominal wall function following abdominal flaps for postmastectomy breast reconstruction. Ann Plast Surg 2009 Aug;63(2):222-30

Bak M, Rostkowska E. The influence of using breast prosthesis during the night on the changes of body posture among woman after mastectomy. Physioth 2000;8(4):11–5.

Bąk M, Cieśla S. Assessment of postural disorders in women after radical mastectomy followed by immediate breast Reconstruction. Physioth 2009;17(1)30-37.

Blondeel PN, Vanderstraeten GG, Monstrey SJ, et al. The donor site morbidity of free DIEP flaps and free TRAM flaps for breast reconstruction. Br J Plast Surg 1997; 50:322.

Brackley PT, Mishra A, Sigaroudina M, Iqbal A. Modified muscle sparing latissimus dorsi with implant for total breast reconstruction - extending the boundaries. J Plast Reconstr Aesthet Surg 2010 Sep;63(9):1495-502.

Breuing KH, Warren SM. Immediate bilateral breast reconstruction with implants and AlloDerm slings. Ann Plast Surg. 2005;55:232–239.

Cieśla S, Bąk M : Disorders of body posture on women after mastectomy in photogrammetric estimation. Eur J Cancer 2004; 2(3): S167 - 4th European Breast Cancer Conference. Hamburg 2004

Cieśla S, Bąk M. (2004) The influence of immediate breast reconstruction with the use of the Becker prosthesis on body posture estimation at women after mastectomy for cancer. Eur J Cancer 2004; 2(3): S168 -4 th Europen Breast Cancer Conference Hamburg 2004.

Cieśla S, Immediate breast reconstruction after skin sparing mastectomy-102 cases. Eur J Surg Oncol, 2006;(32), Suppl 1,91

Ciesla S, Bąk M. The influence of immediate breast reconstruction on proper body posture on women after mastectomy for cancer. Eur J Surg Oncol 2006; 32(1): S99

Cieśla S., Połom K. The effect of immediate breast reconstruction with Becker-25 prosthesis on the preservation of propter body posture in patients after mastectomy. Eur J Surg Oncol 2010; (36), 7:625-631.

Cordeiro PG. Breast reconstruction after surgery for breast cancer. N Engl J Med 2008;359:1590–601.

Cordeiro PG, McCarthy CM. A single surgeon's 12-year experience with tissue expander/implant breast reconstruction: II. A prospective analysis of long-term complications, aesthetic outcomes and patients satisfaction. Plast Reconstr Surg 2006;118:832–9.

Daltrey I, Thomson H, Hussien M, Krishna K, Rayter Z, Winters ZE. Randomized clinical trial of the effect of quilting latissimus dorsi flap donor site on seroma formation. B J Surg 2006 Jul;93(7):825-30.

Elder EE, Brandberg Y, Bjorklund T, et al. Quality of life and patient satisfaction in breast cancer patients after immediate breast reconstruction: a prospective study. Breast 2005;14:201–18.

Ferlay J, Autier P, Boniol M, Heanue M, Colombet M, Boyle P (2007) Estimates of the cancer incidence and mortality in Europe in 2006. Ann Oncol 18(3): 581-592

Findikcioglu K, Ozmen S, Guclu T. The impact of breast size on the vertebral column: a radiologic study. Aesthetic Plast Surg 2007;31: 23–7.

Janni W, Rjosk D, Dimpfl TH, et al. Quality of life influenced by primary surgical treatment for stage I-III breast cancer. Long term follow up of a matched pair analysis. Ann Surg Oncol 2001;8: 542–8.

Kopanski Z, Wojewoda T, Wojewoda A, et al. Influence of some anthropometric parameters on the risk of development of distal complications after mastectomy carried out because of breast carcinoma. Am J Human Biol 2003;15(3):433–9.

Meadows DM, Johnson WO, Allen JB. Generation of surface contours by Moire´ patterns. Appl Opt 1970;9:942–7.

Mojallal A, Saint-Cyr M, Wong C, Veber M, Braye F, Rohrich R. Muscle-sparing latissimus dorsi flap. Vascular anatomy and indications in breast reconstruction. Ann Chir Plast Esthet 2010 Apr; 55(2).87-96.

Morrow M, Scott SK, Menck HR, Mustoe TA, Winchester DP. Factors influencing the use of breast reconstruction postmastectomy: a National Cancer Database Study. J Am Coll Surg 2001;192:1–8.

Nava MB, Ottolenghi J, Pennati A, Spano A, Bruno N, Catanuto G, Boliglowa D, Visintini V, Santoro S, Folli S. Skin/nipple sparing mastectomies and implant-based breast reconstruction in patients with large and ptotic breast: Oncological and reconstructive results. Breast. 2011 Mar 22.

Parker PA, Youssef A, Walker S, et al. Short-term and long-term psychosocial adjustment and quality of life in women undergoing different surgical procedures for breast cancer. Ann Surg Oncol 2007;14:3078–89.

Rietman JS, Dijkstra PU, Hoekstra HJ, et al. Late morbidity after treatment of breast cancer in relation to daily activities and quality of life: a systemic review. EJSO 2003;29:229–38.

Rostkowska E, Bak M, Samborski W. Body posture in women after mastectomy and its changes as a result of rehabilitation. Adv Med Sci 2006;51:287–97.

Takasaki H. Moire´ topography. Appl Opt 1970;9(1457):1472.

Wong H-K, Balasubramaniam P, Rajan U, Chng S-Y. Direct spinal curvature digitization in scoliosis screening e a comparative study with Moire conturography. J Spinal Disord 1997;10(3):185–92.

Part 3

Autogenous Breast Reconstruction

5

Modified Extended Latissimus Dorsi Myocutaneous Flap with Added Vascularised Chest Wall Fat in Immediate Breast Reconstruction After Conservative (Sparing) Mastectomies

Adel Denewer and Omar Farouk
Surgical Oncology Department, Oncology Center, Mansoura University, Egypt

1. Introduction

Breasts are symbols of feminity rather than feeding young. This physiological fact is eclipsed by the emotional and cultural values placed on the breast which minimizes its basic function and emphasizes femininity and sexuality.

In the light of the above, it is not surprising that many women have concerns about the size, shape and appearance of their breasts ranging from mild satisfaction to severe anxiety and depressive neurosis.

In surgical treatment of the breast cancer, it is obvious that removing a breast leads to grieving for loss while conservative treatment provokes mistrust about that breast with a fear that cancer is still lurking and a mastectomy will prove inevitable. Women with breast cancer are conscious of inevitable death, humiliation, shame, loss of dignity and loss of control (Denewer et al., 2011).

In North Africa, the incidence of breast cancer was similar to that in Europe and slightly less than USA. There was a significant difference as regard younger age incidence by about ten (10) years (Denewer et al., 2010).

The primary goal of breast reconstruction is to recreate form and symmetry by correcting the anatomic defect while preserving patients' safety and health. Breast reconstruction is performed in several stages: restoration of the breast contour, revisions, and reconstruction of the nipple-areola complex. Many options for breast reconstruction exist, which are typically grouped into alloplastic, autologous and a combination of both. The choice of technique is directed by several factors that include the size and shape of the native breast, the location and type of cancer, the quantity and quality of tissues around the breast and at the other donor sites, the patients' demographic information and whether adjuvant therapy is warranted. Breast mound reconstruction can be performed immediately, at the time of mastectomy, or can be delayed for several weeks or months (Hu & Alderman, 2007).

In keeping with the Hippocratic Oath, one of the goals of breast reconstruction is "first do no harm". Reconstruction after mastectomy should not impede the patients' oncologic treatment (i.e., delay administration of chemotherapy or radiation therapy), also it should not add an unacceptable increase in operative morbidity or mortality. Current data indicate that reconstruction is safe and does not delay adjuvant therapy or detection of cancer recurrence (Alderman et al., 2002; Wilson et al., 2004).

Most predictable results in breast reconstruction involve the use of autologous tissue. Many surgeons prefer to use autogenous tissue (i.e., LDF), in part because of greater patient satisfaction with these techniques. In general, it involves the use of the patients' own tissue resulting in a reconstruction that can closely match the opposite breast in size, shape and texture. Depending on the volume of the tissue transferred and the volume of contralateral breast, autologous tissue breast reconstruction sometimes also requires an implant (Patrek & Disa, 2005).

Breast reconstruction is becoming increasingly important due to change in patient expectations and demand. There is growing recognition that immediate reconstruction in appropriately selected women can combine an oncological and aesthetic procedure in one operation with excellent results. Because most breast surgery is performed by general surgeons, most reconstructions were performed as delayed procedures by plastic surgeons. Increasingly, breast surgery is being performed by breast surgeons trained in oncoplastic techniques who can offer immediate reconstruction with both therapeutic and economic benefits (Khoo et al., 1998; Baildam, 2002).

2. Immediate autologous breast reconstruction

Immediate autologous breast reconstruction yields the most durable and natural appearing results with the greatest consistency (Patrek & Disa, 2005).

The aesthetic results from autologous reconstruction are superior to those of implant based reconstruction due to their versatility, their more natural appearance, consistency and durability. Autologous tissue can better withstand radiotherapy.

Although reconstruction with implants can produce good cosmetic outcomes, complications requiring additional surgery occur in 34% of patients over the first 5 years after reconstruction. Problems such as infection, implant exposure, capsular contracture, seroma and rupture or deflation of the implant can occur and can adversely affect the cosmetic outcome and increase the long-term costs by necessitating further surgery and hospitalization (Chevray & Robb, 2007).

Delgado and his co-workers published a study in 2007, whose results showed that the most frequent complications were cutaneous necrosis, some of which was accompanied by seroma. In all the cases that had a seroma, the devices were explanted because of the exposure of the prosthesis (Delgado et al., 2007).

The commonest and least predictable complication of breast implant surgery is capsular contracture in many series. Submuscular placement of silicone gel-filled implants consistently decreases the incidence of significant contracture from 60 to 30%, although this often may be confounded by the effect of preoperative or postoperative irradiation (Salgarello & Farallo, 2005).

Capsular contracture refers to tightening of the implant capsule over time. In mild cases, this causes the reconstructed breast to become more firm and stiff. In moderate cases, capsular contracture can make the reconstructed breast become more round, spherical and rise in position on the chest wall. In severe cases, capsular contracture can cause breast and chest wall pain and restrict shoulder and arm range of motion (Chevray & Robb, 2007).

Autologous Reconstruction can be achieved by:

i. L.D. with added vascularised fat flap (Denewer & Farouk, 2007; Denewer et al., 2008)
ii. Myomammary flap from other breast (in huge pendulous breast) (Denewer, 1997; Denewer et al., 2007)
iii. TRAM flaps; pedicled, free with microvascular, DIEP, SIEP (Hartrampf, 1988).
iv. Others; superior gluteal artery perforator flap (SGAP) (Allen & Tucker, 1995), the lateral thigh flap (Elliot et al., 1990), The Rubens flap, or deep circumflex iliac soft tissue flap (Tachi & Yamada, 2005).

Surgical treatment of breast cancer has evolved from radical mastectomy with routine removal of the nipple-areolar complex (NAC) to breast conservative therapy with preservation of the breast and NAC. When breast conservation is not appropriate or the patient desires mastectomy for risk reduction, conventional therapy still consists of mastectomy with or without removal of the NAC, followed by reconstruction (Chung & Sacchini, 2008).

3. Modified extended latissimus dorsi myocutaneous flap with added vascularised chest wall fat

3.1 Anatomy of latissimus dorsi muscle

It is a type V flap according to Mathes and Nahai's classification of muscle vascularisation, which means that it can survive solely on its principal pedicle (Mathes & Nahai, 1982).

The latissimus dorsi, the broadest muscle of the back consists of two triangular shaped muscles with fascial origins from the spinous processes of the lower six thoracic, lumbar and sacral vertebrae, and from the iliac crest. Additionally, there are muscular origins from the anterolateral aspect of the lower four ribs as well as the external oblique and tip of the scapula.

The fibers converge superiolaterally and twist 180° before inserting into the intertubercular groove of the humerus. The muscle, which is largely expendable, functions to extend, adduct and medially rotate the arm.

The lateral part of the muscle is closely associated with the serratus anterior muscle on its deep aspect. The latissimus dorsi muscle has two free borders, (i) an upper border passing from the posterior axillary line to the sixth thoracic spine and (ii) a lateral border demarcating the midaxillary line

3.2 Surgical anatomy of the added vascularised chest wall fat

The third part of axillary artery contributes in blood supply to lateral chest wall via its largest branch; the subscapular artery, which further gives the thoracodorsal branch. Fat over serratus anterior muscle is supplied by a small branch of the thoracic part of thoracodorsal artery and in some instances by another branch of the dorsal part.

The technique involves meticulous dissection of the thoracic branch of the thoracodorsal vessels, which supplies the fat and superficial part of the underlying serratus anterior muscle, with transfer of the superficial fibres of the lower three digitations of the serratus anterior muscle to get the benefit of preservation of the blood supply to the overlying fat that dissected and remained attached to latissimus dorsi muscle in continuity (Figures 1&2) at its anterior border (Denewer et al., 2008).

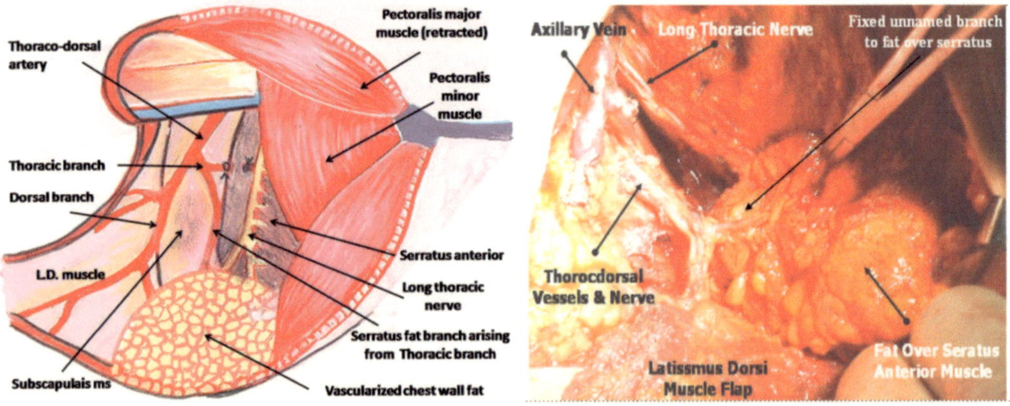

Fig. 1. The vascularized fat over the serratus muscle is supplied constantly by branches from both thoracic branch & dorsal branch which are called serratus branches.

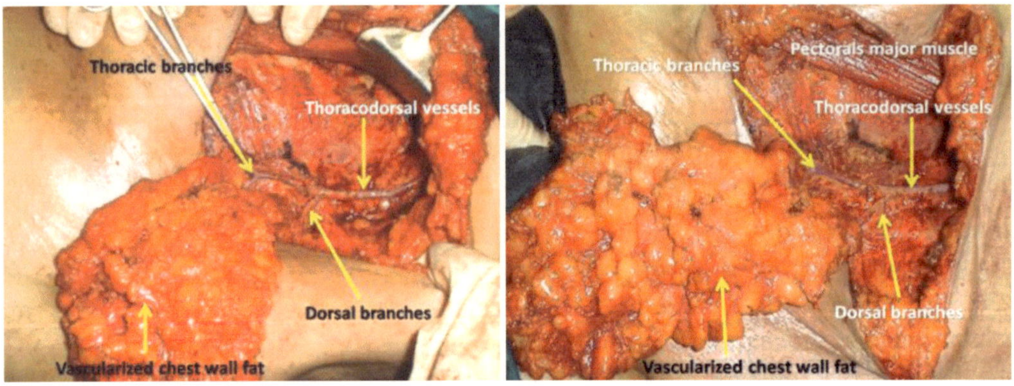

Fig. 2. The vascularised chest wall fat

3.3 The concept of oncological safety of SSM

The development of skin-sparing mastectomy (SSM) with immediate reconstruction achieved the goal of radical excision of the tumor with improved cosmetic outcome. In addition, the overall survival and local recurrence rates were similar to cases of modified radical mastectomy (Carlson et al, 2001; Denewer & Farouk, 2007).

The main oncological concern in both SSM and non-skin sparing mastectomy (NSSM) relates to the possibility of leaving residual tumor within the skin envelope which may manifest later as local recurrence (LR). Indeed, Ho et al. performed histological examinations of the skin and subcutaneous tissue of 30 NSSM specimens and found that the skin flaps (excluding the NAC) were involved in 23% (7 of 30) of cases. In five cases, the skin involved was situated directly over the tumor (Ho et al, 2003). Importantly, long-term follow-up of selected patients has not shown a difference in local recurrence rates after skin-sparing mastectomy versus traditional mastectomy (Hidalgo et al, 1998).

Unfortunately, many of the studies addressing the issue of LR following SSM have not followed-up patients long enough for it to be seen. In addition, there is a significant lack of prospective data and nearly all studies are from single institutions (Cunnick & Mokbel, 2006).

3.4 Technique

Skin incisions are generally conservative and in the most favourable cases a small circular incision around the areola will suffice with preservation of the inframammary fold and limited dissection of the skin flaps beyond the breast tissue. Either formal axillary dissection or sentinel node biopsy can be performed at the same time through either the areolar incision, a lateral extension thereof or a separate axillary incision (Nair et al., 2010).

3.4.1 Technical aspects of SSM

Peri-areolar incision (5 mm away from areola) is designed either alone (Figure 3) or with lateral extension rising towards the axilla (tennis racket incision) in order to facilitate mastectomy and axillary dissection (Figure 4). Inferolateral incision may be utilized for its higher cosmetic result (Figure 5).

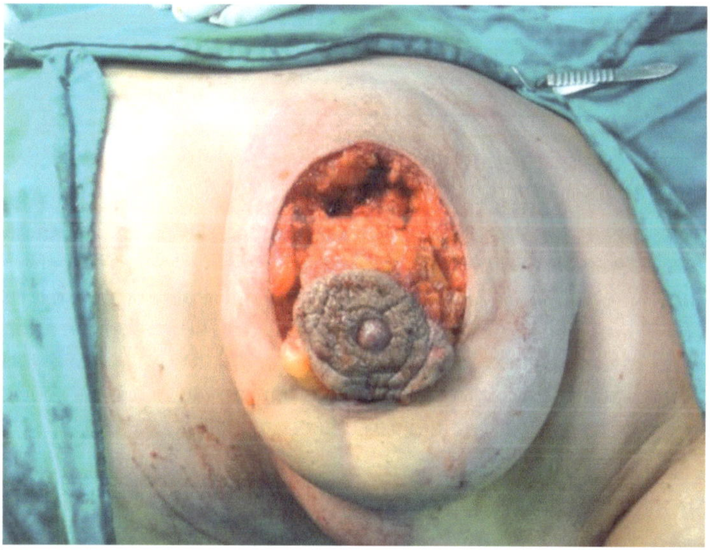

Fig. 3. Peri-aereolar incision in SSM.

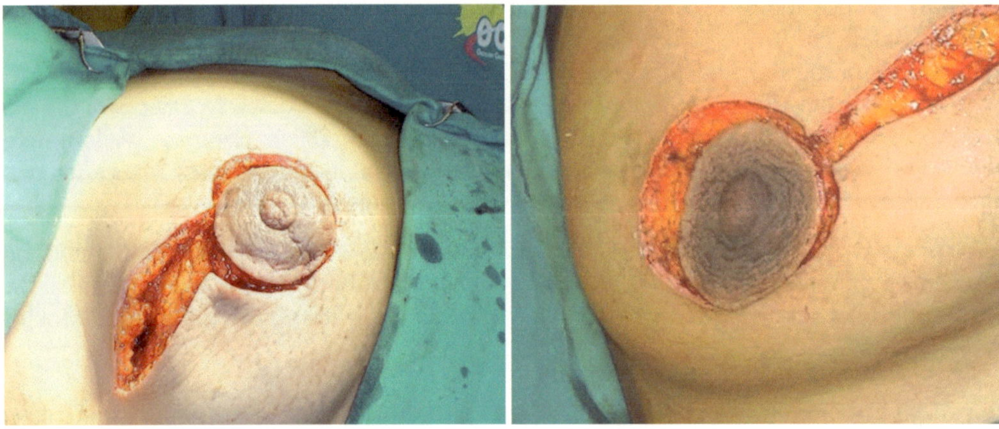

Fig. 4. Peri-aereolar incision in SSM, with lateral extension rising towards the axilla (tennis racket incision). (Denewer & Farouk, 2007).

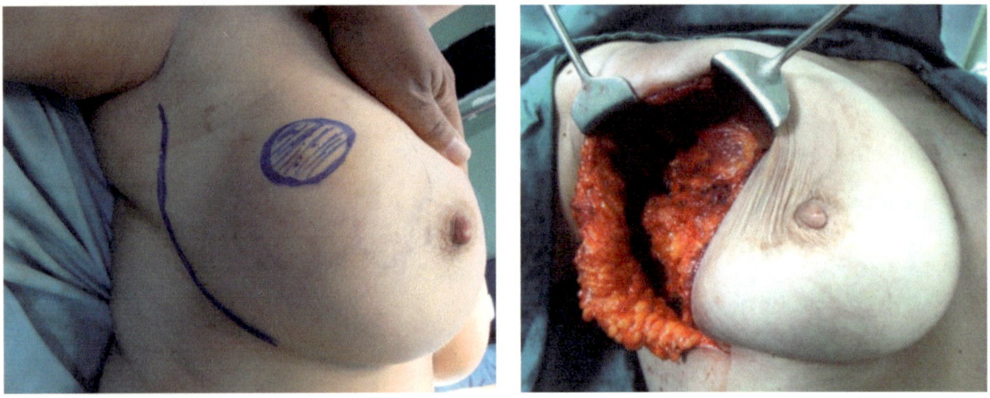

Fig. 5. Infero-lateral incision.

The native skin envelope flaps are dissected and elevated, which should be meticulous in the fatty layer between the dermis and the glandular tissue so as not to jeopardize skin vascularity (Figure 6).

The dissection plane of SSM advances between the breast parenchyma and the subcutaneous fat. Scissors are conventionally used for the sharp dissection and bleeding vessels are typically cauterized using electric bipolar diathermy. This element of the procedure is of vital importance in avoiding later SSM skin-flap complications, given that a solid hemostasis is essential. However, thermal injury to the skin needs to be avoided. In addition, blood supply to the skin should not be compromised, and the perforating arteries should be preserved whenever possible (Meretoja et al., 2008).

To maximize a good cosmetic outcome, the dissection of the lower skin flap should not continue beyond the inframammary fold (Figure 7), so that the final aesthetic shape of the immediate breast reconstruction (IBR) will be very similar to the original breast. The breast tissue is then removed off the pectoralis major muscle as in a (NSM).

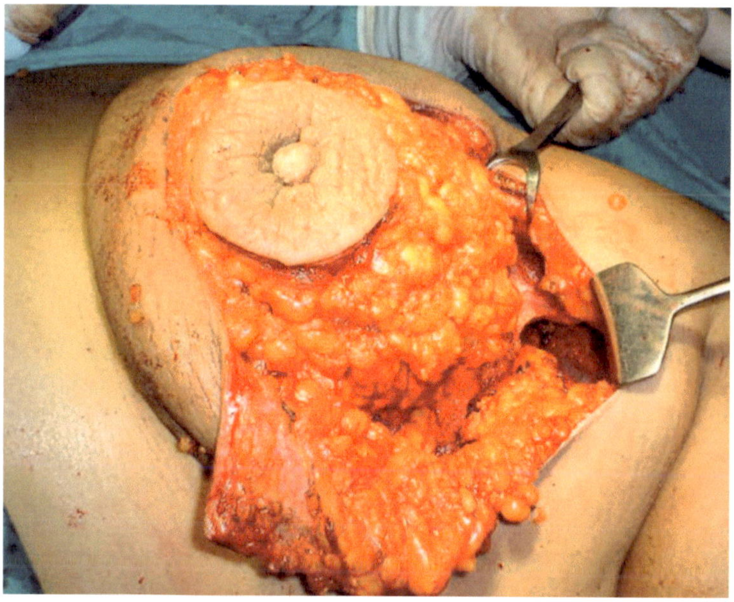

Fig. 6. The native skin envelope flaps are dissected and elevated (Denewer et al., 2008).

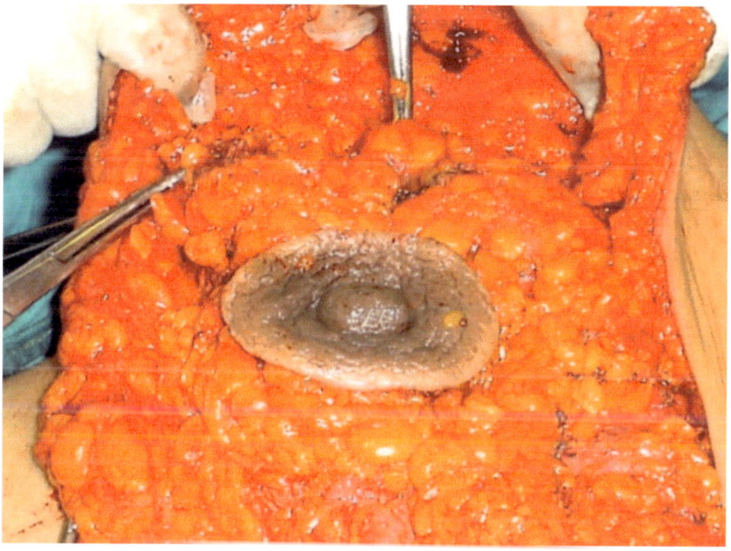

Fig. 7. The dissection of the lower skin flap, with preservation of the inframammary fold (Denewer et al., 2008).

Axillary dissection (level I and II) is then performed through the same incision, with preservation of thoracodorsal vessels and both pectoralis major and minor (Figure 8). Finally the whole breast parenchyma, nipple, areola, and axillary lymph nodes are removed completely as a whole specimen (Figure 9) (Denewer et al., 2008).

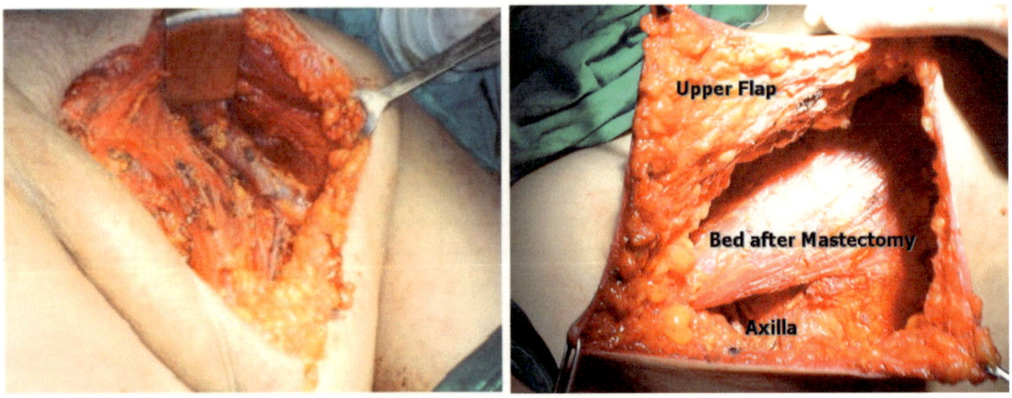

Fig. 8. The breast bed after complete SSM & The axilla after complete axillary dissection (level I and II).

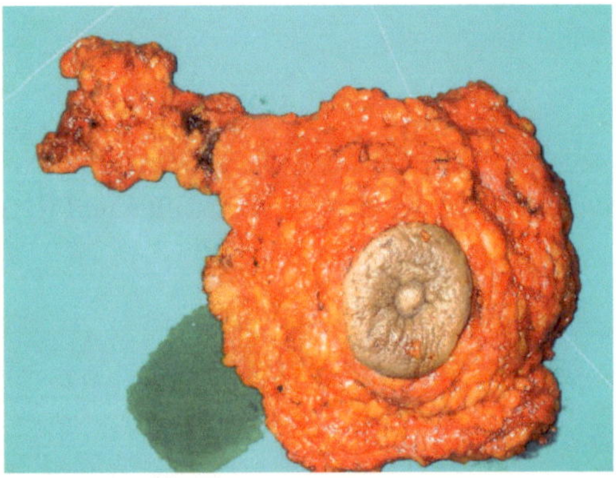

Fig. 9. Specimen appearance after complete resection of the whole breast parenchymal tissue and NAC, with level I and II axillary dissection (in SSM).

3.4.2 Technical aspects of L.D. flap

A transverse skin puddle incision with its long axis centered over the seventh rib extending from the posterior axillary line to the parascapular line is marked. The LD muscle with overlying fat is elevated and transected near the iliac crest inferiorly and tendon of insertion is separated from the humerus superiorly (Figure 10). After complete dissection of LD muscle, the back incision is closed (Figure 11).

Where autologous tissue has been imported as part of a myocutaneous flap, a disc of skin can be used from the donor site to replace the defect resulting from excision of the nipple-areola complex. Under these circumstances the skin is closed in a circumferential fashion to yield a scar of dimensions similar to the contralateral areola.

After dissection of the thoracodorsal vessels; the upper branch of the thoracic artery is cut and ligated in order to protect the long thoracic nerve, while the lower branches are preserved to supply the chest wall fat over the serratus anterior muscle, in addition to preservation of the terminal branches of the dorsal artery that supply this fat which remains attached to the anterior border of L.D.

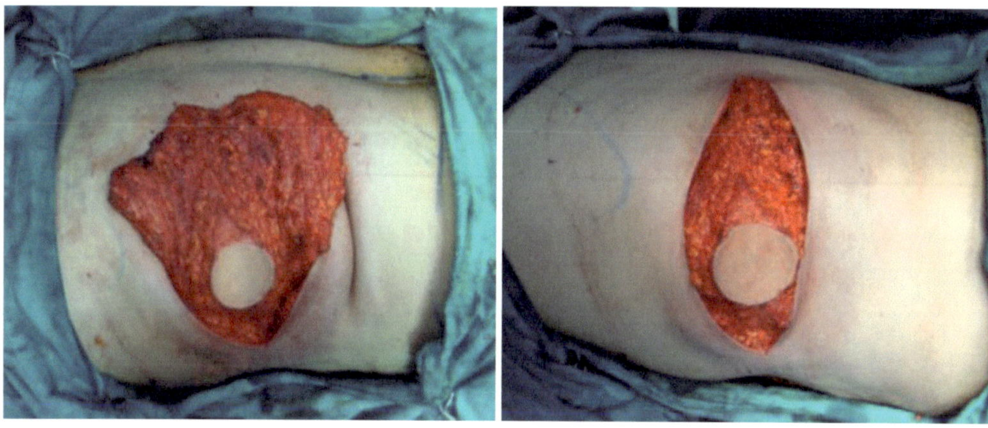

Fig. 10. Dissection of the LD flap.

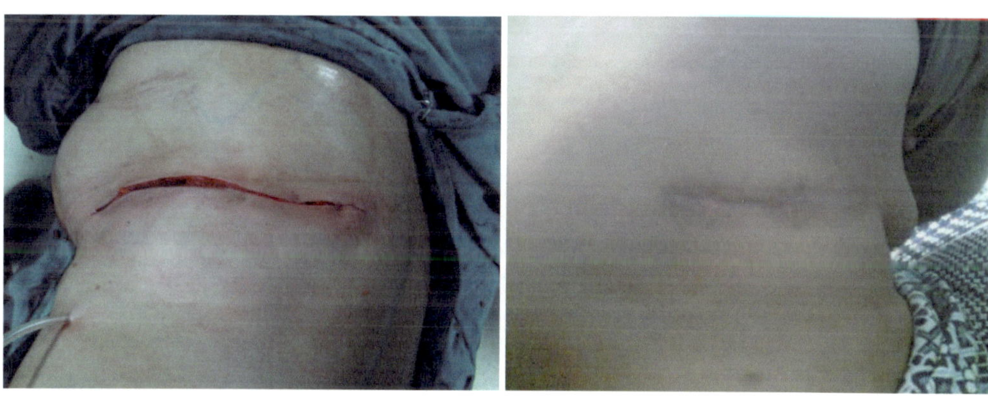

Fig. 11. Closure of the back wound.

This amount of fat is harvested from the chest wall and now is attached to the upper-anterior border of L.D. the vascularisation of this fat is entailed through the terminal branches of both thoracic & dorsal arteries (serratus branches).

Now the modified extended LD myocutaneous flap together with the added vascularized chest wall fat are tunneled through the axilla to be transposed to the breast bed under the skin envelop (Figure 12) (Denewer et al., 2008)

The vascularized fat is fixed to the pectoralis major muscle, forming the first layer of the reconstructed breast (Figure 12c), and then the flap is folded on itself to form the second layer of the desired reconstructed mound, fixed with a few absorbable sutures, and then the skin envelop is closed (Figure 13) to yield the final view of the reconstructed breast (Figures 14 - 16).

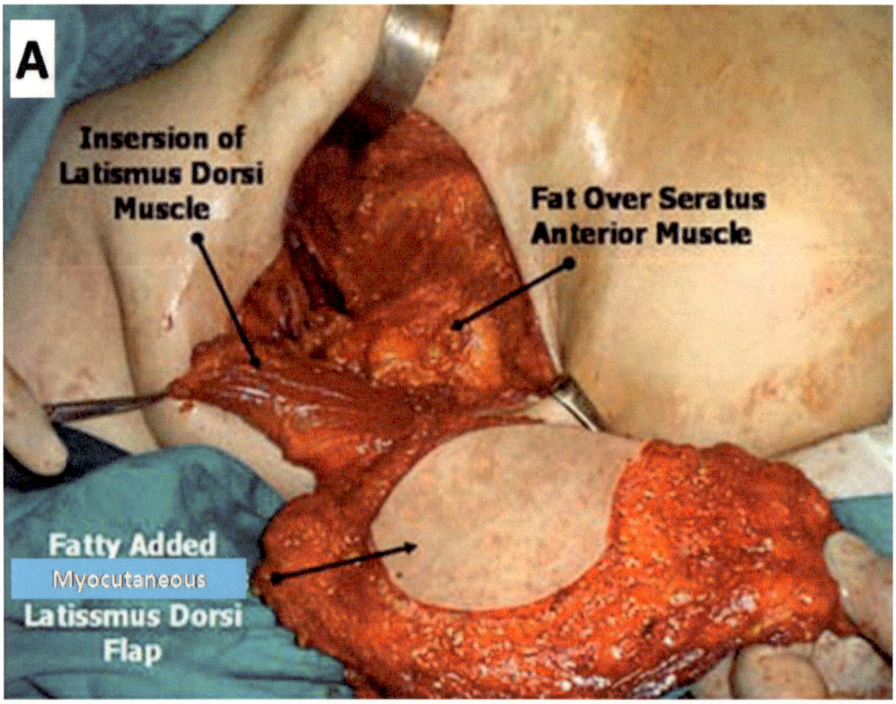

Fig. 12 (A). Dorsal view of the flap after its dissection and transposition through the axilla.

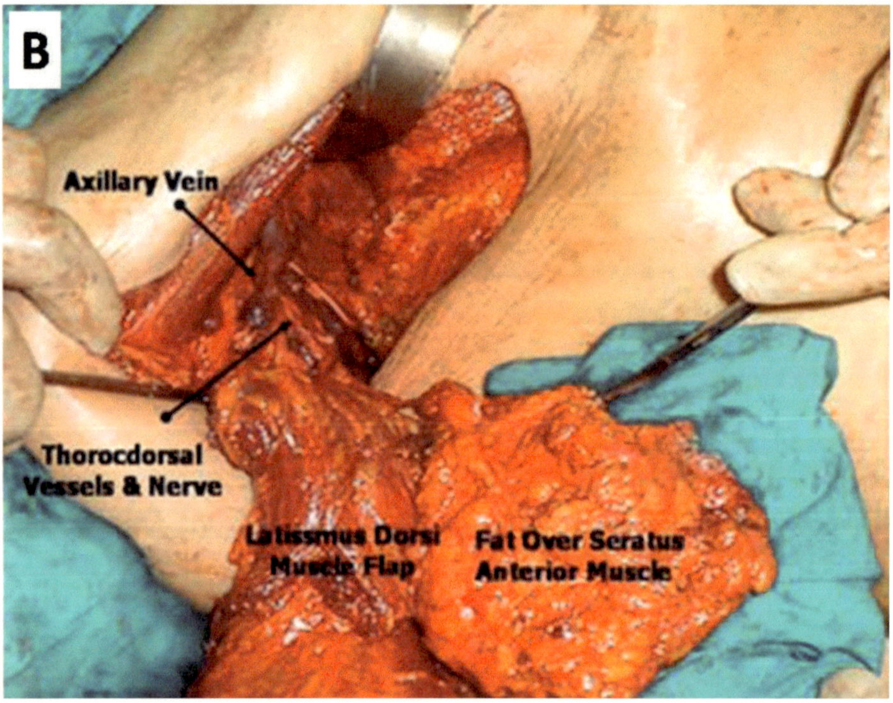

Fig. 12. (B) Ventral view of the flap with the attached fat over seratus anterior muscle.

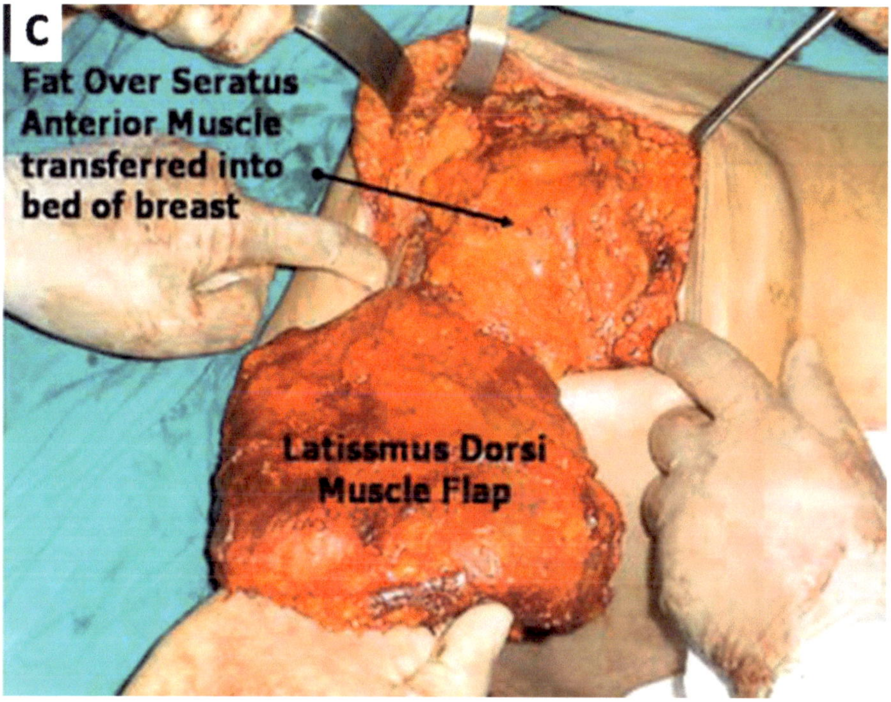

Fig. 12 (C). Fixation of the added vascularized fat to the pectoralis major muscle forming the first layer of the reconstructed breast (Denewer & Farouk, 2007).

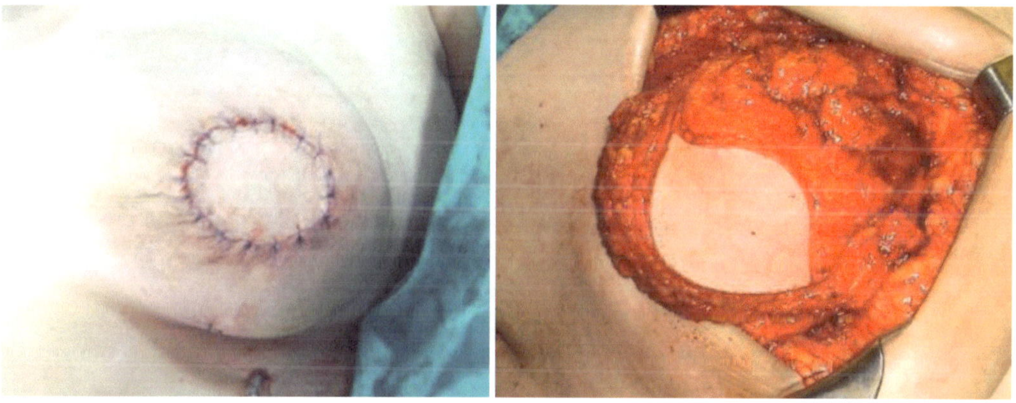

Fig. 13. The remaining of the flap is folded to complete the breast mound with closure of the wounds.

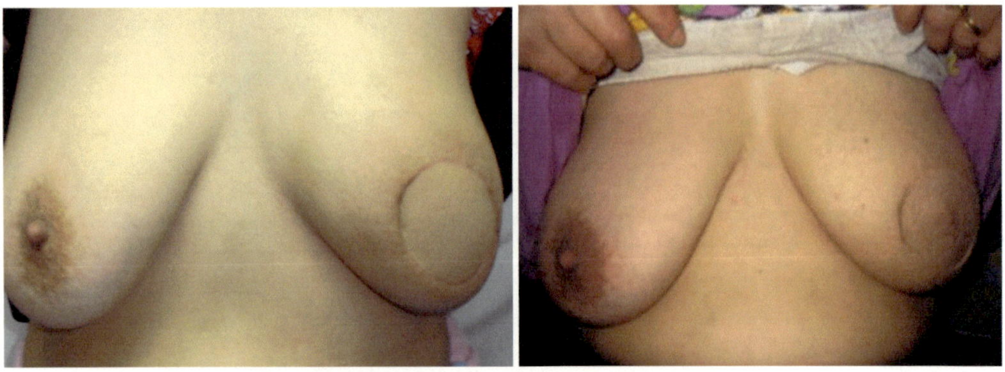

Fig. 14. SSM with modified latissimus dorsi vascularized fat-added flap after 6 months.

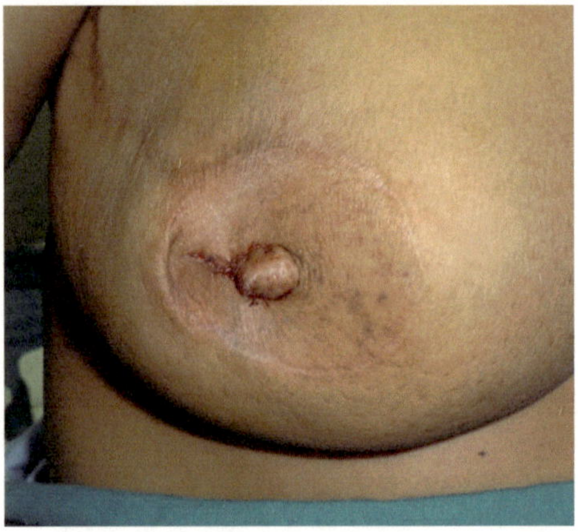

Fig. 15. Nipple reconstruction & first stage tattooing.

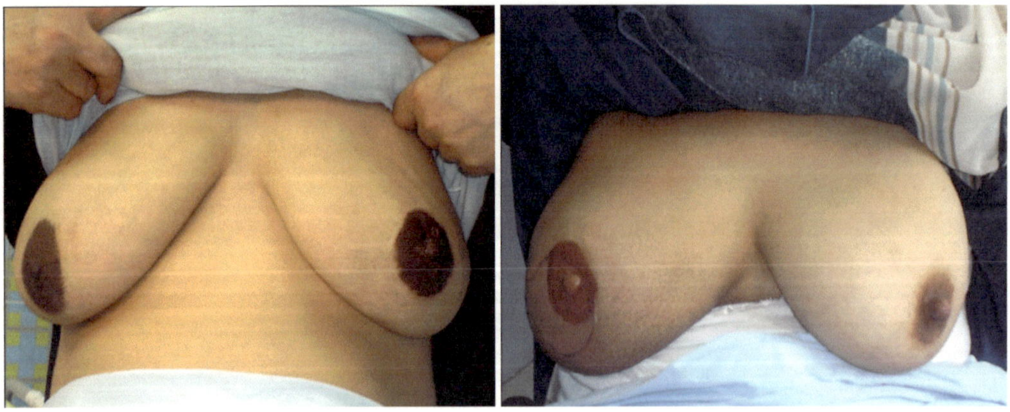

Fig. 16. Final appearance of areola tattooing after nipple reconstruction.

3.4.3 Technical aspects of NSM

Rising interest in improved cosmesis has led to the introduction of Nipple sparing mastectomy as potential alternatives to mastectomy (Chung & Sacchini, 2008). Nipple sparing mastectomy combines skin-sparing mastectomy with preservation of the nipple-areolar complex (NAC) and intraoperative pathologic assessment of the nipple core. This approach preserves the dermis and epidermis of the NAC but removes major ducts from within the nipple (Sookhan et al., 2008).

NSM may be performed according to total mastectomy indications if an intraoperative frozen section (and the corresponding HE histopathology) of the tissue next to the nipple-areola skin is free of tumor. The remaining contraindications for NSM are: extensive tumor involvement of the skin, inflammatory breast cancer, and a clinically suspicious nipple.

In a study, representing OCMU experience, Denewer and Farouk concluded that nipple-sparing mastectomy provides a good cosmetic result with a low risk of postoperative complications. The additional volume obtained by using a new modification of latissimus dorsi fat-added flap allows single-stage NSM with immediate autologous breast reconstruction without implant insertion and without contralateral operations in medium and large-sized breasts (Denewer & Farouk, 2007).

A claw like incision encompassing the lateral half circle of NAC with lateral extension rising towards the axilla is performed. The incision did not involve the NAC in any breast (Figure 17). Inferolateral incision may be utilized for its higher cosmetic result (Figure 5).

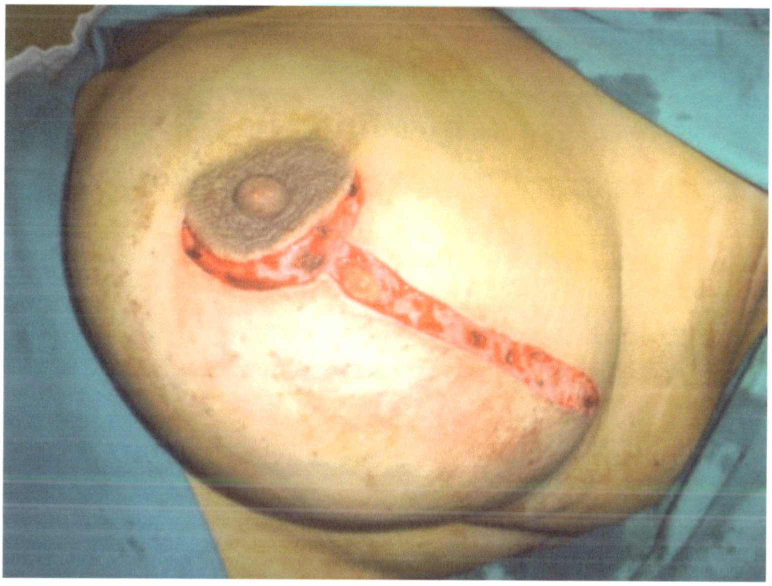

Fig. 17. Claw like incision with lateral extension rising towards the axilla (Denewer & Farouk, 2007).

The NAC is dissected and elevated. At least 3-mm thick nipple-areola flap should remain (so as not to jeopardize its vascularity). An intraoperative frozen section analysis (FSA) of both the undersurface of the nipple itself and the en face retroareolar margin of the resected breast mound is obtained to verify the absence of neoplasia or atypia. The remaining steps of dissection, reconstruction & follow-up are the same as performed in SSM (Figures 18 - 22).

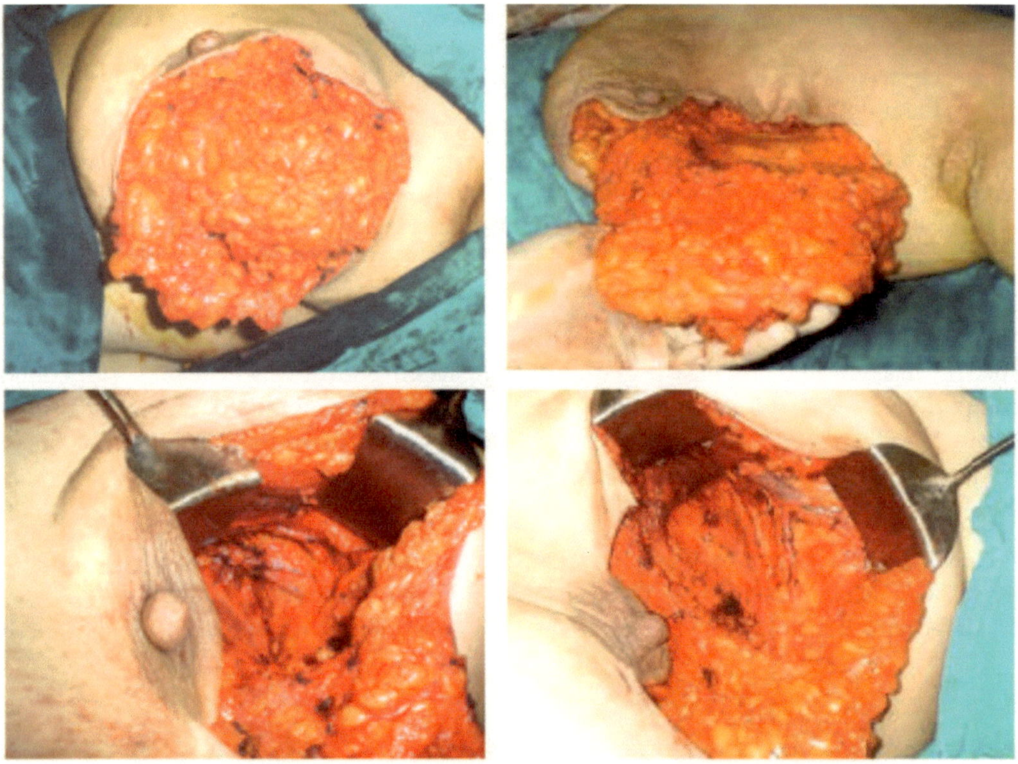

Fig. 18. Standard NSM with level I and II axillary dissection, with preservation of NAC.

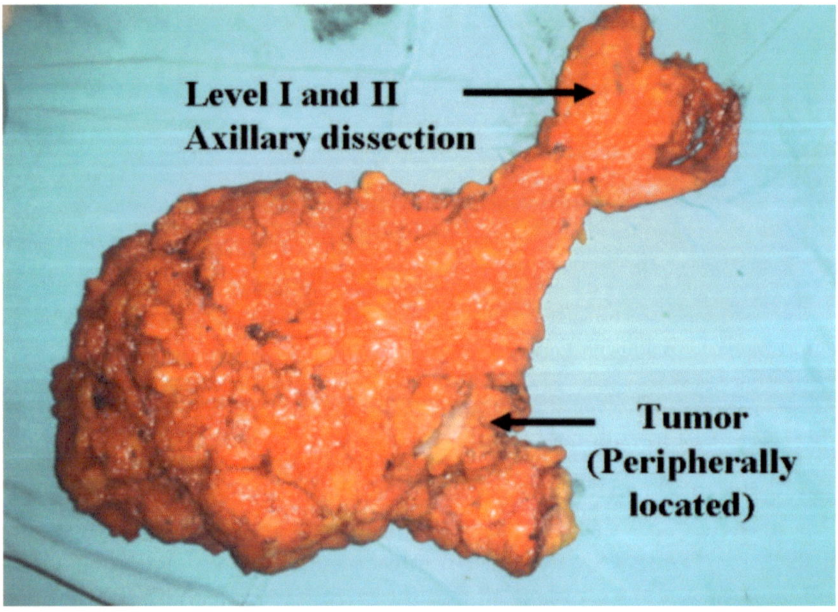

Fig. 19. Gross specimen appearance after complete resection of the whole breast parenchymal tissue with level I and II axillary dissection (in NSM).

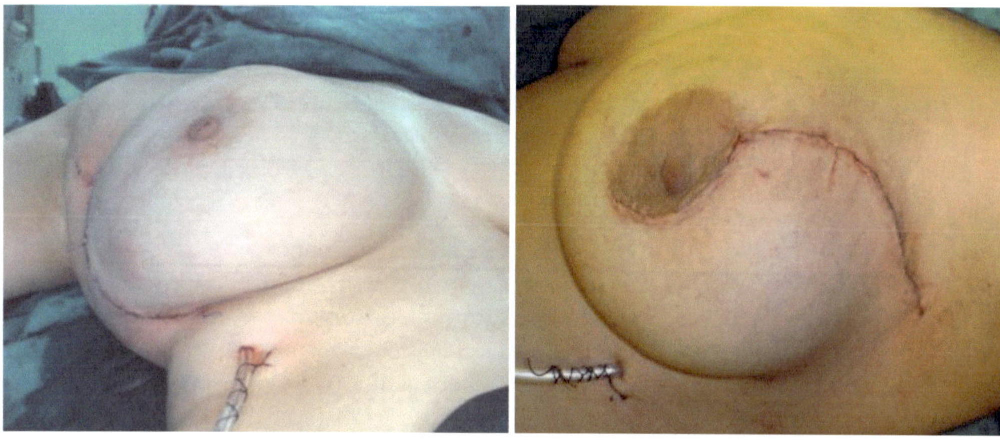

Fig. 20. Single-stage NSM with modified latissimus dorsi vascularized fat-added flap

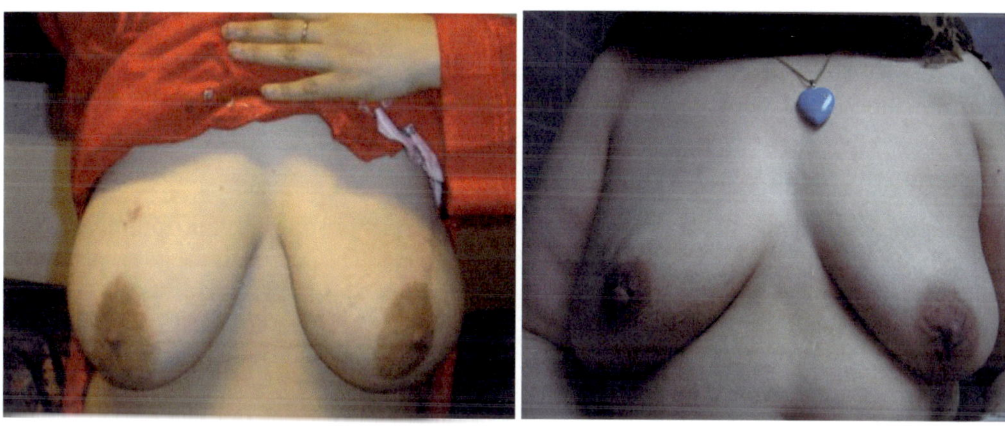

Fig. 21. NSM with modified latissimus dorsi vascularized fat-added flap after 6 months

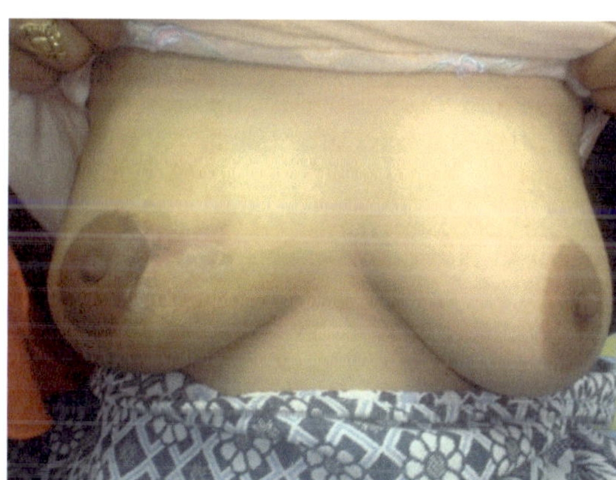

Fig. 22. Another NSM with modified latissimus dorsi vascularized fat-added flap after 5 months in lady with previous unplanned resected tumor in the upper inner quadrant of the right breast.

3.5 Oncological safety of nipple and areola sparing mastectomy

NSM appears to be oncologically safe for appropriately selected patients, although additional long-term follow-up is needed, and these patients should be followed with special surveillance following NSM (Benediktsson & Perbeck, 2008). However, 5 years follow up in our series proved to be oncologically safe. In this period of follow up, the rate of local recurrence is 3.8% & the distant metastasis is 3.2%.

It was found that nipple and areolar invasion with malignancy is a rare event in the presence of an early peripherally located tumor; with a clinically normal NAC, this incidence dropped to 1.2 % in peripherally located tumor. Skin & nipple sparing mastectomy is technically feasible in spite of the relatively large size of the breast, with low morbidity & very satisfactory cosmetic results (Stance et al., 2003; Crowe et al., 2004)

When the malignant involvement of the areola versus nipple was analyzed separately, areola involvement was detected in <1% of patients & only in those with central/retroareolar/diffuse invasive carcinomas, large (>5) tumors & multiple positive axillary lymph nodes. No patient with stage 0, I, or II breast carcinoma had areolar involvement. Only patients with stage III had areolar involvement. All patients with areolar involvement also had involvement of nipple (Simmons et al, 2002)

3.6 Current status & overall views

Immediate reconstruction does not delay the administration of adjuvant radiotherapy or chemotherapy (Yule et al, 1996). Significant additional morbidity with delay of chemotherapy has not been noted with either breast implants or autogenous tissue (Hidalgo et al, 1998). The overall complication rate of RT following autologous breast reconstruction ranges from 5% to 16%. Following breast reconstruction using the transverse rectus abdominis myocutaneous (TRAM) flap, the most common complications of RT include fat necrosis (16%) and radiation fibrosis (11%), which may cause shrinkage and deformation of the reconstructed breast (Patani et al., 2008).

In our series; five hundred & seventy patients of stage I to III breast carcinoma have autologous breast reconstruction. Age ranges from 23 to 53 years (median = 40.5) have modified extended LDF 47% had SSM and the remaining had NSM. Subjective patient satisfaction was excellent in 71%, good in 20%, fair in 7% & poor in 2% of cases. Bilateral size & shape symmetry are excellent in 56%, good in 26%, fair in 12% & poor in 6% patient. The overall RT-related complications are 9 %, the most common complications are skin burns (5%) & fat necrosis (4%). Patients are followed for mean follow up of 75.5 months (2-96).

Several studies with extended follow up have corroborated the earlier findings .In a 15-year retrospective series of women with stage 0-2 IBC, 225 patients undergoing SSM and IBR were compared to 1022 patients treated by conventional mastectomy .after an average follow -up of 49 months, there was found to be no significance difference in LR (Greenway et al., 2005).

The overall survival and local recurrence rates were similar to cases of modified radical mastectomy (Denewer & Farouk, 2007).

4. Comparison of extended LDF with added vascularized chest wall fat after S.S.M. & N.S.M. versus myocutaneous flap from the contralateral breast versus therapeutic mammoplasty in the management of breast cancer in huge breast

The initial results in three hundreds of huge breast cancer management:

1. Extended LDF with added vascularized chest wall fat.
2. Myomammary flap from other breast.
3. Therapeutic reduction mammoplasty.

The oncologic outcome of extended LDF with added vascularized chest wall fat in the reconstruction of the huge breast (Figure 29 & 30) was superior to myomammary flap (Figures 23 & 24) with near equal oncologic outcome. NSM is better cosmetically than SSM, as there is no need for NAC reconstruction, moreover in good selected cases there is no difference in oncologic safety.

In special situation in management of huge breast cancer; the therapeutic reduction mammoplasty is employed with better outcome than conventional conservative breast surgery as the safety margin which in the first is wider (5-10 cm) and more confidential than the conventional conservative breast surgery (CBS), the aesthetic outcome is better than CBS (Figures 25 - 28) but the operative time and hospital stay are longer than CBS. In comparison to SSM and NSM which are aesthetically near equal to therapeutic mammoplasty, however the oncologic outcome is better than therapeutic mammoplasty. Table (1) summarize the main surgical characteristics of each technique.

Method	Average operative time	Oncologic outcome	Aesthetic outcome	Feasibility of operative technique	Contralateral Surgery
L.D. with vascularized fat	3 hours	++++ (As M.R.M.)	++++	+++	- -
Myomammary Flap	2. 5 hours	++++ (As M.R.M.)	++	+	++++
Therapeutic reduction mammoplasty	3 hours	++ (Less than M.R.M. & better than CBS.	++++	++	++++

Table 1. Comparison of the three methods in immediate reconstruction of huge breast.

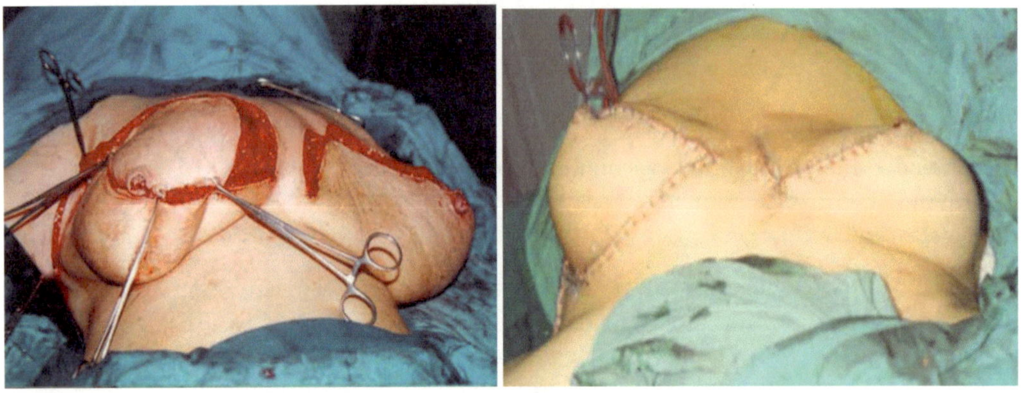

Fig. 23. Operative views of myomammry flap.

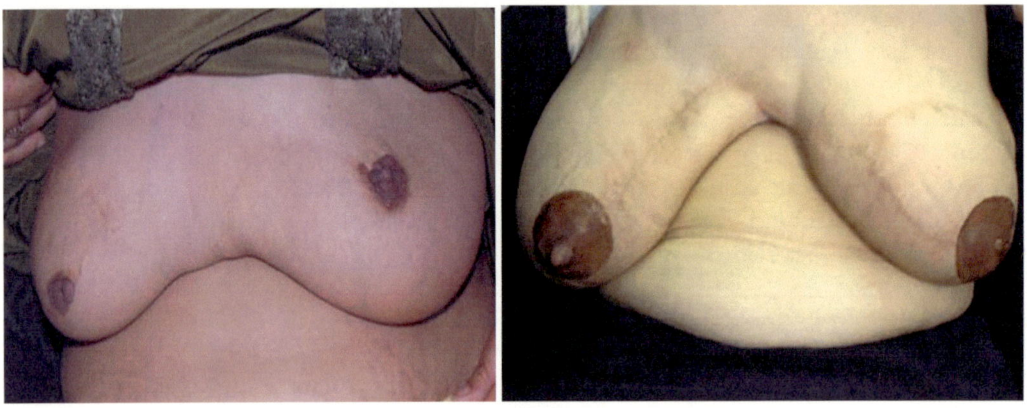

Fig. 24. Post-operative view of patients with myomammary flap reconstruction. Right photo shows bilateral temporary symmetrical tattooing.

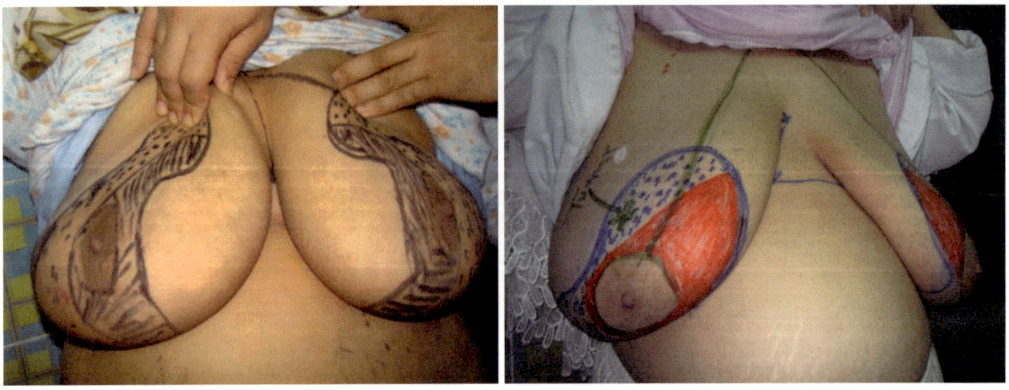

Fig. 25. Preoperative marking of patients with huge breasts, who are planned for therapeutic reduction mammoplasty.

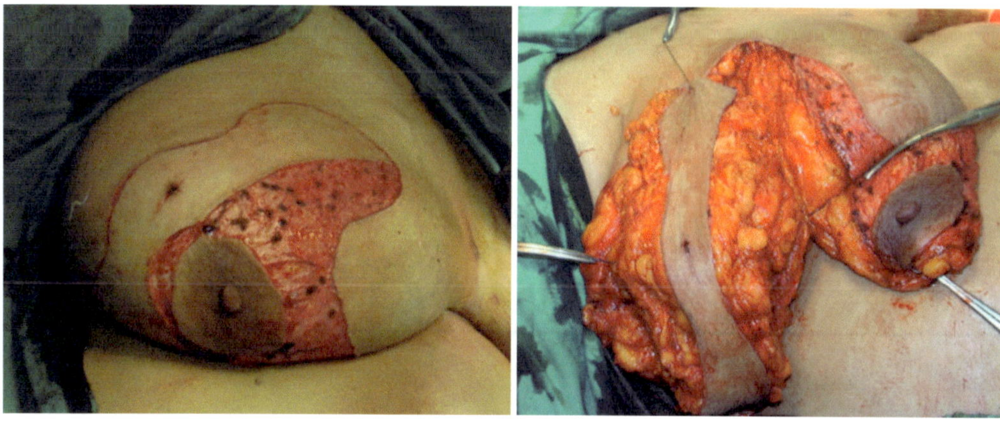

Fig. 26. Operative views of therapeutic reduction mammoplasty; the tumor safety margin is ranged from 5 - 11 cm all-around.

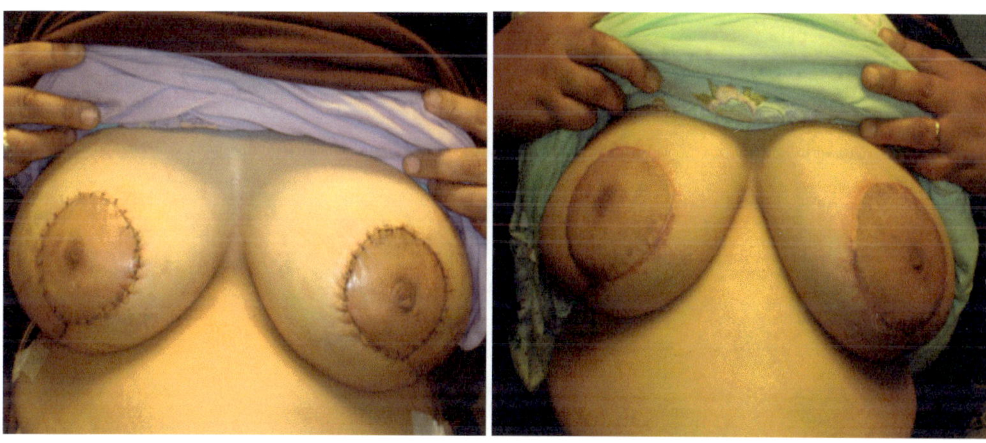

Fig. 27. Early Postoperative views of therapeutic reduction mammoplasty.

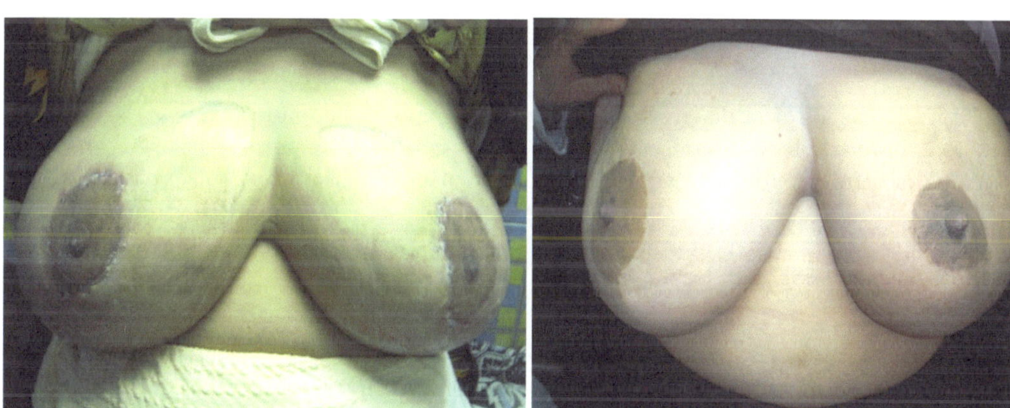

Fig. 28. Late postoperative views of therapeutic reduction mammoplasty; Left photo after 6 months & Right photo shows another patient after 2 years.

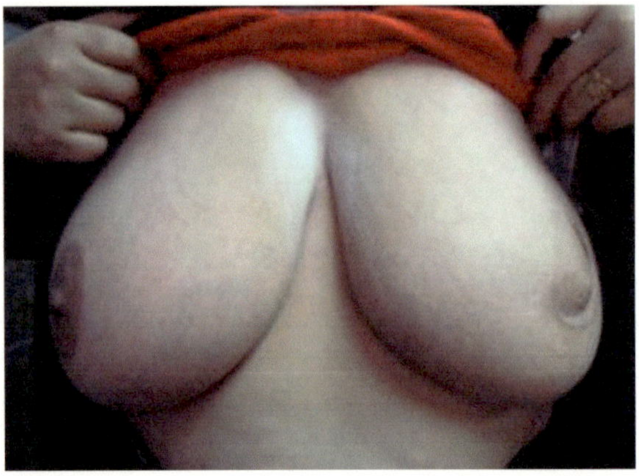

Fig. 29. Immediate breast reconstruction of huge breast with SSM using modified latissimus dorsi vascularized fat-added flap with SSM & nipple reconstruction and waiting areolar tattooing.

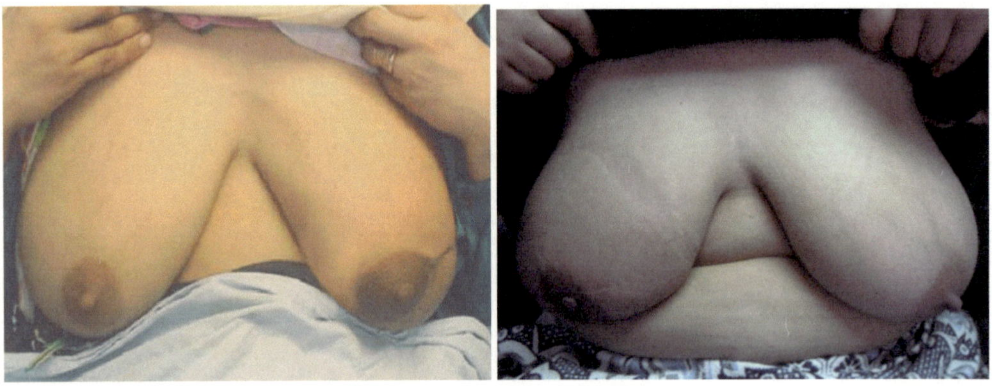

Fig. 30. Immediate breast reconstruction of huge breast with NSM using modified latissimus dorsi vascularized fat-added flap.

5. Conclusion

The trend in the surgical management of breast carcinoma has moved toward less radical surgery & has become more conservative. Although conservative surgery has been shown to be an oncologically sound strategy for most early stage breast cancer, mastectomy remains the treatment of choice for many women, either because of patient preference or because of tumor characteristics that are not compatible with a more conservative approach, in addition to consideration of local recurrence.

The development of SSM & NSM with immediate breast reconstruction achieved the goal of radical excision of the tumor with improved cosmetic outcome. Because the NAC area typically has been included in the resection(SSM) ,cosmetic approaches have involved nipple - areola reconstruction . Although this approach can give excellent cosmetic results ,it has potential disadvantages in the form of loss of nipple sensation ,pale color ,and possible loss of projection as the scars soften over time (Denewer & Farouk, 2007)

Single stage totally autologous breast reconstruction allows reconstruction without the additional cost of an implant, many complications of synthetic implants, micro vascular procedure second stage surgery or surgical manipulation in the other breast. In addition the overall survival & local recurrence rates were similar to MRM.

In conclusion, conservative mastectomy (sparing mastectomy; SSM & NSM) is oncologically as safe as MRM and better oncologic outcome than conservative breast surgery. Aesthetically the immediate reconstruction after these two techniques is superior to delayed reconstruction after MRM & immediate oncoplastic conserveative breast surgery.

The new technique of vascularized chest wall fat added to LDF can allow immediate autologous breast reconstruction after SSM & NSM in all breast sizes even the huge breast without any synthetic implant with excellent aesthetic and oncologic outcome. This immediate breast reconstruction can avoid contralateral operation in medium and huge breast of cup C and D brassier sizes, moreover avoidance of psychological trauma of mastectomy and postoperative depression, anexiety and obsessions.

In the past three decades, there has been a gradual significant shift in breast cancer management which is the restoration of patient psychological, physical well-being as well as quality of life and body image. This is now considered as paramount importance in overall treatment of breast cancer.

For more efficient outcome, it is mandatory to achieve the following;

1. Pre-operative counseling of the patient
2. Patient selection as regards the disease stage, comorbidity and radiation therapy.
3. Good refinement and understanding of anatomical basis of autologous flaps.
4. Oncoplastic experience
5. Geometrical surgical imagination.
6. Consideration the immediate breast reconstruction
7. Skin sparing mastectomy and nipple sparing mastectomy have the least revision procedures necessary for perfection of breast shape and symmetry.
8. Ensure good vascularization of autologous tissue to decrease complications like fat necrosis, fibrosis and skin necrosis.

6. Acknowledgment

The authors gratefully acknowledge the contribution of Dr. Osama El-Damshety, Dr. Mohammed Tharwat, Dr. Hossam Elfeki and stuff members of surgical oncology department.

7. References

Alderman A.K., Wilkins E., Kim M. (2002). Complications in post-mastectomy breast reconstruction: two year results of the Michigan breast reconstruction outcome study. *Plast Reconstr Surg* Vol.109, pp. 2265–2274, ISSN 0032-1052 Online ISSN 1529-4242.

Allen R.J., Tucker C. (1995). Superior gluteal artery perforator free flap for breast reconstruction. *Plast Reconstr Surg* Vol.95, pp. 1207–1212, ISSN 0032-1052 Online ISSN 1529-4242.

Baildam AD. (2002). Oncoplastic surgery of the breast. *Br. J. Surg.* Vol.89, pp. 532–533, ISSN: 0007-1323, Online ISSN: 1365-2168.

Benediktsson KP, Perbeck L. (2008). Survival in breast cancer after nipple-sparing subcutaneous mastectomy and immediate reconstruction with implants: a prospective trial with 13 years median follow-up in 216 patients. *Eur J Surg Oncol.* Vol.34, No.2, pp. 143-148, ISSN 0748-7983.

Carlson GW, Moore B, Thornton JF, Elliott M, Bolitho G. (2001). Breast cancer after augmentation mammaplasty: treatment by skin-sparing mastectomy and immediate reconstruction. *Plast Reconstr Surg* Vol.107, No.3, pp. 687–692, ISSN 0032-1052 Online ISSN 1529-4242.

Chevray PM. (2004). Breast reconstruction with superficial inferior epigastric artery flaps: a prospective comparison with TRAM and DIEP flaps. *Plast Reconstr Surg*; Vol.114, pp. 1077–1083, ISSN: 0032-1052 Online ISSN 1529-4242.

Chevray P, Robb RL (2007). Breast Reconstruction. In: *M.D. Anderson Cancer Care Series: Breast Cancer (Second Edition)*, Hunt KK, Robb GL, Strom EA, Ueno NT, Robb GL., (Ed.), pp. 235-270, Springer, ISBN-13:978-0-387-34950-3 e-ISBN-13:978-0-387-34952-7, New York.

Chevray PM, Robb GL (2008). Breast Reconstruction. In: *Breast Reconstruction*, Kelly K. Hunt, pp. (2nd edn). New York, Springer 2008.

Chun YS, Verma K, Rosen H, Lipsitz S, Morris D, Kenney P (2010). Implant-based breast reconstruction using acellular dermal matrix and the risk of postoperative complications. *Plast Reconstr Surg.* Vol.125, pp. 429–436, ISSN 0032-1052 Online ISSN 1529-4242.

Chung AP and Sacchini V (2008). Nipple-sparing mastectomy: Where are we now? *Surgical Oncology* Vol.17, pp. 261-266, ISSN 0960-7404.

Cunnick GH and Mokbel K. (2006). Oncological considerations of skin-sparing mastectomy; Review. *International Seminars in Surgical Oncology.* Vol.3, pp. 14, ISSN 1477-7800.

Crowe JP, Kim JA, Yetman R. (2004). Nipple-sparing mastectomy: technique and results of 54 procedures. *Arch Surg.* Vol.139, pp. 148–150, ISSN (printed): 0004-0010. ISSN (electronic): 0096-6908

Delgado JM, Martinez-Mendez JR, de Santiago J. (2007). Immediate breast reconstruction (IBR) with direct, anatomic, extra-projection prosthesis:102 cases. *Ann Plast Surg* Vol. 58, pp. 99-104, ISSN 0148-7043.

Denewer A (1997) Myomammary Flap of Pectoralis Major Muscle for Breast Reconstruction: New Technique. *World J. Surg.* Vol.21, pp. 57-61, ISSN 0364-2313 electronic ISSN 1432-2323.

Denewer A. & Farouk O. (2007). Can Nipple-sparing Mastectomy and Immediate Breast Reconstruction with Modified Extended Latissimus Dorsi Muscular Flap Improve the Cosmetic and Functional Outcome among Patients with Breast Carcinoma? *World J Surg* Vol.31, pp. 1169–1177, ISSN 0364-2313 electronic ISSN 1432-2323.

Denewer A., Setit A. and Farouk O. (2007). Outcome of Pectoralis Major Myomammary Flap for Post-mastectomy Breast Reconstruction: Extended Experience. *World J Surg.* Vol.31, pp. 1382–1386, ISSN 0364-2313 electronic ISSN 1432-2323.

Denewer A., Setit A., Hussein O., Farouk O. (2008). Skin-Sparing Mastectomy with Immediate Breast Reconstruction by a New Modification of Extended Latissimus Dorsi Myocutaneous Flap. *World J Surg*. Vol.32, pp. 2586–2592, ISSN 0364-2313 electronic ISSN 1432-2323.

Dnewer A, Hussein O, Farouk O, Elnahas W, Khater A and El-Saed A (2010). Cost-effectiveness of clinical breast assessment-based screening in rural Egypt. *World J. Surg*. Vol. 34, No.9, (September 2010), pp. 2204-2210, ISSN 0364-2313 electronic ISSN 1432-2323.

Denewer A., Farouk O., Mostafa W. and Elshamy K. (2011). Social support and hope among Egyptian women with breast cancer after mastectomy: *breast cancer; basic and clinical research* Vol.5, pp. 93 - 103, ISSN: 1178-2234

Elliot L.F., Beegle P.H., Hartrampf C.R. (1990). The lateral transverse thigh free flap: an alternative for autogenous-tissue breast reconstruction. *Plast Reconstr Surg* Vol.85, pp. 169–178, ISSN: 0032-1052 Online ISSN 1529-4242

Hartrampf C.R. (1988). The transverse abdominal island flap for breast reconstruction. A 7-year experience. *Clin Plast Surg*. Vol.15, No.4, pp. 703, ISSN 0094-1298.

Hidalgo DA, Borgen PJ, Petrek JA, Heerdt AH, Cody HS, and Disa JJ (1998). Immediate reconstruction after complete skin sparing mastectomy with autologous tissue. *J Am Coll Surg*; Vol.187, pp. 17-21, ISSN 1072-7515.

Ho CM, Mak CK, Lau Y, Cheung WY, Chan MC, and Hung WK. (2003). Skin involvement in invasive breast carcinoma: safety of skin sparing mastectomy. *Ann Surg Oncol* Vol.10, pp.102-107, ISSN 0148-7043.

Hu E. and Alderman A.K. (2007). Breast reconstruction. In: *Surgical clinics of north America (87)*. Martin R.F. & Newman L.A., (Ed.), 453- 467, Elsevier Inc., ISBN 978-1-4160-5125-1, Michigan.

Khoo A., Kroll S.S., Reece G.P. (1998). A comparison of resource costs of immediate and delayed breast reconstruction. *Plast Reconstr Surg*. Vol.101, No.4, pp. 964–968, ISSN 0032-1052 Online ISSN 1529-4242.

Mathes SJ and Nahai F. Breast (Ed.), (1982). A systematic approach to flap selection. In: *clinical application for muscle and musclo-cutaneous flaps*, pp.285, Mosby co., ISBN 0801631645, St. Louis.

Meretoja TJ, von Smitten KA, Kuokkanen HO, Suominen SH, Jahkola TA. (2008). Complications of Skin-Sparing Mastectomy Followed by Immediate Breast Reconstruction. *Ann Plast Surg*, Vol.60, pp. 24–28, ISSN 0148-7043.

Nair A, Jaleel S, Abbott N, Buxton P, Matey P (2010). Skin Reducing Mastectomy With Immediate Implant Reconstruction as an Indispensable Tool in the Provision of Oncoplastic Breast Services. *Ann Surg Oncol* Vol.17, No.9, pp. 2480-2485, ISSN 0148-7043.

Petrek J A, and Disa J J (2005). Rehabilitation after Treatment for Cancer of the Breast; Part of "Chapter 33 - Cancer of the Breast" In: *Cancer: Principles & Practice of Oncology (7th edition)*. Devita VT, Hellman JS and Rosenberg SA, (Eds), pp. 1478- 1488, Lippincott Williams & Wilkins, ISBN 0-718-74450-4 .

Sacchini V, Pinotti JA, Barros AC. (2006). Nipple sparing mastectomies for breast cancer and risk reduction: oncological or technical problem? *J Am Coll Surg* Vol.203, pp. 704–714, ISSN 1072-7515 Online ISSN: 1365-2168.

Salgarello M & Farallo F. (2005). Immediate breast reconstruction with definitive anatomical implants after skin-sparing mastectomy. *Br J Plast Surg* Vol.58, pp. 216–222, ISSN 0007-1323.

Simmons RM, Brennan M, Christos P, King V, and Osborne M. (2002). Analysis of nipple/areolar involvement with mastectomy: can the areola be preserved? *Ann Surg Oncol* Vol.9, pp. 165–168, ISSN (printed): 1068-9265. ISSN (electronic): 1534-4681.

Sookhan N, Boughey JC, Walsh MF, Degnim AC (2008). Nipple-sparing mastectomy—initial experience at a tertiary center. *The American Journal of Surgery* Vol.196, pp.575–577, ISSN 0002-9610.

Tachi M. and Yamada A. Choice of flaps for breast reconstruction (2005). *Int J Clin Oncol.* Vol.10, pp. 289–297, ISSN (printed): 1341-9625. ISSN (electronic): 1437-7772.

Wilson CR, Brown IM, Weiller-Mithoff E. (2004). Immediate breast reconstruction does not lead to a delay in the delivery of adjuvant chemotherapy. *Eur J Surg Oncol* Vol. 30, No.6, pp.624–627, ISSN: 0748-7983; Electronic ISSN: 1532-2157.

Breast Reconstruction with DIEP and S/IGAP

Maria M. LoTempio, Grace Lucta Gerald and Robert J. Allen
Medical University of South Carolina, USA

1. Introduction

Breast reconstruction is an essential component in the treatment of breast cancer patients. It is being performed with increasingly sophisticated techniques to optimize the appearance and feel of the reconstructed breast and to decrease donor site morbidity. The use of autologous tissue allows the reconstruction of a breast which looks and feels more like a natural breast.

The abdomen is an ideal source of tissue for breast reconstruction. Most patients who develop breast cancer are at an age when they also have excess abdominal skin and fat. The fat is typically soft and easy for the surgeon to shape and closely approximate the look and feel of a native breast. In addition, an added bonus of an abdominal donor site for most patients is improved abdominal contour after flap harvest, with results similar to that of an abdominoplasty or "tummy tuck." However, women who have had abdominal surgeries in the past may not be candidates for abdominal free tissue transfer depending on the placement of the scar and the extent of their prior surgery.

Patient preference and body habitus play a role in determining the location from where autologous tissue is harvested. Some women do not like the long scar of the DIEP and prefer not to have surgery on their abdomen. Most women can be categorized into two main body shapes: pear and apple. The women who are apple shaped predominantly have fat in their abdomen whereas, women who are pear shaped have more fat in their thighs and buttock. The surgeon needs to take all of this into consideration before determining the appropriate donor site for a woman's breast reconstruction.

In this chapter we will review the deep inferior epigastric perforator flap (DIEP) and the superior/inferior gluteal artery perforator (S/IGAP) flap for breast reconstruction. We will also discuss the superior and inferior gluteal artery perforator flaps with the septocutaneous variations.

Our hope for the reader is to gain a knowledge base of the normal anatomy, the patient selection, surgical technique, post-operative management and potential complications one may encounter in pursuing this type of surgery. We will also include clinical examples.

2. DIEP

The deep inferior epigastric artery perforator (DIEP) flap is usually our first choice flap from the abdomen. It allows for the ease of transfer of skin and fat from the abdomen for the reconstruction of a new breast without the sacrifice of rectus muscle or fascia.

3. History

The modern era of autogenous breast reconstruction began with the TRAM flap, popularized by Carl Hartrampf. In 1982, he used the pedicle flap concept to transfer abdominal tissue to the chest for breast reconstruction using the superior epigastric artery and the rectus abdominus muscle as a carrier.[1] This flap came to be known as the transverse rectus abdominus myocutaneous, or TRAM, flap.

In 1973, the term "Free Flap"was used by Taylor and Daniel to describe the distant transfer of an island flap by microvascular anastomosis.[2,3] Two years later, they documented a detailed anatomical description of many of the more common free flap donor sites still in use today.[4]

The concept of donor site muscle sparing techniques were then embarked upon, as represented by Elliott with the split latissimus and by Feller with the partial rectus abdominus muscle transfer.[5,6] Koshima took this concept one step further and used the skin territory overlying the rectus abdominus muscle for reconstruction of head and neck defects.[7] The flaps were based on a single paraumbilical perforating vessel from the deep inferior epigastric artery.

The goal of muscle preservation became more apparent and in the early 1990's our group at Louisiana State University made the next significant advance in perforator flap breast reconstruction. By injecting fresh abdominoplasty specimens, it was determined that the skin and fat could be transferred without sacrifice of the rectus abdominus muscle. This led to the first DIEP flap for breast reconstruction by Allen in 1992.[8] The inception of free tissue transfer allowed an infinite range of possibilities to appropriately match donor and recipient sites.[9]

4. Indications

Most women who have had or will have mastectomies for breast cancer are possible candidates for a DIEP flap.[10] Absolute contraindications specific to abdominal perforator flap breast reconstruction in our practice include history of previous abdominoplasty, abdominal liposuction, or active smoking (within 1 month prior to surgery). A relative contraindication is previous large transverse or oblique abdominal incisions.

If the patient is undergoing radiation therapy we have them complete it six months prior to surgical breast reconstruction and if they are having chemotherapy we usually wait six weeks to obtain normal blood chemistries before proceeding to surgical breast reconstruction. This time allows radiation effects to stabilize and allows for the removal of damaged chest wall skin so that it can be replaced with soft, unirradiated abdominal skin and tissue.[11]

5. Anatomy

Like a TRAM flap, the DIEP flap is based on the deep inferior epigastric artery and vein. One, two, or three rows of perforating arteries and veins penetrate the rectus muscle on each side of the abdomen to provide the blood supply for the overlying skin and fat. The deep inferior epigastric artery is typically between 2 and 3 mm in diameter and the accompanying veins are between 2 and 3.5 mm in size.

In contrast to a TRAM flap, no rectus muscle or fascia must be sacrificed. Instead, the perforating vessels which supply the overlying skin and fat are dissected through the rectus muscle to their origins from the deep inferior epigastric vessels. The rectus muscle is spread apart in the direction of the muscle fibers during the dissection with minimal damage to the muscle. When nerves are encountered they are preserved to the best of our ability.

6. Surgical technique

All of our patients undergo a pre-operative CTA or MRA of the abdomen to determine the perforator vessels location, size, and intramuscular course. This study also allows us to differentiate between a musculocutaneous versus a septocutaneous variation of the DIEP and to assess the superficial inferior epigastric artery (SIEA) system. By knowing the specifics of the perforating vessels, the operating time is shortened by an hour.

The patient is usually seen in the office one day prior to surgery. The surgical plan is reviewed with the patient and any remaining questions are answered. Standard abdominoplasty markings are made in the sitting or standing position based around the selected perforator. The side of the abdomen contralateral to the side to be reconstructed is preferred, as this provides for easier insetting at the time of surgery. However, because a very long pedicle may be harvested, insetting typically is not a problem with either an ipsilateral or contralateral pedicle. Flaps are marked with their superior border just above the umbilicus and their inferior border approximately 12 cm below the umbilicus. The lateral flap markings extend approximately 22 to 24 cm from the midline. Then, with the patient in a supine position, a Doppler probe is used to audibly hear the main perforator selected by CTA/MRA. The superficial inferior epigastric artery and vein are likewise found with the Doppler probe and marked.

On the chest, the midline and the bilateral inframammary folds are marked. For patients undergoing immediate breast reconstruction, suggested skin markings for the surgical oncologist are drawn on the breast. If the patient is undergoing nipple-sparing procedures (usually BRCA patients), the incision mark is drawn from the inferior portion of the nipple straight down to the inframammary fold. In patients with cancer the lollypop incision marks are placed onto the breasts.

The operating room table is turned 180° to allow the surgeons to sit comfortably with legs under the table during the microvascular anastomosis. The morning of surgery, the patient receives 5000 units of heparin subcutaneously and sequential compression hose are placed prior to general anesthesia for deep vein thrombosis prophylaxis. Under general anesthesia, the patient is prepped and draped from the chin to the upper thighs. The ipsilateral arm may be prepped and included in the field if an immediate sentinel node biopsy or axillary node dissection is to be performed in addition to the mastectomy.

A two team approach is used with simultaneous raising of the flap and preparation of the recipient vessels. The internal mammary artery (IMA) and vein (IMV) are used in over 90% of our cases. The thoracodorsal vessels are our second choice and are used when the internal mammaries are not available.

We approach the IMA in the second or third intercostal space. Occasionally, a large perforating artery and vein from the internal mammary vessels may be found emanating from the second interspace and these vessels may be used as the recipients in the chest. The IMA and IMV are usually between 2.5 and 3 mm in size. Sometimes a second vein between 1.5 and 3 mm may be encountered. In the case of a narrow intercostal space a small portion of the rib cartilage above and below may be removed for better exposure and insetting of the pedicle.

When we perform a DIEP flap, the superior and inferior skin incisions are made and the superficial inferior epigastric vessels are first approached. If these are found to be of significant size and quality, they are followed down to their origin from the superficial femoral artery and an SIEA flap is performed instead. This avoids dissection of the fascia and any possible nerve injury. Often only the superficial inferior epigastric vein is present and this is dissected free for several centimeters. This can be used as a backup for the venous drainage of the flap if venous congestion is present after the anastomosis is performed in the chest. In our experience, this vein can prove invaluable in the rare case where congestion is present due to insufficient drainage through the deep system.

The abdominal skin island is carefully elevated from lateral to medial or medial to lateral based on the selected perforator from the CTA/MRA. When a large lateral perforator is selected, the flap may be based on this vessel. Additional perforators in the same row may also be dissected and included with the flap for additional perfusion. If no single dominant perforator is found two or even three smaller perforators in the same lateral or medial row may be taken to carry the flap, however this is all decided in most cases before the patient is in the operating room. In our experience, approximately 25% of flaps are based on one perforator, 50% on two perforators, and 25% on three or more perforators.[12]

Once the appropriate perforators are chosen, the anterior rectus sheath is opened around the perforators and the vessels are carefully dissected down through the rectus muscle to the deep inferior epigastric artery and vein. The muscle is spread apart in the direction of the fibers and care is taken to identify and preserve any intercostal nerves innervating the medial aspect of the muscle that might cross the pedicle. Dissection continues until the pedicle is of sufficient length, typically eight to ten cm long, and the vessels are of sufficient caliber to match the recipient vessels in the chest. It is often easier to dissect the two veins and artery free from one another before ligating them. We use methylene blue to mark the pedicle to prevent distortion and twisting when performing the anastomosis. High power loupe magnification and careful microsurgical technique are essential during this dissection.

Pure sensory nerves, which innervate the flap skin paddle, typically run with the perforators and may also be dissected free for anastomosis into divided recipient sensory nerves in the chest.

Once the recipient vessels are ready, the artery and then veins of the pedicle are ligated and the pedicle slid out from underneath any crossing intercostal nerves. The flap is then weighed and transferred to the anterior chest wall. Great care is taken to align the flap pedicle with that of the recipient vessels without any twists or kinks. While vascular problems occur rarely with these flaps, many of the venous difficulties that do occur result from a twist or a kink in the pedicle. Temporary stay sutures are placed in the flap and the operating microscope is brought into position.

Under magnification, the anterior surface of the recipient artery and vein are also labeled with a surgical marker and the larger vein is ligated distally. An anastomotic coupling device is typically used to connect the recipient and flap veins. A coupling device makes the anastomosis easier and faster and has the additional benefit of stenting the vein open after the vessels are joined. Typically, the arterial anastomosis is performed with a nylon 9-0 suture. In the case of a good size match between the flap and recipient arteries, a running suture is employed. Otherwise, interrupted 9-0 nylon sutures are usually used. After the anastomosis is complete the flap is checked for bleeding and capillary refill.

The abdominal fascia is closed and securely tied with interrupted 2-0 vicryls and a running size 0 PDS suture. Mesh or other synthetic materials are not required for the abdominal wall closure. The edges of the umbilicus are tacked down to the fascia with a 2-0 vicryl suture. The upper abdominal flap is elevated and the patient is flexed and the wound is closed in layers over two closed suction drains. Care is taken to approximate Scarpa's fascia with 2-0 interrupted vicryl sutures. As in an abdominoplasty, the umbilicus is brought out through the abdominal flap and secured in place.

The flap is typically inset with the narrower, more lateral portion of the flap placed up towards the axilla and the thicker, more medial aspect of the flap placed inferiorly and medially. The flap can be further medialized and kept from falling laterally into the axilla by suturing the superior, inferior medial, and lateral flap aspects to portions of the pectoralis major muscle. A minimal number of sutures should be considered for this as the sutures have a propensity to contribute to fat necrosis. The flap may also be folded over onto itself inferiorly to provide more natural looking inferior ptosis and fullness for the reconstructed breast. The insetting and closure are performed over a suction drain and great care is used to monitor the integrity of the pedicle at all times during the insetting. Excess skin is de-epithelialized and the flap is inset with a visible skin paddle left in place. The skin paddle allows easier postoperative monitoring for signs of venous congestion and provides tissue for the construction of a nipple at this time or at a later second stage revision.

6.1 Post-operative care

Postoperatively, the patient is observed in the recovery room for a few hours and then transferred to their private room where they will remain for the duration of their hospitalization. Postoperative pain is significantly less with the DIEP flap than with a TRAM flap reconstruction and so it is managed with oral pain medications beginning on postoperative day 1.[13] The patient's urinary catheter, IV, BP cuff, and oxygen are discontinued on day 1 and the patient begins to ambulate. She is discharged home on postoperative day 3 or 4 depending on her recovery.

A second stage revision and nipple creation are performed in the operating room between 8 and 12 weeks after the initial surgery to further refine and finish the appearance of the breast. We often use fat grafting to fill in any defects and to increase the volume of a flap if it initially falls short in volume. Any revisions at the donor site, such as dog-ear removal or liposuction, are also performed at this time.

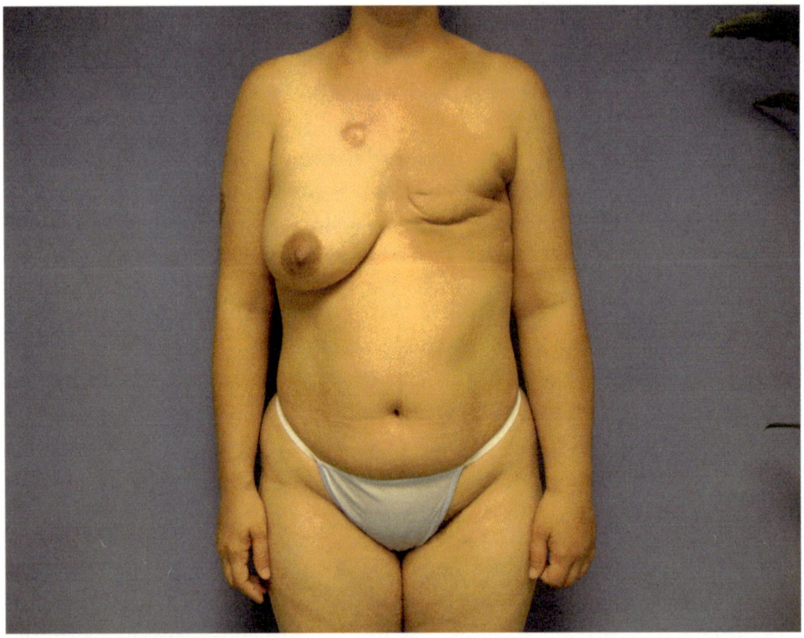

Fig. 1a. 38 year old female with a history of left breast cancer, s/p left mastectomy.

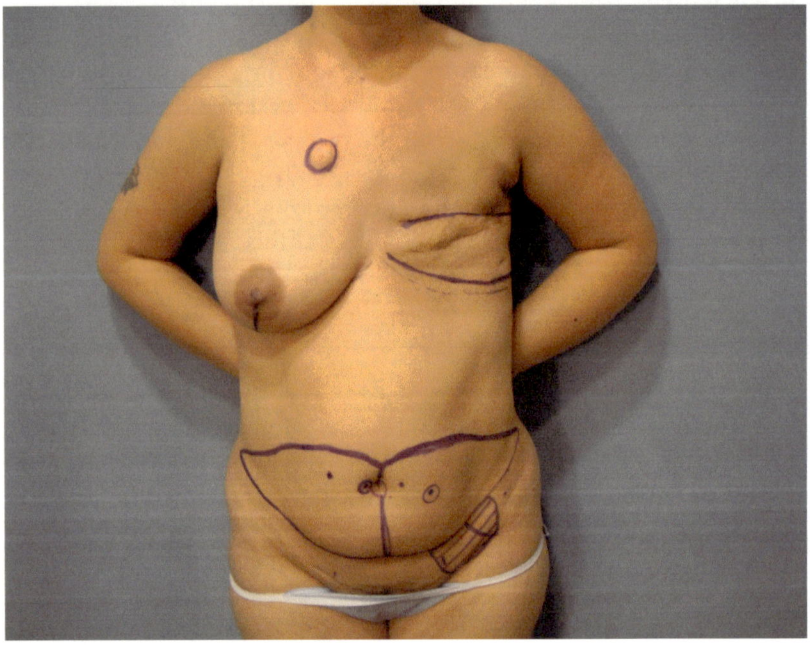

Fig. 1b. Pre-operative markings for the Bilateral DIEP with vascularized lymph node transfer. The right breast will undergo a nipple sparing mastectomy with DIEP, the left breast will have a DIEP with lymph nodes harvested from the groin and placed into the axilla for left arm lymphedema. The marks on the abdomen circled, are the perforators chosen for surgery.

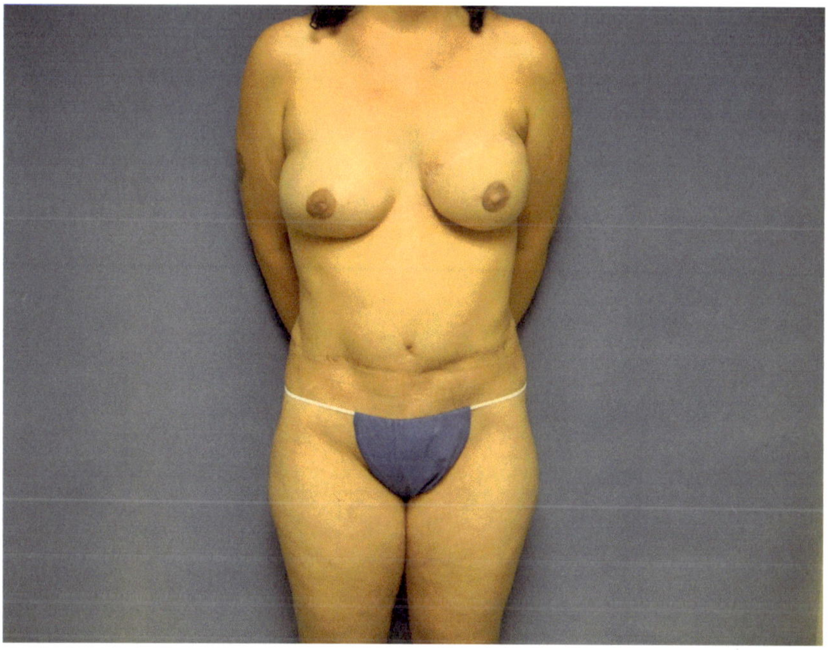

Fig. 1c. Ten months post-operative.

6.2 Complications

Complications are infrequent. In a 10-year retrospective review of 758 DIEP flaps by our unit, 6% of patients returned to the operating room for flap related problems. Partial flap loss occurred in 2.5% while total flap loss occurred in less than 1% of all cases. Problems with the vein or venous anastomosis were almost 8 times more likely than problems with the artery or arterial anastomosis. Fat necrosis appeared in 13% of flaps. Seroma formation at the abdominal donor site occurred in approximately 5% of cases and abdominal hernia occurred in 0.7% of cases.[12]

7. Pearls

Pre-operative CT/MRA and reviewing with the radiologist the location of the perforator on an X/Y axis will decrease intra-operative time by at least an hour. Things to note are the intramuscular course, the type of branching pattern of the deep inferior epigastric artery, and where the perforator enters the main branch. Even though one large perforator is all that is needed to carry the vascular supply of the flap, a back up is necessary when choosing the perforators. The SIEA system is important because often when the deep inferior epigrastric perforators are small, less than 2 mm, the dominant supply to the flap is the SIEA system. Have the radiologist give you the coordinates and size of these vessels.

When beginning the dissection, beveling above the incision line is necessary in the thin person to obtain appropriate volume. Avoid midline beveling since this will decrease the vascularity of this region and when the abdomen is closed the tension can lead to an open wound.

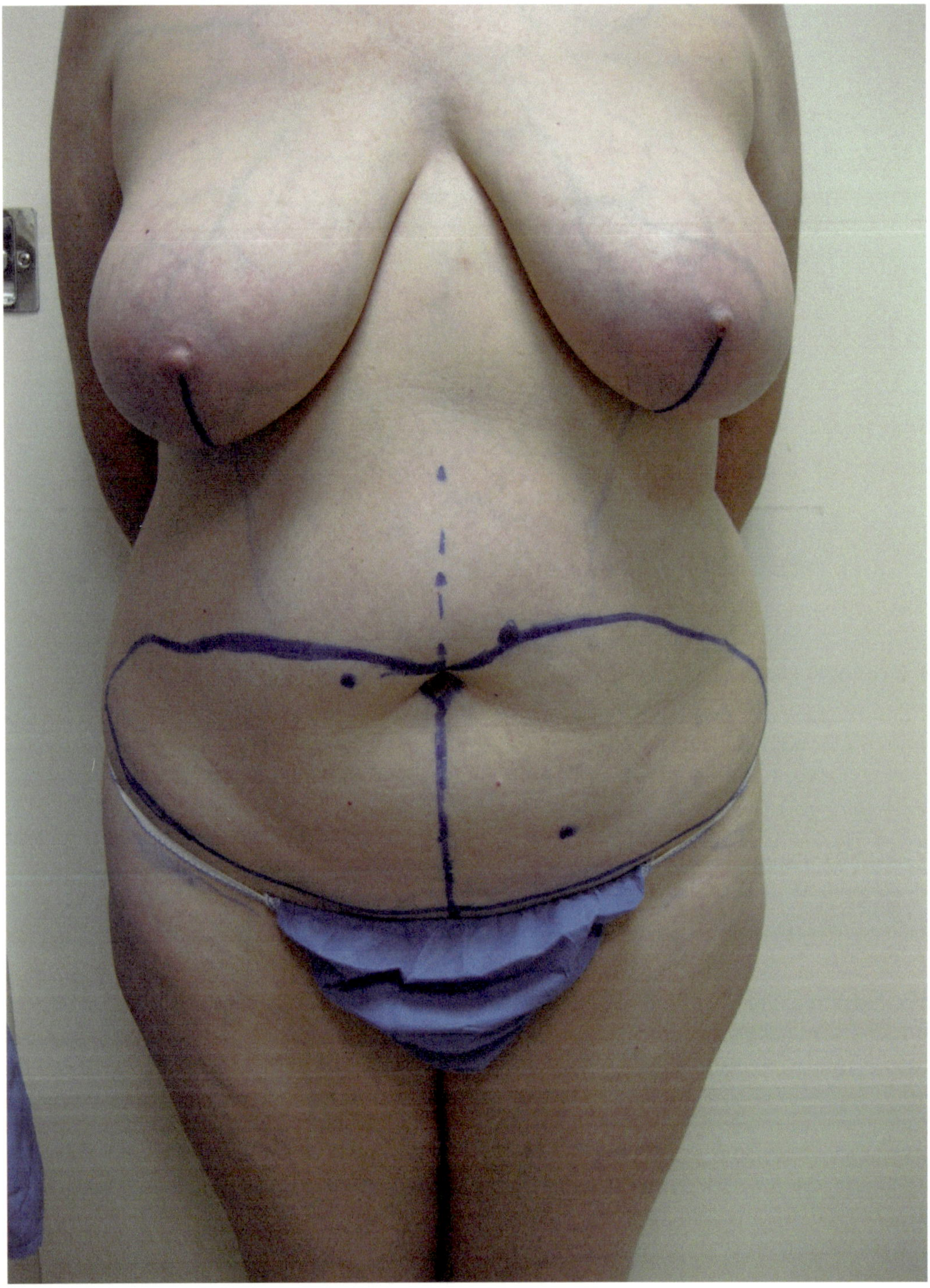

Fig. 2a. 55 year old woman, undergoing bilateral nipple sparing mastectomies with immediate reconstruction with B DIEP.

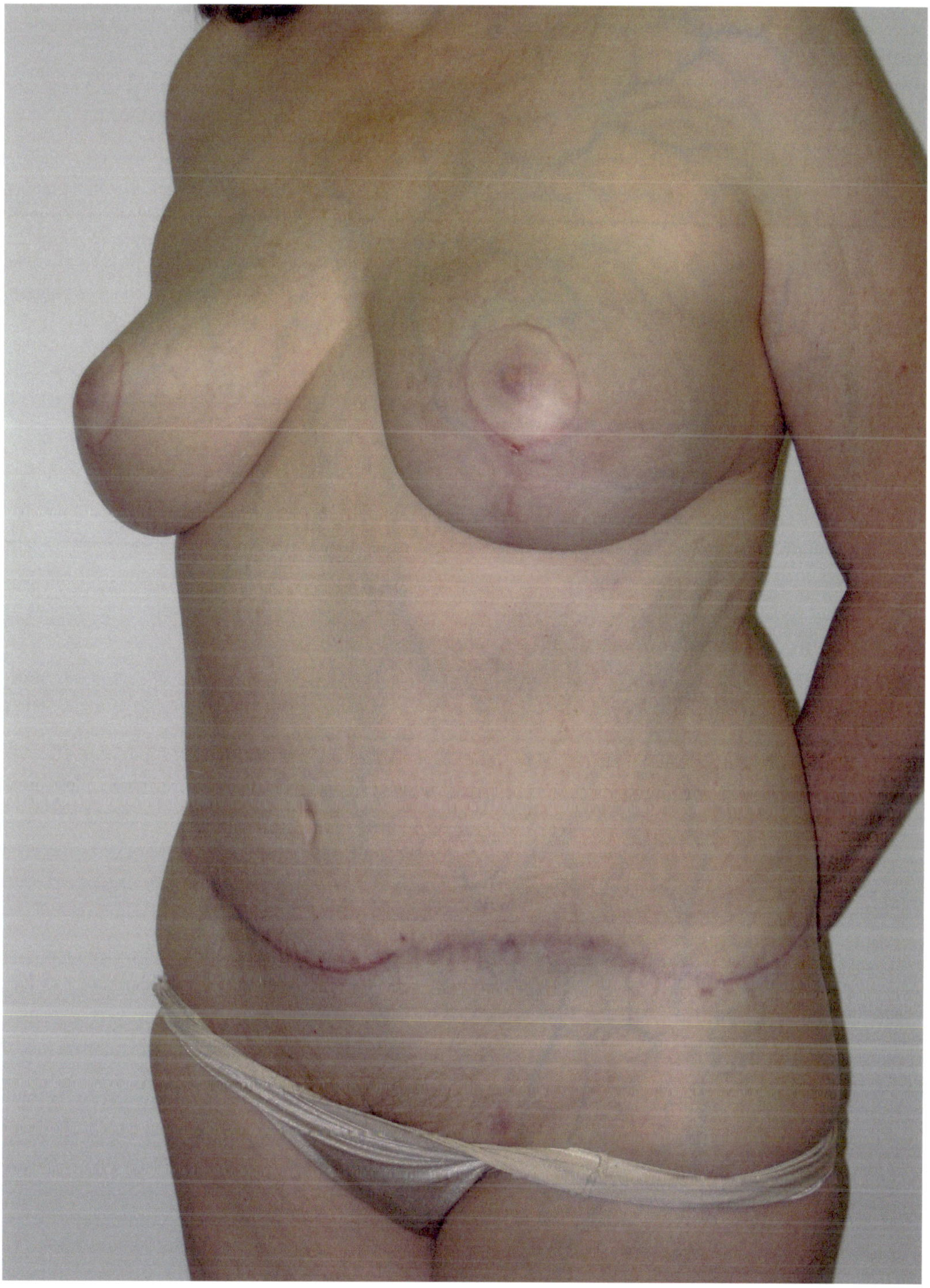

Fig. 2b. Post-operative B DIEP-2 months.

Find the medial vein immediately when dissecting the lower limits of your dissection. This is your lifeboat if the flap is congested. A length of 6 cm is usually adequate. The perforator can be approached either medially or laterally. If done medially the lateral row can be preserved and may be evaluated later if a problem arises. Often the surgeon should already know the anatomy based on the CT/MRA, however inspection is the final course.

Once the perforator is identified, use only Westcott or similar scissors when dissecting through the fascia because using the bipolar may transmit heat and injure the small vessels. This is the most critical part of the dissection, go slow!

Once through the fascia, the bipolar can be used for ligations of small vessels but be careful not to tug on the vessels, just cauterize them and then ligate them with microscissors. Ligature clips should be used for medium or large vessels.

Always be gentle when holding the vessel; try not to manipulate the vessel directly but rather grab surrounding adventitia if possible. If your vessel goes into spasm use papervine and wait a few minutes before proceeding.

Always use the Doppler to check the vessel patency; this will help you localize the problem if you think you are in trouble.

If you encounter bleeding on the perforator, apply pressure with a moist gauze pad. Using the bipolar will transmit heat and damage the vessel.

Once in the main vessel, dissect for a total of 6 cm to give yourself enough room to position the flap on the chest wall for the anastomosis. Often times, it is easier to skeletonize the two veins and artery in-situ. The lateral vein should be clipped and the artery and medial vein on the flap side should be open after ligating the pedicle. Mark the artery and vein with methylene blue. Often times after transfer the pedicle will rotate.

When ligating the IMV, mark with methylene blue to avoid twisting when placing it into the coupler. Have the blue mark anterior to make sure alignment matches.

After the anastomosis, when placing the flap into the pocket, make sure the pocket is not too tight and check to see that the pedicle is lying in a comfortable position. Some of the pectoralis may need to be scored.

When securing the flap into the pocket, make sure the defect created by removing the rib and dissecting the vessels is completely covered by the flap. This contour deficiency post-operatively is difficult to rectify and the patient will comment on it.

Use minimal sutures to secure the flap because this can cause fat necrosis and become apparent to the patient later on.

7.1 S/IGAP history

In 1975, Fujino described the superior gluteal myocutaneous flap for breast reconstruction. The myocutaneous superior gluteal artery free flap for breast reconstruction was popularized by Dr. Bill Shaw.[14-18] The main limitation of this flap is the short vascular pedicle, which frequently requires vein grafting, increasing the difficulty, complications, and the time required for this technique. Le Quang performed the first breast reconstruction with an inferior gluteal myocutaneous flap in 1978.[19]

The superior and inferior gluteal artery perforator flaps for breast reconstruction were described by our group in 1993.[20] Advantages of the gluteal artery perforator flaps versus the previous myocutaneous gluteal flaps include preservation of the gluteus maximus muscle and additional length of the pedicle, negating the use of vein grafts. Bilateral simultaneous S/IGAPS are often done by our group but require two skilled microsurgeons in order to minimize operating time and ischemia time for the flaps.[21,22] Pre-operative CT/MRI angiograms allow identification of the septocutaneous variants of the S/IGAPS for breast reconstruction.[23,24] The angiograms identify the key perforators as being musculocutaneous or septocutaneous as well as their caliber, location, and course, allowing pre-operative mapping. As with other perforator flaps, donor site morbidity is minimal and no sacrifice of muscle is required. Overall the SGAP is slightly more popular than the IGAP, but the upper buttock donor site may have a scooped out appearance. When a patient has a saddlebag deformity, the IGAP is a good choice because of an improved donor site contour and a hidden scar, which lays in the crease.[20,25,26] These techniques can be difficult and complicated.

7.2 Patient selection

Some patients have more skin and fat in the gluteal region than the abdominal area. In this subset of patients, a gluteal artery perforator (GAP) flap may be used as a first choice for breast reconstruction.

Most women who have undergone or will undergo mastectomies and wish to be reconstructed with autologous tissue are potential candidates for SGAP/IGAP flaps. If the abdomen cannot be used as a donor site either due to previous abdominoplasty, liposuction, or the presence of multiple surgical scars, then the buttock should be considered. Also patients with excess tissue in the buttock versus the abdomen are ideal candidates. In general the buttock has a high fat to skin ratio, whereas the abdomen has a high skin to fat ratio. Patients who require mostly fat and little skin may be candidates for SGAP/IGAPS flaps. A significant amount of tissue may be harvested and, in our series, the average final inset weights of our GAP flaps were slightly greater than the weights of the mastectomy specimens removed.

Absolute contraindications specific to SGAP/IGAP flap breast reconstruction include previous liposuction at the donor site or active smoking within 1 month prior to surgery. Liposuction of the upper buttock is rare and so it doesn't often affect harvesting of the SGAP, but liposuction of the saddlebag area can affect the IGAP flap volume and circulation.

7.3 Anatomy

The superior gluteal artery is a continuation of the posterior division of the internal iliac artery. The artery has a limited length, which runs dorsally between the lumbosacral trunk and the first sacral nerve. It exits from the pelvis above the upper border of the piriformis muscle, where it quickly divides into both a superficial and deep branch. The deep branch travels between the iliac bone and gluteus medius muscle. The superficial branch continues to give off contributions to the upper portion of the gluteus muscle and overlying fat and skin. Anatomic location is planned when the femur is slightly flexed and rotated inward; a line is drawn from the posterior superior iliac spine to the posterior superior angle of the greater trochanter. The point of entrance of the superior gluteal artery from the upper part of the greater sciatic foramen corresponds to the junction of the upper and middle thirds of this line. Perforating vessels are found off of the superior branch of the superior gluteal artery.[27,28] Pre-operatively CTA or MRA has greatly impacted planning of this procedure.

The inferior gluteal artery is a terminal branch of the anterior division of the internal iliac artery and exits the pelvis through the greater sciatic foramen.[29,30] A line is drawn from the posterior superior iliac spine to the outer part of the ischial tuberosity; the junction of its lower with its middle third marks the point of emergence of the inferior gluteal and its surrounding vessels from the lower part of the greater sciatic foramen. The artery accompanies the greater sciatic nerve, internal pudendal vessels, and the posterior femoral cutaneous nerve. In this sub-fascial recess, the inferior gluteal vein will receive tributaries from other pelvic veins. The inferior gluteal vasculature continues towards the surface by perforating the sacral fascia. It exits the pelvis caudal to the piriformis muscle. Once under the inferior portion of the gluteus maximus, perforating vessels are seen branching out through the substance of the muscle to feed the overlying skin and fat. The course of the inferior gluteal artery perforating vessels are more oblique through the gluteus maximus muscle than the course of the superior gluteal artery perforators, which tend to travel more directly to the superficial tissue up through the muscle. Thus, the length of the inferior gluteal artery perforator and the resultant pedicle length for the IGAP flap is 7-10cm while the SGAP pedicle is 5-8 cm in length. Because the skin island is placed inferior to the origin of the inferior gluteal vessels, a longer pedicle is usually obtained.

The direction of the perforating vessels can be superior, lateral, or inferior. Perforating vessels that nourish the medial and inferior portions of the buttock have relatively short intramuscular lengths, between 5 to 7 centimeters, depending on the thickness of the muscle. Perforators, which nourish the lateral portions of the overlying skin paddle, are observed traveling through the muscle substance in an oblique manner 4 to 6 centimeters before turning upwards towards the skin surface. By traveling through the muscle for relatively long distances, these vessels are longer than their medially based counterparts. The perforating vessels can be separated from the underlying gluteus maximus muscle and fascia and traced down to the parent vessel, forming the basis for the inferior gluteal artery perforator flap. Between 2 to 4 perforating vessels originating from the inferior gluteal artery will be located in the lower half of the gluteus maximus.[24]

After giving off perforators in the buttocks, the inferior gluteal artery descends into the thigh accompanied by the posterior femoral cutaneous nerve and follows a long course, eventually surfacing to supply the skin of the posterior thigh.[26] The branches of the inferior gluteal nerve (L5, S1-2) supply the skin of the inferior buttock. A neurosensory flap can be elevated if these nerves are preserved in the dissection of the flap.[31,32]

The superior gluteal nerve arises from the dorsal divisions of the fourth and fifth lumbar and first sacral nerves. It exits the pelvis through the greater sciatic foramen above the piriformis muscle, accompanied by the superior gluteal vessels, and divides into both superior and inferior branches. The superior and inferior branches of the nerves travel with their corresponding arterial branches to end up in the gluteus medius, gluteus minimus, and tensor fasciae lata, respectively.

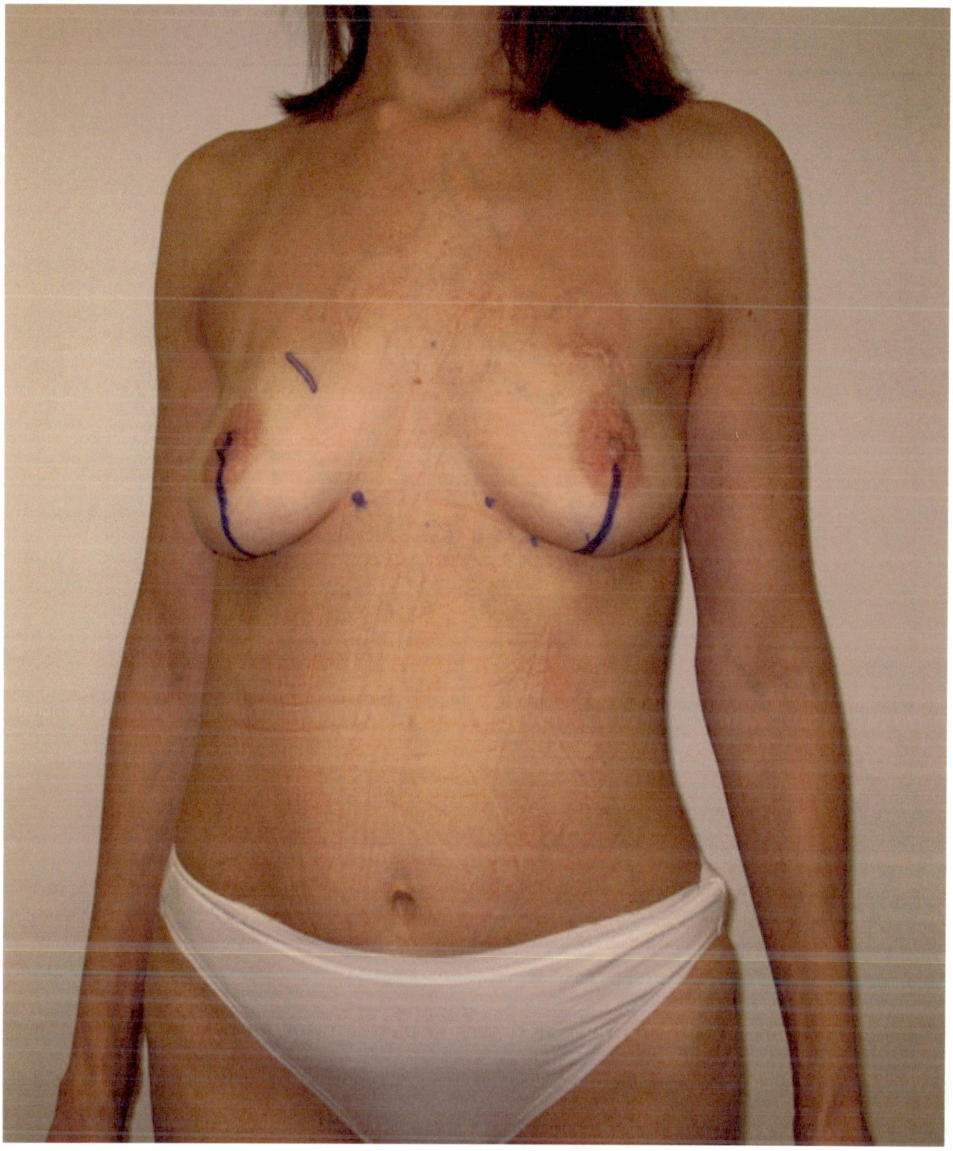

Fig. 3a. 45 year old women with BRCA positive gene. Pre-operative markings for nipple sparing mastectomies.

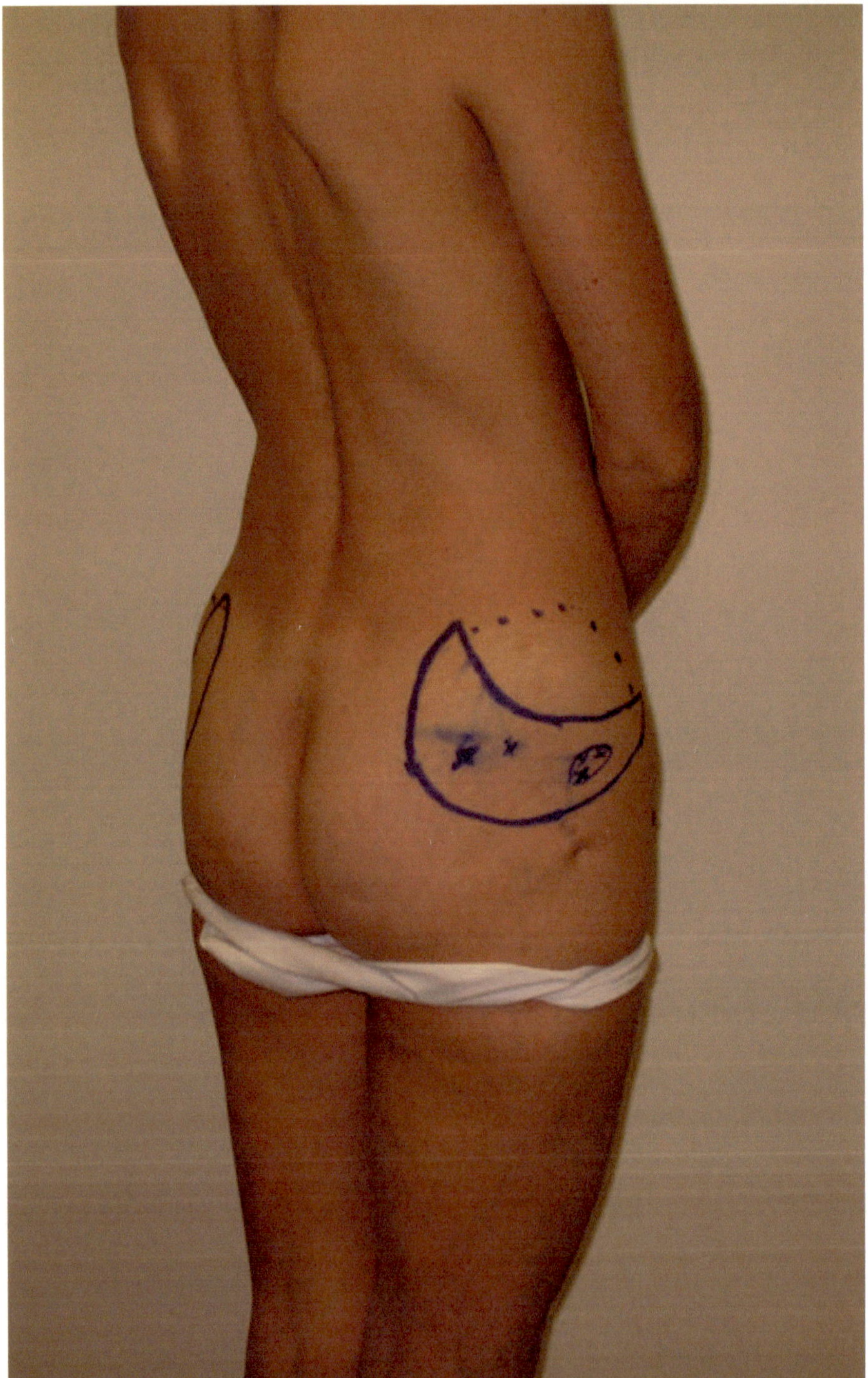

Fig. 3b. Pre-operative marking for the SGAP-crescent pattern. The perforator chosen is marked with the large X.

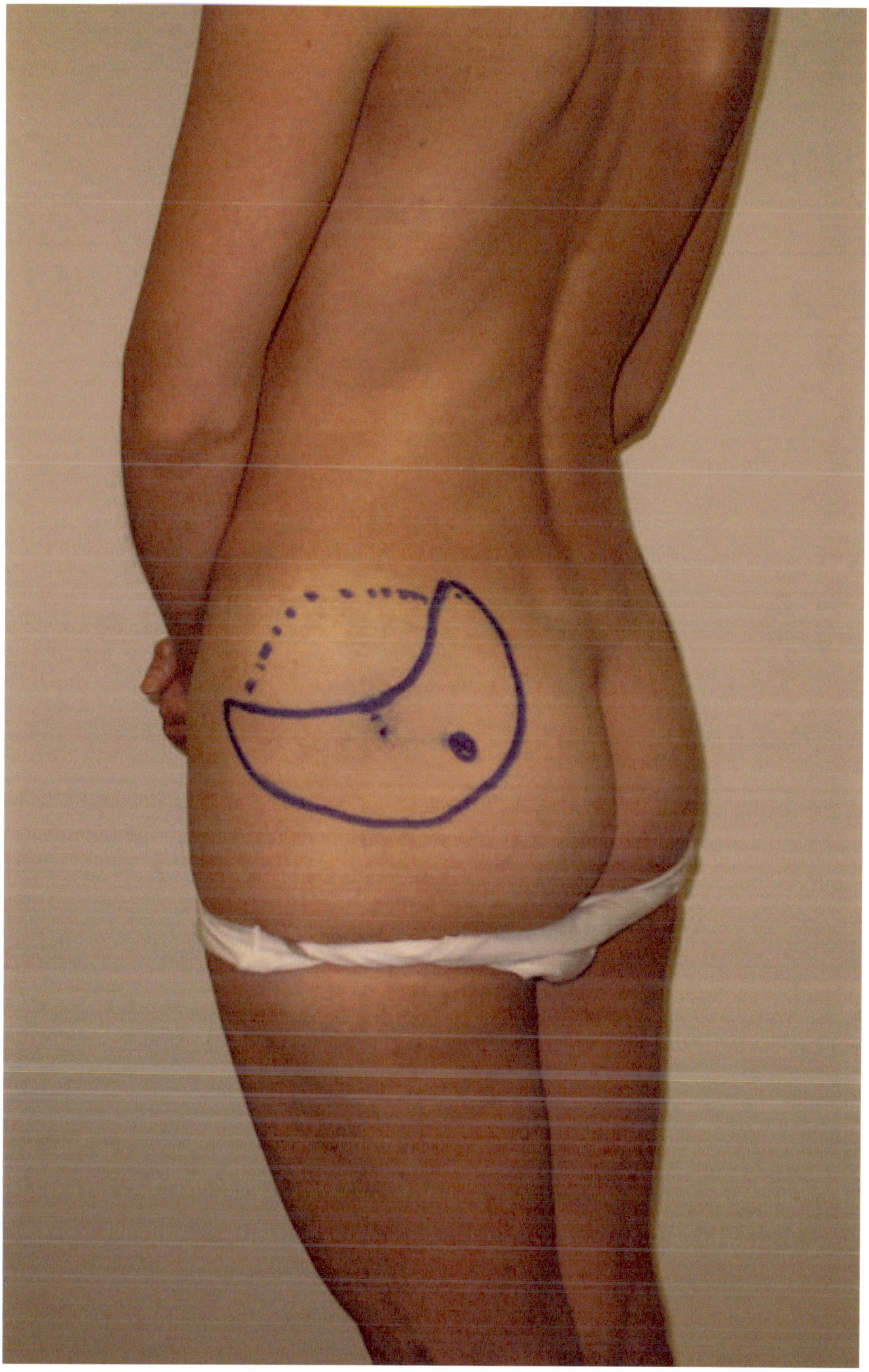

Fig. 3c. Pre-operative marking for the SGAP- crescent pattern.

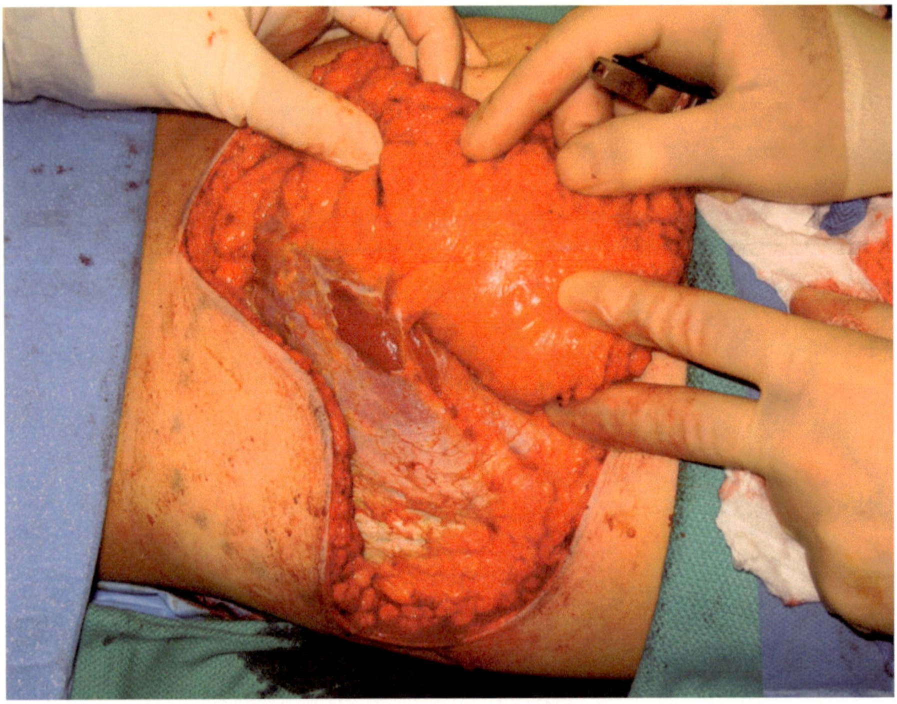

Fig. 3d. Intra-operative dissection showing the perforator.

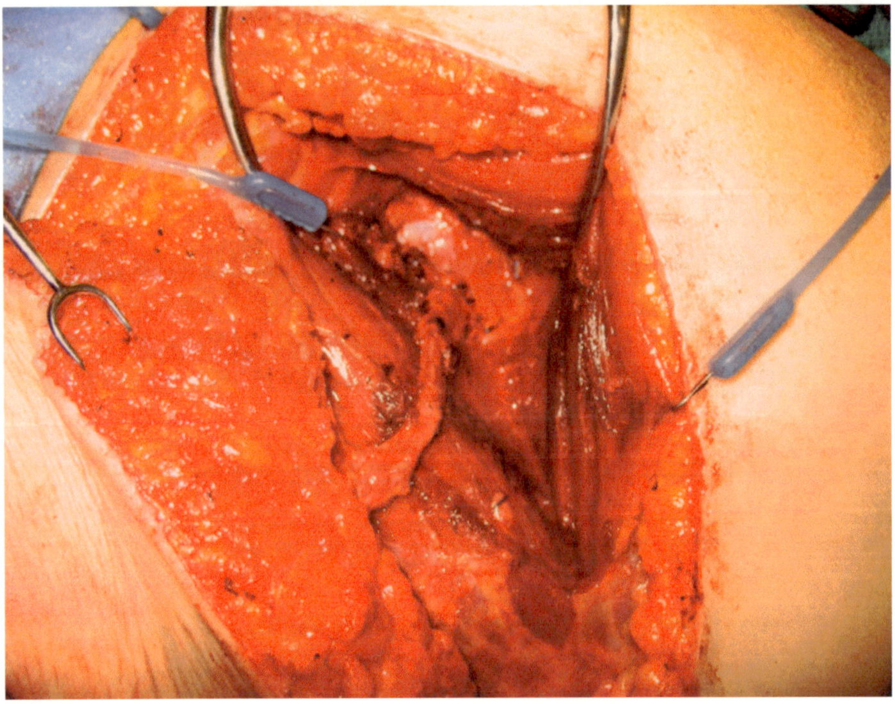

Fig. 3e. Intra-operative dissection showing the perforator leading into the main pedicle.

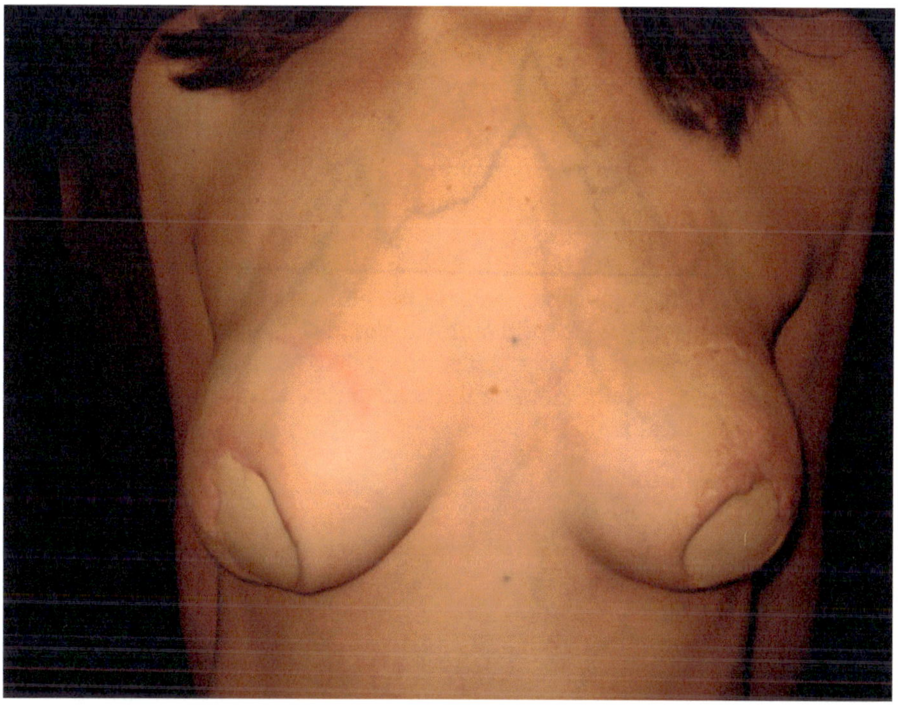

Fig. 3f. Three months post-operative photo before the nipple/areola reconstruction.

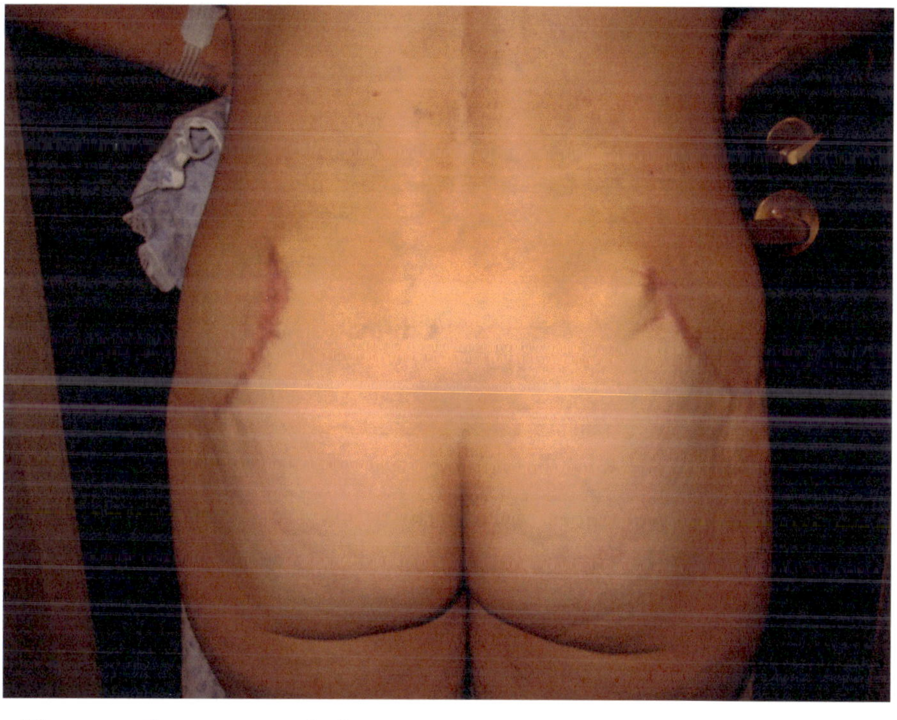

Fig. 3g. Three months post-operatively.

The inferior gluteal nerve arises from the dorsal divisions of the fifth lumbar and first and second sacral nerves. It exits the pelvis through the greater sciatic foramen, below the piriformis muscle, and divides into branches that enter the deep surface of the gluteus maximus.

The posterior femoral cutaneous nerve innervates the skin of the perineum and posterior surface of the thigh and leg. It arises partly from the dorsal divisions of the first and second, and from the ventral divisions of the second and third sacral nerves, and issues from the pelvis through the greater sciatic foramen below the piriformis muscle, along with the inferior gluteal artery. It then descends beneath the gluteus maximus and the fascia lata to travel over the long head of the biceps femoris to the posterior knee. Finally, it pierces the deep fascia and accompanies the lesser saphenous vein to the middle of the posterior leg. Some terminal branches communicate with the sural nerve. All of its branches are cutaneous and distributed to the gluteal region, the perineum, and the posterior thigh and leg.

7.4 Surgical technique

The chest is marked in a sitting position. The midline and the inframammary crease on both sides are marked to be at the same level. If a patient is undergoing immediate breast reconstruction, skin markings are drawn on the breast, which include marks for the mastectomy as well as marking of the inframammary fold. In patients who are undergoing a nipple-sparring mastectomy vertical, lateral, or an inframammary incision is marked.

For unilateral SGAP flap markings, the patient is placed in a lateral decubitus position. Pre-operative CT or MR angiography along with the hand held Doppler probe are used to locate perforating vessels from the superior gluteal artery. These are usually located approximately one third of the distance on a line from the posterior superior iliac crest to the greater trochanter. Additional perforators may be found slightly more lateral from above. It should be noted that more laterally located perforators produce longer pedicles thus allowing for easier anastomosis. Septocutaneous perforators are the most lateral and course between the gluteal maximus and medius. The skin paddle is marked in an oblique pattern from inferior medial to superior lateral that includes these perforators. On average, the flap height and length is 7-10 cm and 18-24 cm, respectively. For bilateral SGAP planning, the patient is marked in the prone position.

For the IGAP flap, the gluteal fold is noted with the patient in a standing position. The inferior limit of the flap is marked 1 cm inferior and parallel to the gluteal fold. CT or MRA and the hand held Doppler probe are used to locate perforating vessels from the inferior gluteal artery. An ellipse is drawn for the skin paddle to include these perforators, which roughly parallels the gluteal fold with dimensions of approximately 7 x 18 cm. To include the "saddle bag" deformity, the skin pattern is shifted more laterally. This prevents harvesting of the fat pad over the ischial tuberosity just medial to the gluteus maximus muscle in order to prevent discomfort with sitting.

For unilateral procedures the patient is placed in the lateral decubitus position and a two-team approach is used. The recipient vessels are prepared, while the SGAP/IGAP flap is harvested. For breast reconstruction, the internal mammary vessels or internal mammary perforators are preferred for anastomosis to the superior or inferior gluteal vessels allowing easier medialization of the flap when it is inset. Often we need to remove some rib cartilage in order to gain length necessary to perform the anastomosis. The IGAP flap often has a long enough pedicle to reach the thoracodorsal vessels, however the SGAP may be challenging due to a shorter pedicle length. For bilateral simultaneous GAP flap reconstruction the procedure is started supine. After mastectomy and recipient vessel preparation the patient is repositioned prone for flap harvest. Then the patient is returned to the supine position for anastomosis and insetting.

The skin incisions are made and dissection down to the gluteus maximus is performed circumferentially. Beveling is performed as needed, particularly lateral to the muscle in the superior and inferior direction to harvest enough tissue for width and volume to create a natural breast shape. The flap is elevated from the muscle in the subfascial plane and the perforators approached beginning from lateral to medial or medial to lateral. It is preferred to use a single large perforator, if present, but two perforators in the same plane and direction of the gluteus maximus muscle fibers can be taken together as well. The muscle is then spread in the direction of the muscle fibers and the perforators are followed through the muscle. The dissection continues until both the artery and the vein are of sufficient size to be anastomosed to the recipient vessels in the chest. Usually, the artery is the limiting factor in this dissection. The arterial perforator is visualized and preserved as it enters the main ascending superior gluteal artery or the descending inferior gluteal artery. The preferable artery and vein diameter for anastomosis is 2.0-2.5 mm and 3.0-4.0 mm, respectively. When using the internal mammary vein (IMV) perforators as recipients a shorter pedicle and smaller artery will suffice thereby simplifying flap harvest.

When the recipient vessels are ready, the gluteal artery and vein are divided and the flap is weighed. The skin and fat overlying the gluteus maximus muscle and posterior thigh with the IGAP are elevated superiorly and inferiorly to allow layered approximation of the fat of the donor site to prevent a contour deformity. The donor site is closed in several layers over a suction drain. Adding permanent removable skin sutures increases the strength of the skin closure.

The anastomosis is performed to the recipient vessels under the operating microscope. The flap is inset over a suction drain into the breast pocket with care taken not to twist or kink the pedicle. To create a spherical flap the ends of the ellipse are excised or approximated. The flap may be inset horizontally, vertically, or obliquely depending on the situation.

7.5 Postoperative care

Our patients have a one to two hour stay in the recovery room and then are transferred to their private room with monitoring of the flap circulation every two hours through the night and then every four hours starting on post-operative day one. The ICU is not necessarily needed although in institutions where experienced nursing staff is not available, it may be considered. Patients typically go home on the third or fourth postoperative day. The donor site drain usually remains for a minimum of ten days and is then removed once it is draining less than 40 cc in a twenty-four hour period. Breast drains are usually removed on post-operative day three.

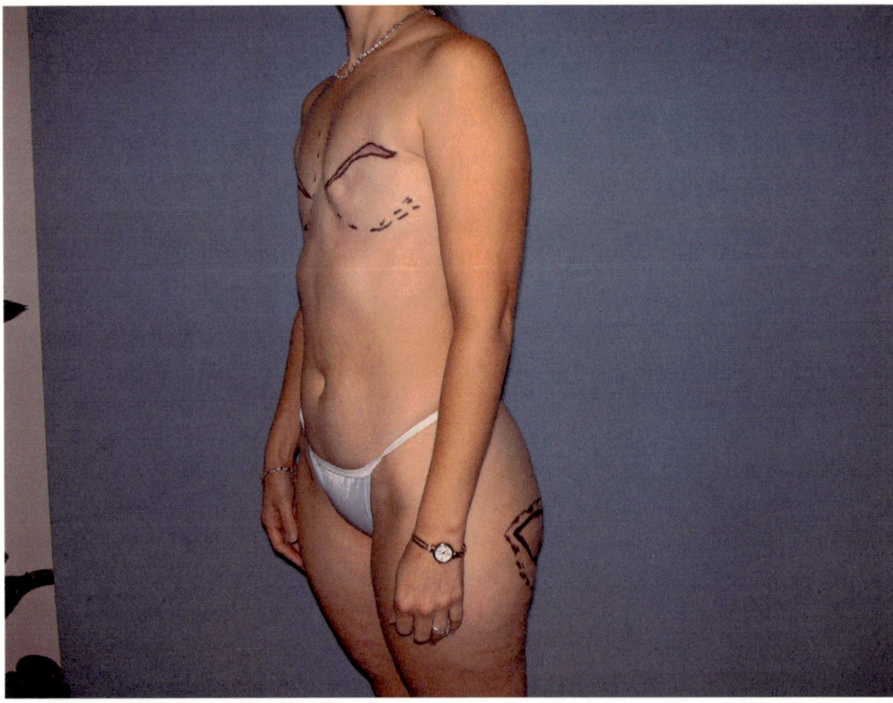

Fig. 4a. Pre-op IGAP markings

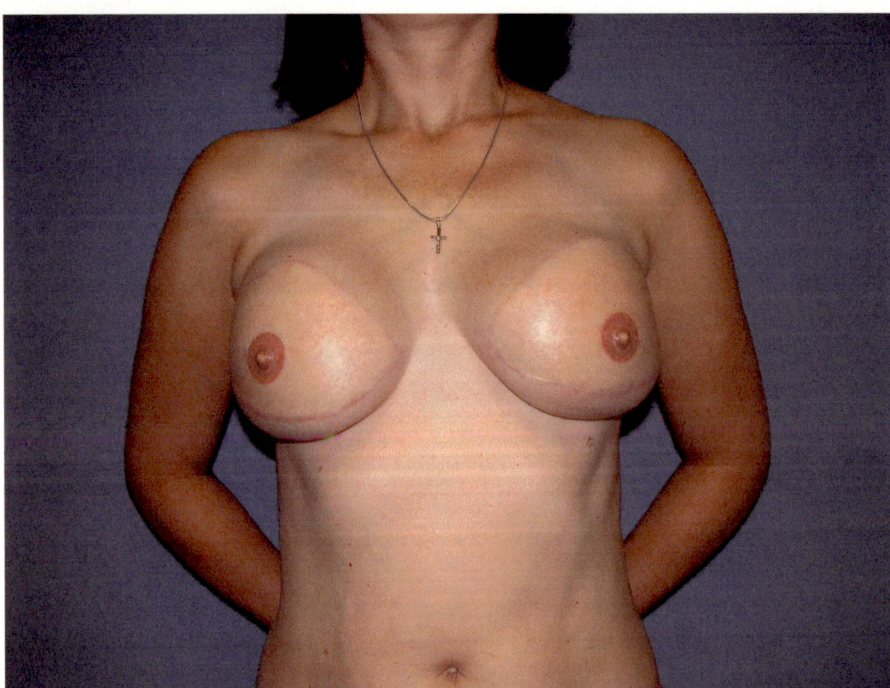

Fig. 4b. Ten months post-operatively from B IGAPS.

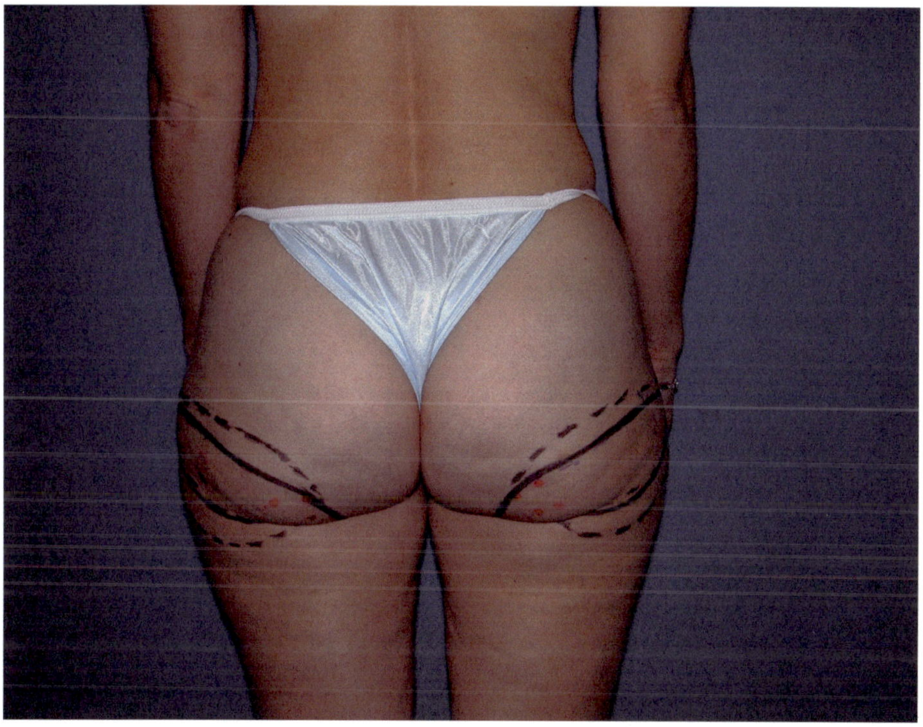

Fig. 4c. IGAP pre-op markings.

7.6 Complications

In a review of 492 GAP flaps performed by our unit for breast reconstruction, the incidence of complications was low. The overall take-back rate for vascular complications was 6%. More commonly there was a venous problem, accounting for 4% with arterial issues only occurring 2% of the time. The total flap failure rate was approximately 2%. Donor site seromas requiring aspiration occurred in 15% of patients. Approximately 20% of patients required revision of the donor site at the second stage of breast reconstruction.[19,21]

The most common reason for donor site revision in a SGAP patient is contour deformity of the upper buttock. The most common revision for the donor site in an IGAP patient is contouring of the lateral trochanteric fat with liposuction. Dog-ear revisions are often done at the time of second stage breast reconstruction in both S/IGAP patients. Recipient site complications include a fat necrosis rate of 8% in both S/IGAP flaps requiring revision. Breast flap contour asymmetry requires fat grafting or revision in approximately 10% of our cases.

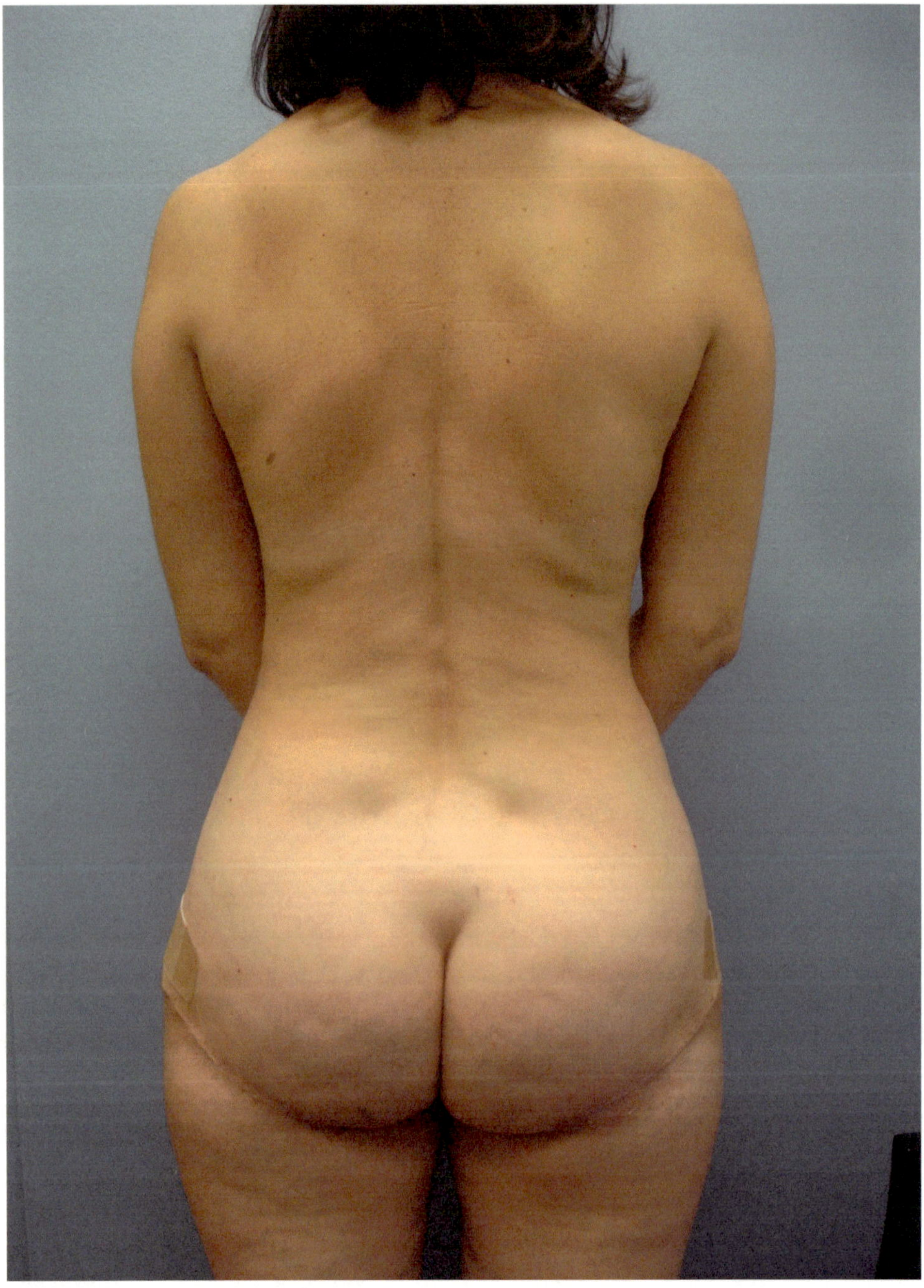

Fig. 4d. Three months status post-operative IGAP

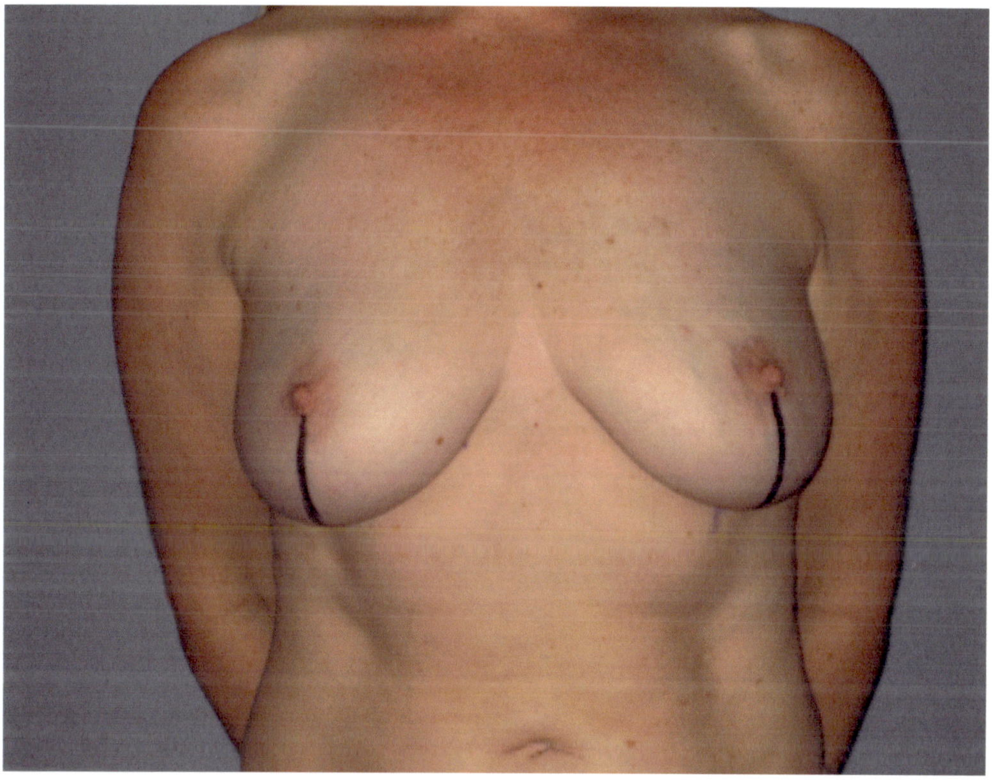

Fig. 5a. Pre-operative markings form nipple sparing with IGAP breast reconstruction.

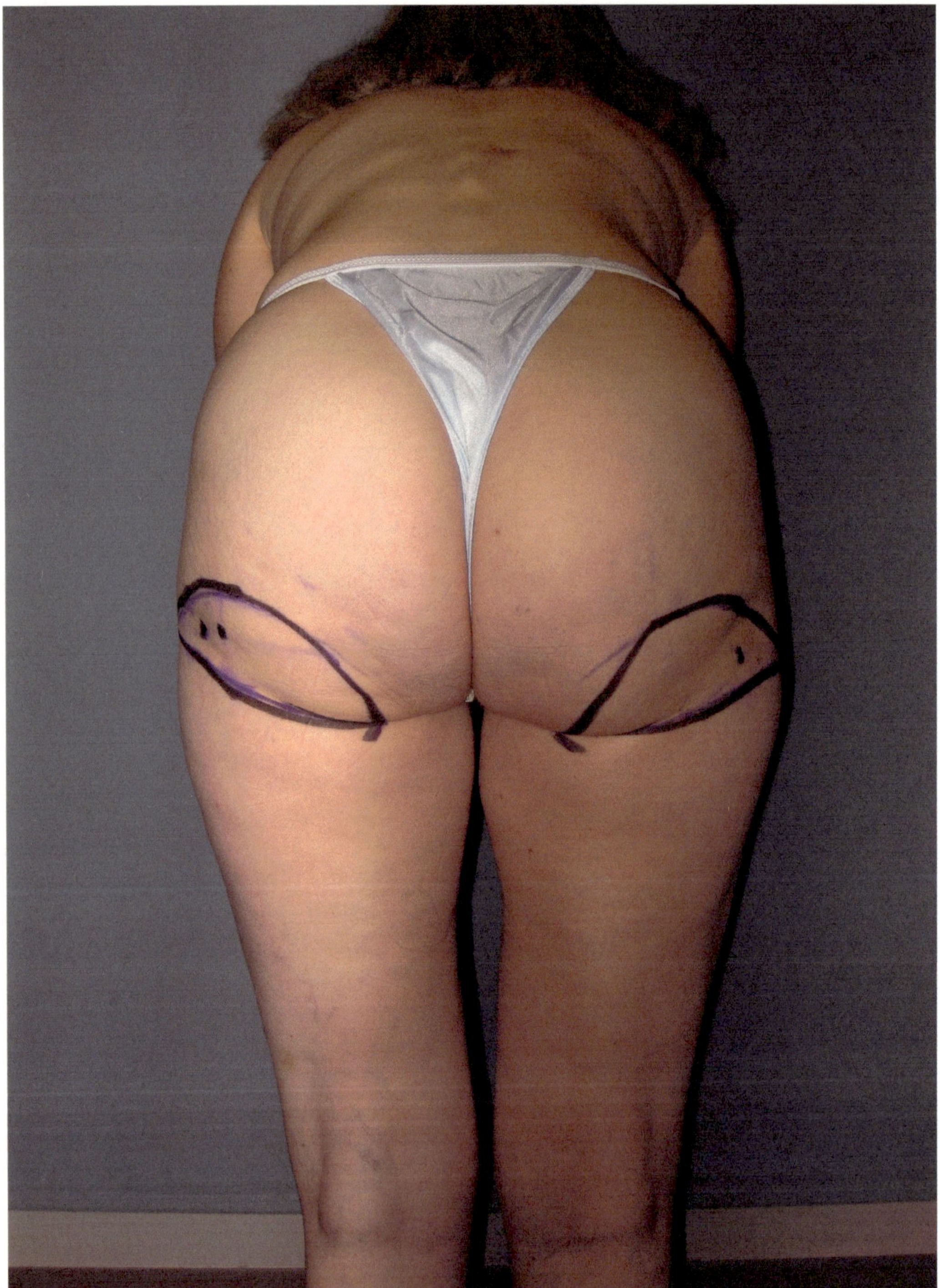

Fig. 5b. Pre-operative markings for B IGAPS. The dots are the selected perforators for surgery.

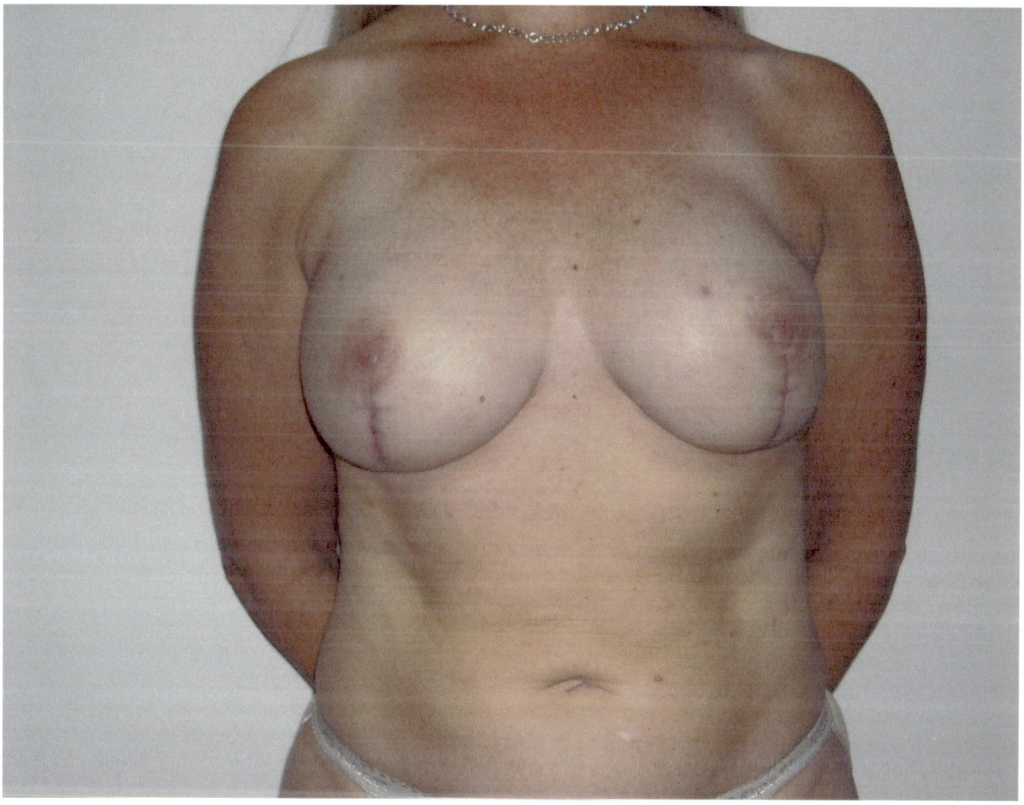

Fig. 5c. Three months post-operative from B IGAPS.

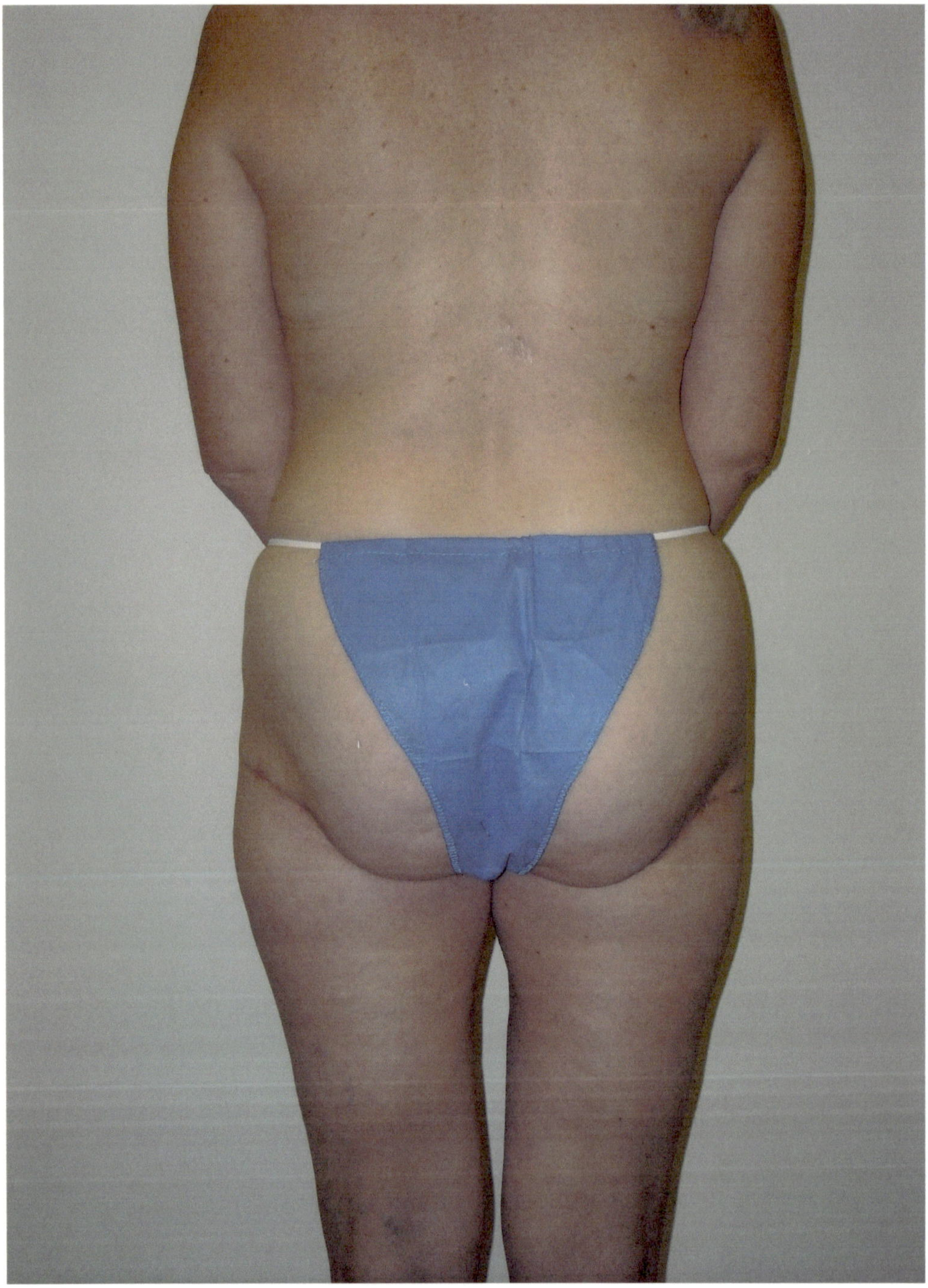

Fig. 5d. Three months post-operative from B IGAPS.

8. Pearls

Review the DIEP pearls, many of these apply to the S/IGAP dissection.

When drawing the markings on the upper or lower buttock, 7 cm should be the width. If this is wider, closure becomes more challenging and dehiscence is a possibility.

Beveling laterally to obtain the saddlebag area is necessary but if too aggressive fat necrosis will ensue.

When obtaining the perforator go layer by layer to find the perforator in the direction of the muscle fibers. This may take some time but with your pre-operative scanning you have a map.

Once the perforator is obtained, the first part of the dissection is straightforward. The last 1 cm of the vessel is the most delicate and tedious. This is where most surgeons run into problems. There is a confluence of vessels here. The problem is finding the main vessels and ligating the ancillary ones. Bleeding is your enemy here, the vessels are often thin walled and any tugging or coarse movement will cause bleeding. This is often difficult to manage without injuring the main vessel needed for anastomosis. Be meticulous at this level.

When the vessels have tributaries, the diameter is usually enlarging. The size of the vessel needed is 2 mm for anastomosis. Once this is obtained, the vessels can be ligated.

Try to skeletonize the vessels in-situ and mark them with methylene blue to be sure of their length. In-situ, the surgeon often feels they have enough length and size but when the flap is transferred to the chest, this is not the case.

The GAP dissections can be very tricky. A single surgeon should not try to perform a bilateral case. There is a learning curve with this flap. The surgeon should assist on as many of these as possible. In our group we always have a second skilled microsurgeon for all of our flaps.

9. General pearls

Pre-operatively discuss with the anesthesiologist about not giving any vasoconstricting agents. Make sure they communicate with you if the systolic blood pressure becomes less than 100 mmHg.

When performing the arterial and venous anastomosis have the blood pressure run high for the artery to remain patent.

Regardless of how well we perform the micro-anastomosis, intra-operatively about 10% will need to be re-done. If the flap shuts down more than two times, check the patient's blood pressure and redo the artery.

The first six hours after surgery is the most critical. This is when we see the most complications. If the artery or vein shuts down, the surgeon must immediately return to the OR to re-evaluate the anastomosis. Let the OR staff know about returns to the operating room during those first six hours. If the surgeons have residents or nurses that communicate to you a problem, notify the OR staff immediately. This will save time arranging the patient's return to the OR.

If the artery has a problem intra-operatively, consider a heparin drip. We use 500-600 units an hour depending on body habitus.

Perforator flap surgery can be very challenging but very rewarding for all parties involved.

There is a learning curve so be patient. Consult with more experienced surgeons if you are encountering difficulties. Good luck!

10. References

[1] Hartrampf CR, Scheflan M, Black PW. Breast reconstruction with a transverse abdominal island flap. Plast Reconstr Surg. 1982 Feb; 69(2): 216-25.

[2] Daniel RK, Taylor GI. Distant transfer of an island flap by microvascular anastomoses. Plas Reconstr Surg 52: 111-117, 1973.

[3] Taylor GI, Daniel RK. The free flap: composite tissue transfer by vascular anastomoses. Australian & New Zealand J. Surg. 43: 1-3, 1973.

[4] Taylor GI, Daniel RK. The anatomy of several free flap donor site. Plas Reconstr Surg. 56(3): 243-253, 1975.

[5] Elliott LF, Raffel B, Wade J: Segmental latissimus dorsi free flap: clinical applications. Ann Plast Surg 1989; 23: 231 -238.

[6] Feller AM: Free TRAM. Results and abdominal wall function. Clin Plast Surg 1994; 21:223- 232.

[7] Koshima I, Moriguchi T, Soeda S, Tanaka H, Umeda N. Free thin paraumbilical perforator-based flaps. Ann Plast Surg. 1992 Jul; 29(1): 12-17.

[8] Allen, R. J., and Treece, P. Deep inferior epigastric perforator flap for breast reconstruction. Ann. Plast. Surg. 32: 32, 1994.

[9] Taylor GI, Daniel RK. The anatomy of f several free flap donor sites. Plast Reconstr Surg. 1975 Sep; 56(3): 243-53.

[10] Allen, R. Heitland, A. Autogenous Augmentation Mammaplasty with Microsurgical Tissue Transfer. Plast Reconstr Surg. 112(1): 91-100, July 2003.

[11] Rogers, N. Allen, R. Radiation Effects on Breast Reconstruction with the Deep Inferior Epigastric Perforator Flap. Plast Reconstr Surg. 109(6): 1919-1924, May 2002.

[12] Gill, P. Hunt, J. Guerra, A. et al. A 10-Year Retrospective Review of 758 DIEP Flaps for Breast Reconstruction. Plast Reconstr Surg. 113(4): 1153-1160, April 1, 2004.

[13] Kroll, S. Sharma, S. Koutz, C. et al. Postoperative morphine requirements of free TRAM and DIEP flaps. Plas Reconstr Surg. 107:338, 2001.

[14] Shaw WW. Breast reconstruction by superior gluteal microvascular free flaps without silicone implants. Plast Reconstr Surg. 1983 Oct; 72(4): 490-501.

[15] Shaw, WW: Microvascular free flap breast reconstruction. Clin. Plast. Surg. 11:333, 1984.

[16] Shaw, WW: Superior Gluteal free flap breast reconstruction. Clin. Plast. Surg. 25:267, 1998.
[17] Codner, MA, Nahai F. The Gluteal artery free flap breast reconstruction: making it work. Clin. Plast. Surg. 24:289, 1994.
[18] Fujino T, Harashina T, Aoyagi F. Reconstruction for aplasia of the breast and pectoral region by microvascular transfer of a free flap from the buttock. Plast Reconstr Surg.1975;56:178-181.
[19] Le-Quang C. Secondary microsurgical reconstruction of the breast and free inferior gluteal flap. Ann Chir Plast Esthet. 1992 Dec;37(6):723-41.
[20] Allen RJ, Tucker C Jr. Superior gluteal artery perforator free flap for breast reconstruction. Plast Reconstr Surg. 1995 Jun;95(7):1207-12.
[21] Guerra AB, Soueid N, Metzinger SE, Levine J, Bidros RS, Erhard H, Allen RJ. Simultaneous bilateral breast reconstruction with superior gluteal artery perforator (SGAP) flaps. Ann Plast Surg. 2004 Oct;53(4):305-10.
[22] DellaCroce FJ, Sullivan SK. Application and refinement of the superior gluteal artery perforator free flap for bilateral simultaneous breast reconstruction. Plast Reconstr Surg. 2005 Jul;116(1):97-103; discussion 104-5.
[23] Vasile JV, Newman T, Rusch DG, Greenspun DT, Allen RJ, Prince M, Levine JL. Anatomic imaging of gluteal perforator flaps without ionizing radiation: seeing is believing with magnetic resonance angiography. J Reconstr Microsurg. 2010 Jan;26(1):45-57.
[24] Tuinder S, Van Der Hulst R, Lataster A, Boeckx W. Superior gluteal artery perforator flap based on septal perforators: preliminary study. Plast Reconstr Surg. 2008 Nov;122(5):146e-148e.
[25] Allen RJ, Levine, JL, Granzow JW. The in-the-crease inferior gluteal artery perforator flap for breast reconstruction. Plast Reconstr Surg 2006 Aug;118(2):333-9.
[26] Granzow JW, Levine JL Chiu ES, Allen RJ. Breast reconstruction with gluteal artery perforator flaps. J Plast Reconstr Aesthet Surg. 2006;59(6):571-9.
[27] Guerra, A. Metzinger, S. Bidros, R. Gill, et al. Breast reconstruction with gluteal artery perforator (GAP) flaps: a critical analysis of 142 cases. Ann Plast Surg. 2004 Feb;52(2):118-25.
[28] Strauch B, Yu HL. Gluteal Region. In Strauch B., Yu H.L. Atlas of Microvascular Surgery: Anatomy and Operative Approaches. New York: Thieme Medical Publishers; 1993, pp102-119.
[29] Ao M, Mae O, Namba Y., and Asagoe, K. Perforator-based flap for coverage of lumbosacral defects. Plast. Reconstr. Surg. 101: 987, 1998.
[30] Roche NA, Van Landuyt K, Blondeel PN, Matton G, and Monstrey S J. The use of pedicled perforator flaps for reconstruction of lumbosacral defects. Ann. Plast. Surg. 45: 7, 2000.
[31] Koshima I., Moriguchi T, Soeda S, Kawata S, Ohta S, Ikeda A. The gluteal perforator-based flap for repair of sacral pressure sores. Plast Reconstr Surg. 91: 678-683, 1993.

[32] Windhofer C., Brenner E., Moriggl B., Papp C. Relationship between the descending branch of the inferior gluteal artery and the posterior femoral cutaneous nerve applicable to flap surgery. Surg Radiol Anat. 24(5): 253-7, 2002.

7

Preoperative Computed Tomographic Angiogram for Deep Inferior Epigastric Artery Perforator Flap for Breast Reconstruction: The Imaging Mapping Era

Jaume Masia[1,*], Carmen Navarro[1], Juan A. Clavero[2] and Xavier Alomar[2]
[1]*Plastic Surgery Department, Hospital de la Santa Creu i Sant Pau (Universidad Autónoma de Barcelona),*
[2]*Radiology Department, Clínica Creu Blanca, Barcelona, Spain*

1. Introduction

Surgical techniques for breast reconstruction have been greatly refined in last decades and important landmarks have been achieved. Autologous reconstruction with microsurgical flaps marked a before and after in breast reconstruction because the aesthetic outcome is improved, a prosthesis is not needed and long-term results are good. Different types of flaps have been used to create a new breast with similar characteristics in shape, size, contour and position to the contralateral one. The preferred donor site for this purpose is the abdominal wall. The deep inferior epigastric artery perforator flap (DIEP) provides fat and skin with characteristics that are very similar to those of the normal breast and spares the rectus abdominis muscle or fascia, thereby minimizing donor site morbidity (1-3). In function of these advantages the DIEP flap has become the gold standard for breast reconstruction in many hospitals (4).

A key point in breast reconstruction with DIEP flap is choosing the best supplying perforator and several factors should be kept in mind when doing so (5). The ideal perforator vessel should have a large right calibre, a short intramuscular course, the easiest dissection, a suitable location within the flap and subcutaneous branching with intraflap axiality. In some cases of DIEP, we can find paramuscular vessels that initially follow a retromuscular plane before piercing the muscular fascia in the exact abdominal mid-line. Many of these perforators have a good caliber and good arborization in the subcutaneous tissue and could be considered to be the ideal perforators because their course facilitates the surgical dissection (6).

After working with perforator flaps for more than 10 years, we can attest that perforator vessels arising from the deep inferior epigastric system are anatomically highly variable regarding their number, location, caliber and relationships with surrounding structures. In

* Corresponding Author

view of this variability, we need a reliable method that will accurately identify and locate the dominant perforator before surgery. This can be achieved through preoperative anatomic images that provide information about the vascularization of the abdomen. Precise imaging can help us to select the best hemiabdomen to raise, to differentiate between superficial and deep epigastric vessels and to combine two or more perforator vessels when there is no dominant vessel. With a precise image we can plan the operative technique, reduce operating time and improve operative outcomes (7). Without a pre-operative investigation, the surgeon may not be aware of previous surgical damage, scar formation or anatomical variants. Using preoperative imaging techniques to study the epigastric vessels we have decreased the number of postoperative complications. An accurate preoperative evaluation by means of imaging of the vascular anatomy of the abdominal wall is extremely valuable for the plastic surgeon as the images provided are easy to interpret and they facilitate safer and faster procedures.

2. Conventional methods for preoperative study of abdominal perforating vessels

Before imaging techniques were described for the study of abdominal perforators, the two most widely used approaches were handheld Doppler ultrasound and color Doppler imaging.

Handheld Doppler ultrasound was the first method described for the study of perforators (8). It is still the most widely used method to locate a perforator, due to its low cost and simplicity of use. However the information it offers is limited. Correlation between the acoustic signal and the diameter of the vessel is unreliable and often imprecise. Furthermore, this technique cannot distinguish perforator vessels from main axial vessels. Besides, this technique has shown an unacceptable number of false positives and tiny vessels can be confused acoustically with a good perforator (9,10). But despite these drawbacks, handheld Doppler ultrasound remains useful in our daily practice and can still be useful for specific indications, such as to assess the location and the course of the superficial epigastric vessels.

Color Doppler imaging provides much more reliable information than Doppler sonography (11). It provides a good evaluation of the main axial vessels and their perforator vessels. It is a highly reliable technique to identify and locate the dominant abdominal perforator vessel. Besides, it provides information about blood flow direction, pattern and velocity. Moreover, the caliber and hemodynamic characteristics of the perforator vessels can be observed directly on color Doppler imaging. The high sensitivity and the 100% predictive value of this technique have made it a good diagnostic tool in the planning of abdominal flaps. However, color Doppler imaging also has some limitations; It is a long test, possibly lasting up to an hour, and this can be uncomfortable for patients as they have to remain in the same position during the procedure. Futhermore, it requires the presence of highly skilled sonographers with knowledge of perforator flap surgery and its results are technician-dependent. In addition, color Doppler imaging does not provide anatomic images that show the surgeon the anatomic relationship between the deep inferior epigastric artery and its perforator branches and other structures along its route. These important limitations have contributed to its relative disuse in microsurgical units.

3. Multidetector-row computed tomography

In 2003 we began to work with CT scan and in 2006 we published the first results where for the first time an imaging technique was used for the visualization and study of abdominal perforator vessels (7). Since then, the multidetector-row computed tomography (MDCT) scan has proved to be highly reliable in preoperative planning of abdominal free flap breast reconstruction and has demonstrated excellent results, significantly reducing operative time and complications (12-16). With the incorporation of the MDCT for mapping the abdominal vascularization, we are not only able to locate the dominant perforators but we also receive extra information about the vessels and the donor area thanks to the anatomical images that these methods provide. Anatomical images inform us about the number of perforators, their location, their intramuscular course and their distribution inside the subcutaneous tissue (figures 1,2: axial MDCT image of an abdominal perforator). They have 100% sensitivity and specificity at the time of locating the dominant perforator, and they are also technically reproducible. This last characteristic is especially handy as it means we can record the information on a CD or pen-drive and have it at our disposition at the moment of surgery. Besides, the increased spatial resolution offered by MDCT allows highly accurate multiplanar and 3D reconstructed images, creating a 3-dimensional map of the perforating vessels. Another advantage is the fact that they provide an anatomical reference of the area. It should also be mentioned that MDCT is very fast to perform and a considerable number of thin sliced CT images are obtained in a short time.

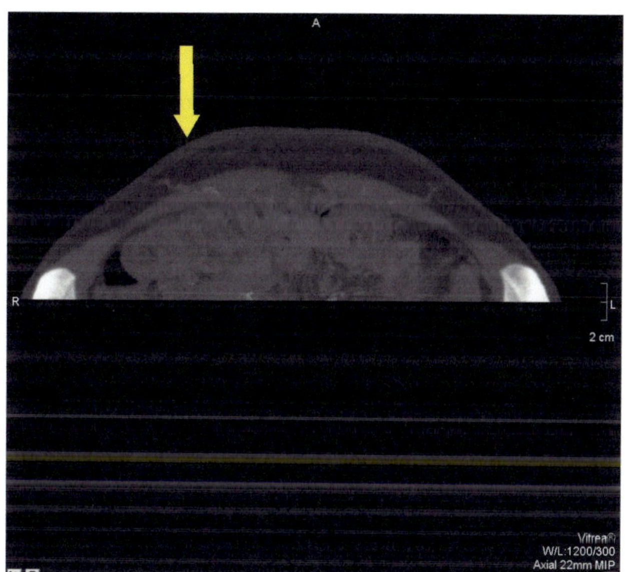

Fig. 1. Axial MCDT image of an intramuscular perforator of the deep epigastric vessels with its branching. Yellow arrow indicates the point in which the perforator pierces the fascia.

In spite of all its advantages, the MDCT has 2 clear drawbacks. The first is the radiation the patient receives when the test is performed (effective dose is 5.6 mSv). However, the effective dose of radiation used with this technique is 5.6mSv which is less than that used for an opaque enema or a conventional abdominal CT scan. The second drawback of the MDCT is the need to administer an intravenous medium; this is uncomfortable for the patient and can cause allergic reactions.

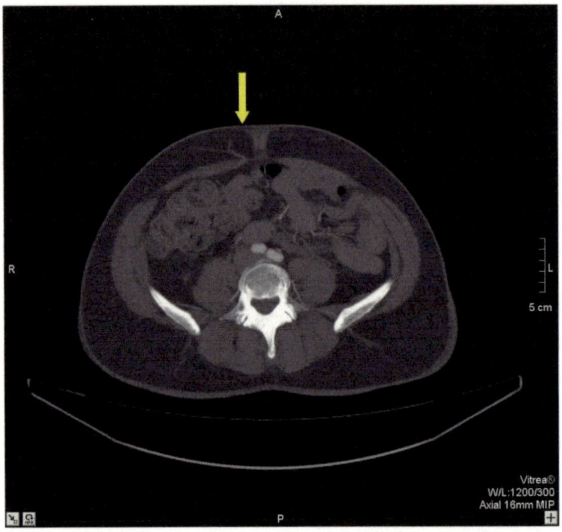

Fig. 2. Axial MCDT image of a paramuscular perforator of the deep epigastric vessels with its branching in the subcutaneous tissue. Yellow arrow indicates the point in which the perforator arises from the fascia.

3.1 MDCT protocol

Nowadays our multidetector computed tomography studies are performed using a 64 or 320detector-row CT scanner with the following parameters: 120 kVp, 80-120 mAs (0.4 sec gantry rotation period), detector configuration 64 x 0;5mm, 54-mm table travel per rotation, 512 x 512 matrix, and a 180 to 240 field of view. All scanning was performed during IV administration of 100 ml of non-ionic iodinated contrast medium with a concentration of 300 mg L/ml (Xenetix 300 [lobitridol]; laboratories Guerbet, Paris, France). The contrast material was mechanically injected (injector TC missori XD 2001); Ulrich GmbH & Co. K, Ulm, Germany) at a rate of 4 ml/sec. through an 18-gauge IV catheter inserted into an antecubital vein.

An important concept to note is that the patient is placed in a supine position on a CT table in the exact manner that will be used on the day of surgery. Sections are obtained from 5 cm above the umbilicus to the lesser trochanter of the hip during a single breath-hold while the patient holds his breath for approximately 10 to 12 seconds. The approximate time of acquisition is 3-4 seconds. The entire procedure takes less than 10 minutes and is therefore very well tolerated by the patient. The volumetric data acquired are then used to reconstruct images with a slice width of 1-millimetre and a reconstruction interval of 0.8-millimetres. The resulting complete set of reconstructed images is automatically transferred to a computer workstation (Vitrea version 4.0.1, Vital Images, Plymouth, MN) which generates the reformatted images in multiple planes (coronal, axial, sagittal and oblique) and in three-dimensional volume rendered images. This system allows measurements to be taken so that different planes of space can be automatically correlated. Data can be stored on a pen drive (e-Film Medical Inc., Toronto, Canada) which can easily be used and managed using a standard computer (17).

4. Non-contrast magnetic resonance imaging

To overcome the limitation of radiation with MDCT-technique, many began to investigate the possibility of using magnetic resonance imaging (MRI) for abdominal perforator mapping (18). For several years, we worked with different kinds of MRI technologies, until we get good results with 1.5T non-contrast magnetic resonance imaging FBI technique (19). In 2010 we published the first results demonstrating that non-contrast magnetic resonance imaging provides reliable information on the vascular anatomy of the abdominal wall. Preoperative magnetic resonance imaging without the contrast showed no false positive or false negative results. This technique provided accurate location of the dominant perforator, good definition of its intramuscular course and excellent evaluation of the superficial inferior epigastric system (figure 3: axial non contrast-MRI image of abdominal perforators). We are also able to define the perforator branching within the subcutaneous abdominal tissue and evaluate the vascular connections between the superficial and the deep inferior epigastric vessels (20).

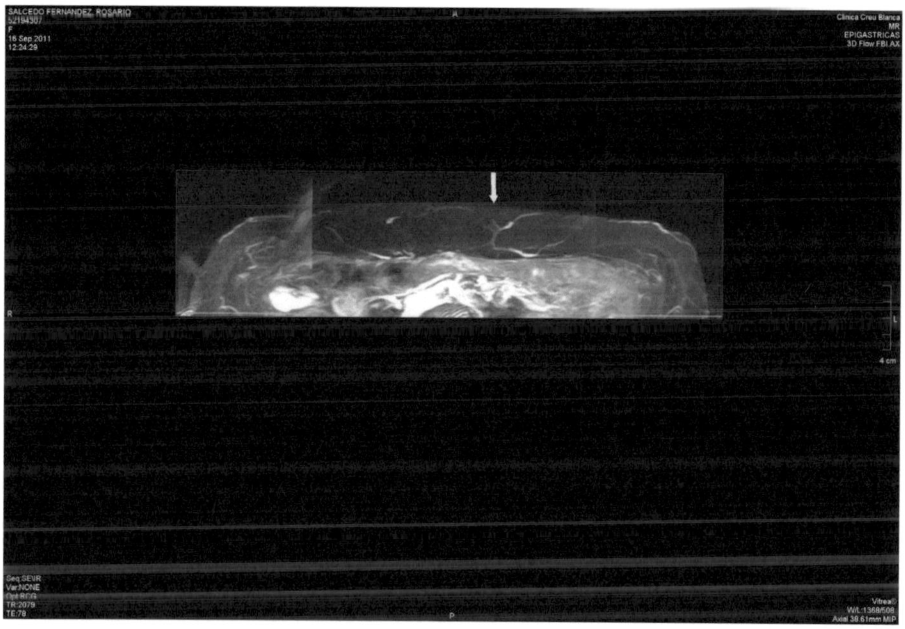

Fig. 3. Axial non contrast-MRI image of abdominal perforators. Yellow arrow indicates the point in which the dominant perforator pierces the fascia.

4.1 Non-contrast MRI protocol

As with MDCT, the first step with this technique is to acquire multiplanar images with the patients in supine in the same position as they will be placed at surgery. In contrast with MDCT, however, no prior patient preparation is needed and nor is contrast medium required, so the patient does not require the 6 hours of fasting before acquisition of images.

We use high speed parallel imaging (speeder technology) to achieve accelerated scan times. Initially, sagittal scouts are acquired to locate the inferior abdominal wall and to delimit the study zone. A sequence phase 3D+5_FSfbi is used in the anterior coronal plane with the following parameters: TR:2694, TE:80, slice thickness 1.5 mm, number of slices: 50, number of acquisition: one, 512x512 matrix, field of view 380x380 mm, TI:160 and resp + ECG gate. A sequence phase 3D+5_FSfbi is then performed in the axial plane with the following parameters: TR:2900, TE:78, slice thickness 3 mm, number of slices: 56, number of acquisition: one, 704x704 matrix, field of view 380x380 mm, TI:160 and resp + ECG gate. The anterior coronal plane phase only includes the anterior abdominal wall, from a plane immediately below the pubis to the xiphoid process of the sternum. The axial plane phase includes the area from the infrapubic zone to 3cm above the umbilicus. The acquisition time ranges from 10 to 20 minutes. Multiplanar formatted images and 3D volume rendered images are regenerated on a Vitrea computer workstation (Vitrea version 3.0.1. Vital Images, Plymouth, MN) (20).

5. Image analysis to select the most suitable perforator

The images obtained are usually interpreted by both the radiologist and the plastic surgeon who is going to harvest the DIEP flap. The team chooses the perforator considered the most suitable according to the following criteria: largest calibre, best location, shortest intramuscular course and also intraflap axiality. The perforator selected gives a pair of x/y coordinates based on an axial system centred on the umbilicus and the flap can be raised based on the dominant perforator. The surgeon is provided with three types of image: axial, sagittal and coronal. The axial views and sagittal reconstructions are of great help in the assessment of the perforator vessel to evaluate its dependence on the main trunk or any direct branch of the deep inferior epigastric artery and to delimit its origin on the fascia and its distribution through subcutaneous fat and skin. Rendered reconstructions allow us to mark on the patient's skin the exact point where the perforator vessel emerges through the fascia of the rectus abdominis muscle.

The image is assessed using the following protocol:

Step 1. In the axial view we study the deep inferior epigastric artery course from its origin, through the muscle, to five centimetres cranial to the umbilicus. We normally identify the two or three best perforators on each side of the abdomen, marking them with an arrow, and classify them according to their external calibre into three categories (small, medium, large). At the suprafascial level we assess the perforator branching in the subcutaneous tissue. We assess the intramuscular course of the deep inferior epigastric artery, defining its relationship to the tendinous intersections and the number of branches. We also study the superficial epigastric system, defining the calibre of the artery at its origin. In our experience vessel size greater than 0.6 mm can potentially be used for raising a SIEA flap if it has a medial distribution on the abdomen. When we choose the best perforator in the imaging technique, we look for the point where it pierces the fascia in the axial view and we mark an arrow on the skin at this level. From there on the arrow will appear in all views. We draw a coordinate x/y axis on the umbilicus and we make measurements to locate the exit of the perforating vessel in relation to the umbilicus. First, we measure the distance from the midline to the perforator in the axial view, and this is given the value "x".

Step 2. We review the sagittal view to double check the quality of the chosen perforators and to place them in three planes. The second measure is done in the sagittal view measuring from the umbilicus level to the exit of the perforator. This will be the "y" value. In the sagittal view we can also assess the interconnections between the superficial and deep systems (figure 4: axial and sagittal views of a dominant perforator).

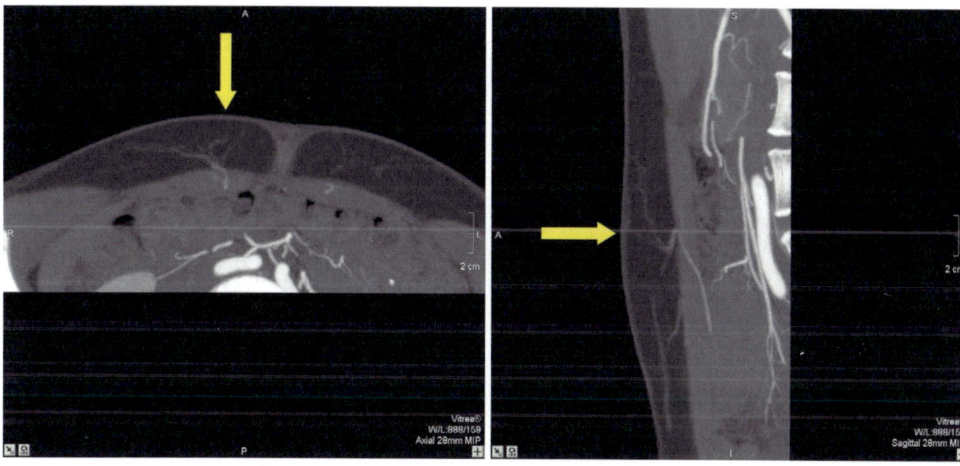

Fig. 4. 4A) Axial MCDT image of an intramuscular perforator of the deep epigastric vessels with its intramuscular course and its branching. 4B) Sagittal view MDCT image of the same patient showing the same perforator with its intramuscular course. Yellow arrow indicates the point in which the perforator pierces the fascia.

Step 3. Then we perform a 3D reconstruction of the abdomen to precisely locate the points on the skin surface where the best perforators emerge from the fascia of the rectus abdominis muscle. Using a virtual coordinate system with the umbilicus at the centre, all information is transferred to a data form sheet so that the perforators are mapped in a format that allows us to transpose their position preoperatively onto the abdominal skin of the patient. If we transfer these values from the computer to paper, we locate the exact point where we will find the perforator when we raise the flap (figures 5a,b,c,d,e,f: protocol for images assesment).

Step 4. Before we complete the study with the radiologist we like to look at the coronal cuts to visualize the subcutaneous and distribution pattern of the superficial inferior epigastric arterial system and assess the connections between the superficial and deep systems (figures 6a,b,c: Coronal images showing the abdominal vascular network).

So therefore, depending on the findings of the images provided by the MDCT or the MRI, we will decide which vessel is going to nourish the flap. The first point to check is the superficial system. If the superficial vessels have a good caliber -that is, more than 0.6mm- and a medial distribution in the abdomen, a SIEA flap could be performed. When there is not a good superficial system, we will consider the deep epigastric system. The second aspect is to search for a good paramuscular perforator. If we find a good one, we will center the flap on it, as its dissection is easier and faster. If we do not find a good paramuscular perforator, we will choose an intramuscular one. Several factors must be taken into account when we are selecting the perforator that is going to nourish the flap. Whenever possible a direct branch from the deep inferior epigastric artery and the one with the shortest intramuscular course will be selected as our perforator. The location of the perforator should be as central as possible within the flap and it should have a good intraflap axiality and subcutaneous branching.

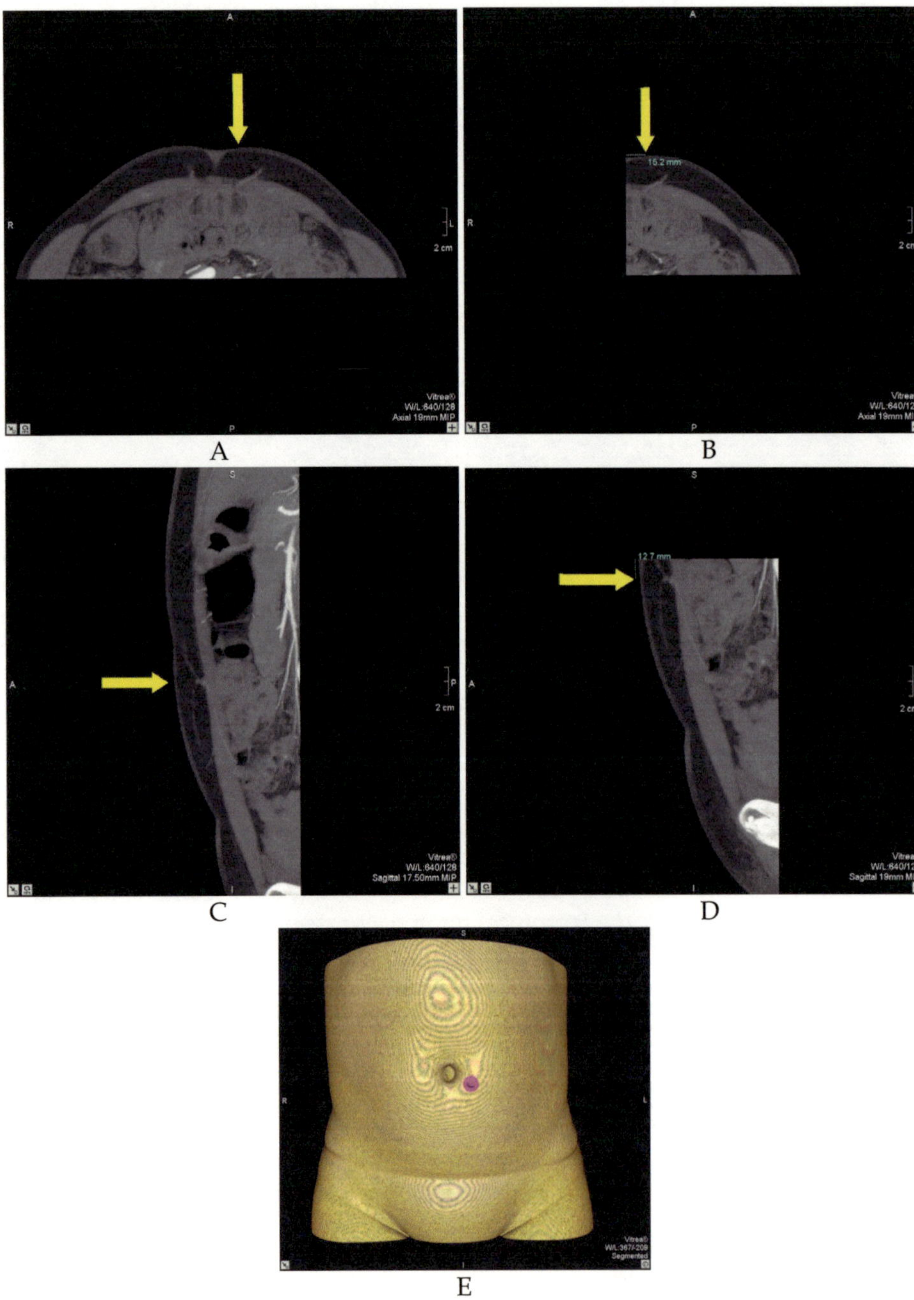

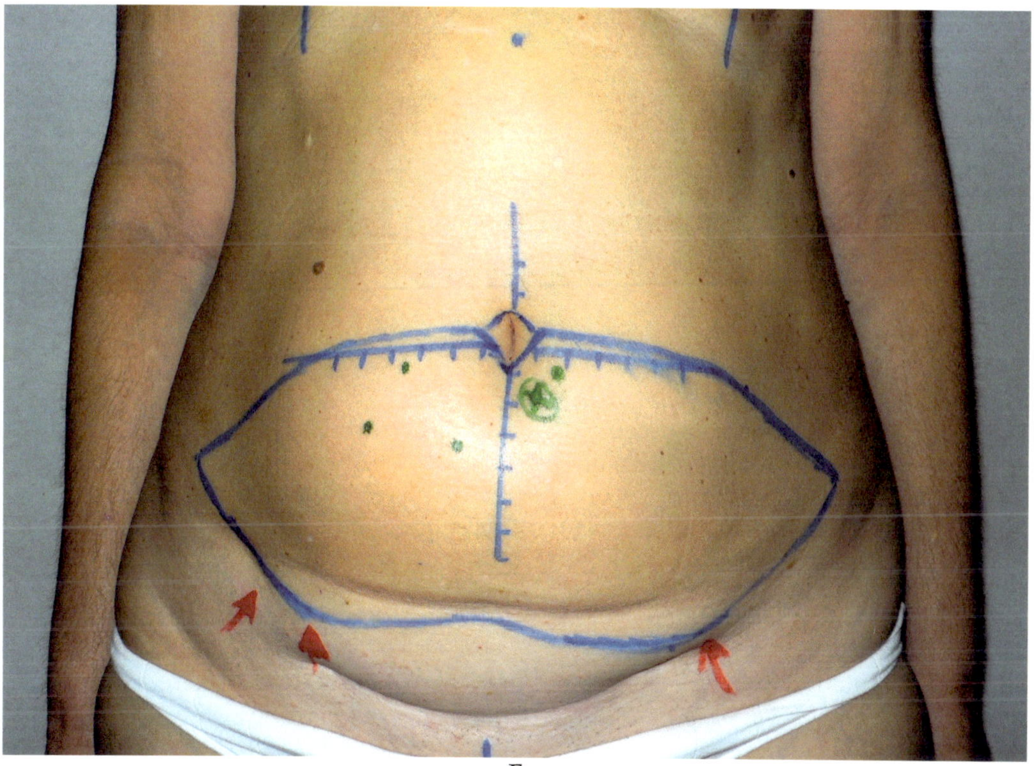

F

Fig. 5. Protocol for images assesment. A) Axial MDCT image showing the most suitable abdominal perforator in this patient. The yellow arrow indicates the point where the paramuscular perforator pierces the fascia. B) We measure the distance from the midline to the perforator in the axial view, and this is given the value of "x". C) Sagittal DMCT image showing the perforator. The yellow arrow indicates the point where the perforator pierces the fascia. D) The second measure is done in the sagittal view measuring from the umbilicus level to the exit of the perforator. This will be the "y" value. E) MDTC 3-D reconstruction for the same patient. The magneta arrow indicates the exactly point where the perforator pierces the fascia. F) Preoperative markings in the patient with the dominant perforator located.

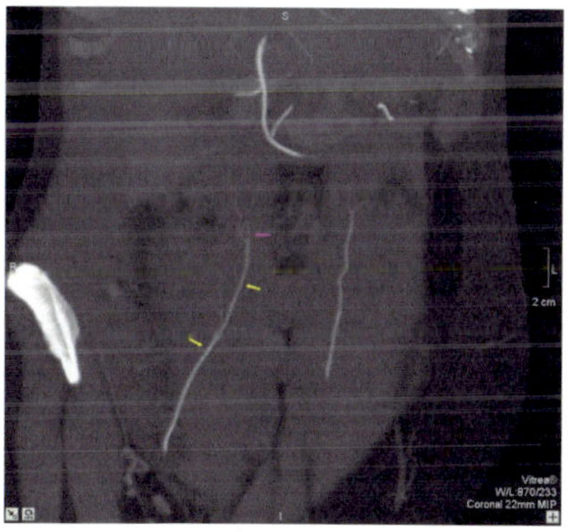

A

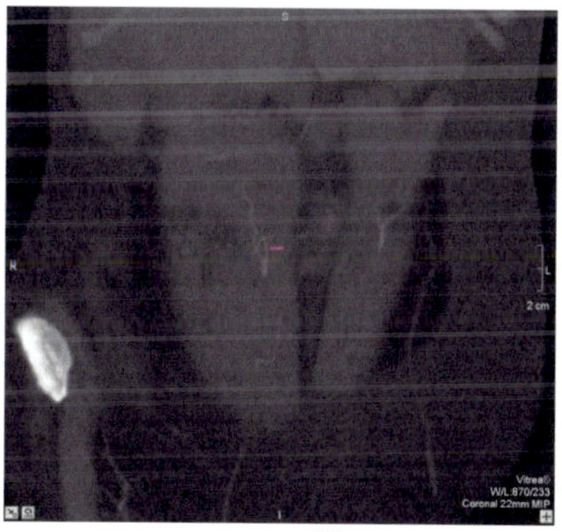

B

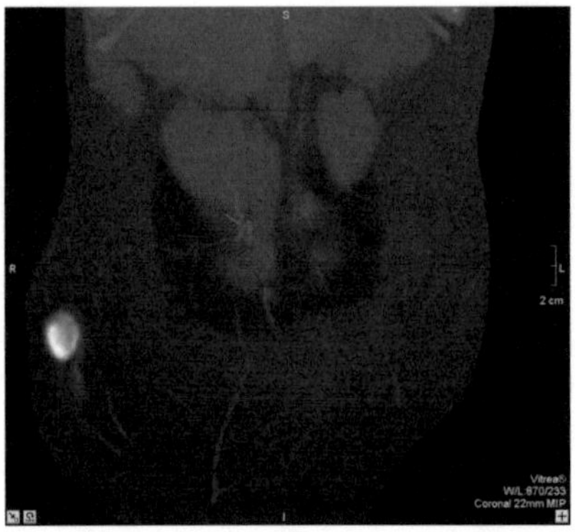

C

Fig. 6. Coronal images showing the abdominal vascular network. A) Deep level: Coronal image showing the course of the deep epigastric vessels (yellow arrows) and the origin of the main perforator (magneta arrow). 6B) Intermediate level. 7B) Superficial level: Coronal image showing the perforator connecting with the superficial vascular network. Magneta arrow marks the same perforator.

6. Discussion

Raising a perforator flap requires meticulous dissection of the perforator vessels, sparing the muscle structure with its segmentary motor nerves. Special skill is needed for such surgical dissection, and the intraoperative time is considerable. Because the vascular anatomy of the abdominal wall varies greatly among individuals and even between one hemi-abdomen and the other in the same individual, establishing a vascular map of each patient before surgery facilitates dissection.

The ability to detect the dominant perforating artery preoperatively saves considerable time for the surgeon. The benefits thus extend to the patient and also to reducing costs and conserving resources. Many techniques have been used to preoperatively map abdominal perforating vessels. The ideal technique should possess low cost, high availability and reproducibility, and high reliability in selecting the dominant perforator. In addition, it should be fast to perform, easy to interpret and free of morbidity.

Since the first reports on MDCT appeared many centers have focused on developing and improving this technique. MDCT today is considered the technique of choice in the preoperative evaluation of patients who are candidates for autologous breast reconstruction (13). In the continuing search for the ideal technique and to minimize the disadvantages of MDCT, many eyes are presently on MRI and results to date seem promising (19,20).

By using imaging techniques to decide preoperatively which perforators are most suitable, we can reduce the amount of stress for the surgeon who can now go straight to the chosen perforator with confidence and can ligate the other perforators safely without wasting time. The amount of time saved in the operating room can be balanced against the extra cost of the investigation. These techniques (MRI and CT) also allow us to plan an optimal design for the flap size the best vascularized tissue supplied by the dominant perforator. As a result, fat necrosis and partial flap loss has been shown to be reduced in our studies when we validated the MDCT that we published in 2006 because it allows the surgeon to choose the best vascularised region of abdominal tissue supplied by the dominant perforator. This information is also extremely valuable if a patient has had previous surgery, such as liposuction or a hysterectomy, in the abdominal area. The high sensitivity, specificity and the 100% positive predictive value of this non-invasive and easy-to-interpret preoperative mapping technique have made it a highly-promising diagnostic tool in the planning of DIEP flaps.

Considerable discussion remains concerning whether MDCT or non-contrast-MRI is the more ideal method for the preoperative study. The answer depends on the facilities of the center, but if we know that we can achieve the same information with both techniques, we should use the one which has less morbidity for the patient. We use MDCT in two main situations: 1) when we can take advantage of the extension study requested by the oncologist in cases of delayed reconstruction and 2) in cases when we need to study a large extension of the body to rule out anatomical abnormalities.

With MDCT and MRI we have achieved a breakthrough in the preoperative evaluation of the perforator surgery. Compared with the handheld Doppler and color Doppler imaging, the advantages are multiple:

- High sensitivity and high specificity
- Good three-dimensional evaluation of quality, course and location of perforators
- Easy interpretation by the radiologist and plastic surgeon
- Easy storage of data on a pendrive, simplifying reproducibility
- Reduction of operating time and complications
- Good patient tolerance
- Reduction of surgeon stress

Day to day progress is being made in the quality of images and radiological equipment. The ideal preoperative method will be that which offers the best quality images with minimal inconvenience to the patient. MDCT and MRI are clearly the best tools available as yet to make a complete preoperative study prior to breast reconstruction. With the application of increasingly sophisticated, faster and less invasive methods, we are getting closer to a virtual dissection of the perforator before surgery. There is still a long road ahead but we have undoubtedly come a long way.

7. Abbreviations

DIEP: Deep Inferior Epigastric Perforator
MDCT: Multidetector Row Computed Tomography
MRI: Magnetic Resonance Imaging
SSFP: steady-state free-precession
T-SLIP: time spatial inversion pulse
FBI: Fresh Blood Imaging

8. References

[1] Allen RJ, Treece P. Deep inferior epigastric perforator flap for breast reconstruction. Ann Plast Surg 1994;32:32-8.
[2] Blondeel PN, Boeckx WD. Refinements in free flap breast reconstruction: The free bilateral deep inferior epigastric perforator flap anastomosed to internal mammary artery. Br J Plast Surg 1994;47:495-501.

[3] Craigie JE, Allen RJ. Autogenous breast reconstruction with the deep inferior epigastric perforator flap. Clin Plast Surg 2003;30:359-69.
[4] Granzow JW, Levine JL. Breast reconstruction with the deep inferior epigastric perforator flap: history and an update on current technique. J Plast Reconstr Aesthet Surg 2006;59:571-9.
[5] Blondeel PN, Neligan PC. Perforator Flaps. Anatomy Technique and Clinical Applications. Vol I Chapter 7: Complications: Avoidance and Treatment. 118-9. Quality Medical Publishin Inc., 2006.
[6] Masia J, Larrañaga J, Clavero JA, Vives L, Pons G, Pons JM. The value of the multidetector row computed tomography for the preoperative planning of deep inferior epigastric artery perforator flap: our experience in 162 cases. Ann Plast Surg 2008; 60:29-36.
[7] Masia J, Clavero JA, Larrañaga JR, Alomar X, Pons G, Serret P. Multidetector-row computed tomography in the planning of abdominal perforator flaps. J Plast Reconstr Aesthet Surg. 2006; 59:594-9.
[8] Taylor, G. I., Doyle, M., and McCarten, G. The Doppler probe for planning flaps: Anatomical study and clinical applications. Br. J. Plast. Surg. 43: 1, 1990.
[9] Blondeel PN, Beyens G, Verhaeghe R, Van Landuyt K, Tonnard P, Monstreny SJ, Matton G. Doppler flowmetry in the planning of perforator flaps. Br J Plast Surg 51:202-209, 1998
[10] Giunta RE, Geisweid A, Feller AM. The value of preoperative Doppler sonography for planning free perforator flaps. Plast Reconstr Surg. 2000 Jun; 105(7):2381-6.
[11] Hallock GG. Doppler sonography and color duplex imaging for planning a perforator flap. Clin Plast Surg 2003 Jul;30(3):347-57, v-vi.
[12] Rajan S. Uppal, Bob Casaer, Koenraad Van Landuyt, Phillip Blondeel. The efficacy of preoperative mapping of perforators in reducing operative times and complications in perforator flap breast reconstruction. J Plast Reconstr Aesthet Surg. 2009 Jul;62(7):859-64.
[13] Mathes DW, Neligan PC. Preoperative imaging techniques for perforator selection in abdomen-based microsurgical breast reconstruction. Clin Plast Surg. 2010 Oct; 37(4):581-91.
[14] Hijjawi JB, Blondeel PN. Advancing deep inferior epigastric artery perforator flap breast reconstruction through multidetector row computed tomography: an evolution in preoperative imaging. J Reconstr Microsurg. 2010 Jan;26(1):11-20.
[15] Hamdi M, Van Landuyt K, Hedent EV,Duyck P. Advances in autogenous breast reconstruction. The role of preoperative perforator mapping. Ann Plast Surg 2007;58:18-26.
[16] Rozen WM, Ashton MW, Grinsell D, Stella DL, Phillips TJ, Taylor GI. Establishing the case for CT angiography in the preoperative imaging of abdominal wall perforators. Microsurgery. 2008;28(5):306-13.
[17] Clavero JA, Masia J, Larrañaga J, Monill JM, Pons G, Siurana S, Alomar X. MDCT in the preoperative planning of abdominal perforator surgery for postmastectomy breast reconstruction. AJR Am J Roentgenol 2008; 191:670-6
[18] Rozen WM, Stella DL, Bowden J, et al. Advances in the pre-operative planning of deep inferior epigastric artery perforator flaps: magnetic resonance angiography. Microsurgery 2009;29:119-23.
[19] Masia J, Kosuotic D, Cervelli D, Clavero JA, Monill JM, Pons G. In search of the ideal method in perforator mapping: noncontrast magnetic resonance imaging. J Reconstr Microsurg. 2010 Jan;26(1):29-35.
[20] Masia J, Navarro C, Clavero JA, Alomar X. Noncontrast magnetic resonante imaging for preoperative perforator mapping. Clin Plast Surg. 2011 Apr; 38(2):253-61.

8

The Superficial Inferior Epigastric Artery (SIEA) Flap and Its Applications in Breast Reconstruction

Zachary Menn and Aldona Spiegel
Weill Cornell Medical College, The Methodist Hospital, Houston, Texas, USA

1. Introduction

The first choice in breast reconstruction is the use of autologous abdominal tissue due to its similar composition and texture. Free tissue transfer of the lower abdominal wall has become a crucial skill for all reconstructive surgeons to develop in order to keep up with the current progress in breast reconstruction. This involves mastery of the free transverse rectus abdominis muscle (free TRAM), deep inferior epigastric perforator (DIEP) and the superficial inferior epigastric perforator (SIEA) flaps, utilizing their donor abdominal tissue to reconstruct a breast defect.

The SIEA flap utilizes the unique characteristics of the lower abdominal tissue, without compromising the strength and integrity of the abdominal wall musculature and fascial layers. In contrast to other abdominal free flaps, the rectus fascia and musculature are left unaltered during elevation of the SIEA flap, and therefore they maintain their preoperative strength. Many patients prefer an abdominal donor site for free tissue transfer for reasons such as improved abdominal contour with the benefits of abdominoplasty, and a low-lying easily hidden scar that can be covered by most swimwear.

The initial published description of the SIEA flap was by Antia and Buch (1971), who used it to reconstruct a soft tissue deformity of the face. The first use of a free SIEA flap for breast reconstruction was reported by Holmström (1979), however Grotting is known for popularizing the SIEA flap for immediate breast reconstruction in 1991.

2. Anatomy

The SIEA flap gets its vascular supply from a more superficial, subdermal vascular plexus system that includes significantly smaller vessels supplied by the superficial inferior epigastric axial vessels. The SIEA flap is a direct axial adipocutaneous flap, unlike the free TRAM and DIEP flaps that are fed by perforating vessels. The superficial inferior epigastric vessels do not actually perforate a muscle or a septum, so it is not classified as a perforator flap.

The origin of the SIEA is 2-5 cm below the inguinal ligament as a branch of the common femoral artery. It most often originates as a shared trunk with the superficial circumflex iliac artery; however it may originate as an individual trunk or an assortment of other alternative origins from the deep femoral artery or even the pudendal artery. The SIEA and its venae commitantes are normally found coursing lateral to the lateral row of deep inferior epigastric perforators. The superficial epigastric artery originates deep to Scarpa's fascia, and as it runs superiorly it penetrates through Scarpa's fascia and continues in the superficial subcutaneous tissue. As for the venous drainage of the SIEA flap, it is primarily from two venae comitantes that run alongside the SIEA before terminating into the femoral vein, and from the superficial inferior epigastric vein (SIEV) which terminates into the saphenous bulb. The arterial diameter ranges from 1.1-1.9 millimeters, with an average pedicle length of 5 - 8 cm. The area of the SIEA flap is lower abdomen that it is perfused by the SIEA; however there is some lateral overlap with the superficial circumflex iliac artery (SCIA). The sensory innervation of the SIEA flap is provided by the 10th to 12th intercostal nerves.

According to a 1975 anatomical investigation of the SIEA by Taylor and Daniels, the SIEA was found to be absent in 35 percent of their subjects. In the remaining subjects, the origins of the SIEA were inspected and discovered to be rather inconsistent, with 48 percent sharing a common trunk with the superficial circumflex artery, whereas 17 percent were found to be direct branches off of the common femoral artery. Our early clinical experience with lower abdominal dissection during breast reconstruction surgery confirmed this finding, showing a lack of an identifiable SIEA in 42 percent of our 278 total patients. These results were published along with data from further investigation of the other 58 percent of patients with an identifiable SIEA, which showed that 54 percent of these patients had arteries with external diameters of 1.5 mm or greater when measured at the level of the lower abdominal incision. This is important when considering our selection criteria for the SIEA flap requires such a diameter. Therefore, only 31 percent of all patients in our study had a SIEA sufficient for use in a free flap.

The tissue perfusion and venous drainage from across the midline of a unipedicled SIEA flap has been a topic of great debate in the literature, the main question being reliability. Some studies reveal the perfusion and drainage across the midline to be unpredictable at best, while others have proven that reliable perfusion across the midline in free flap transfer is indeed, quite possible. The amount of tissue that will dependably perfuse across the midline will differ with each patient and should therefore be determined by intraoperative assessment of cross-flap perfusion.

3. Indications for SIEA flap

For breast reconstruction, we believe the lower abdomen is the ideal site for donor tissue. The SIEA flap is preferred; however we will use the DIEP flap if certain conditions are not met. We have developed and previously published an algorithm for choosing the SIEA flap, and a summary of this algorithm will be presented later on in this chapter. Patients who are not eligible for lower abdominal tissue reconstruction will be reconstructed with either a latissimus dorsi flap (with or without an implant), a superior gluteal artery perforator flap (SGAP), or occasionally with a breast implant alone.

4. Contraindications for the SIEA flap

We will avoid use of the SIEA in certain situations that are counterintuitive to flap survival. We do not routinely operate on patients who are active smokers. Patients are required to quit smoking at least two months prior to surgery and continue to refrain for six weeks after surgery. We will postpone microsurgery on any patient who we believe to be noncompliant with the conditions stated above. Other relative contraindications to our microsurgical reconstruction include BMI greater than 35 kg/m^2, age greater than 65 years, and other medical comorbidities such as a coagulation disorder or uncontrolled diabetes. Finally, we will not use the SIEA flap if the intraoperative criteria of our selection algorithm are not met.

5. Preoperative markings

Vascular imaging may be performed preoperatively to help determine whether or not the diameter of the SIEA is sufficient, as well as to accurately map the path of the vessels. This can be accomplished with contrast enhanced CT scan. Marking begins with the abdominal site while the patient is in the supine position. A pencil Doppler is used to locate and mark the SIEA and its venae commitantes, generally found approximately halfway between the anterior superior iliac spine (ASIS) and the pubic symphysis, slightly superior to the inguinal crease. Second, we mark the SIEV, which is located medial to the SIEA, followed by the arterial and venous periumbilical perforators on both sides of the midline. Next we identify and mark both the medial and lateral row of the deep inferior epigastric perforators. The markings prepare for the possible harvest of both the SIEA flap and the DIEP flap.

It is important to keep in mind when marking the inferior abdominal incision line to keep as low as possible to hopefully encounter the SIEA at an acceptable caliber. If however the SIEA does not meet the 1.5mm diameter required by our algorithm, we then revert to a DIEP flap. Therefore we should be prepared for such a situation by including the periumbilical perforators when designing the flap. The typical dimensions of each SIEA flap is approximately 14 cm vertically and 17 cm from midline to ASIS.

6. Procedural details

To prepare for the procedure, the patient is placed in the supine position, with the arms tucked in to allow for easier microscope positioning over the recipient site. The flap is harvested with Loupe magnification X 5.5, however the microscope is used for the vessel anastomosis. We avoid the use of any vasoconstrictors or local anesthetic at both the donor and recipient sites.

The harvest of the SIEA flap is begun by careful subcutaneous dissection, making sure not to injure the superficially running SIEV. The SIEA and SIEV are then located and dissected away from the adjacent tissue. The size of the SIEA is then examined at the level of the skin incision. There is dual venous drainage, both the SIEV and the venae comitantes of the SIEA, and both are preserved during the dissection.

The algorithm developed and used by our institution for choosing the SIEA flap in breast reconstruction has previously been published. There are three criteria that we use to determine whether the anatomy is suitable for SIEA flap harvest; an arterial vessel diameter that is at least 1.5 millimeters, as well as a visible and a strong palpable pulse. Another key point to note during pedicle dissection is to avoid skeletonizing the vessels. We prefer to leave a small piece of subcutaneous tissue or fat just deep to the vessels to help protect the vascular pedicle from kinking during inset. Caution should be taken though, since adding too much excess tissue around the pedicle could lead to a lingering, unnecessary seroma formation due to elimination of the lymphatics. The only area of the vessel that should be fully skeletonized is the distal most section, in preparation for the anastomosis.

We generally use the ipsilateral side as our hemi-abdomen of choice for unilateral reconstructions. There are several reasons behind our favor of the ipsilateral flap. The SIEA pedicle enters the abdominal flap on its lateral aspect, so when the flap is rotated (180 degrees) for inset, the pedicle and the recipient internal mammary vessels are much closer together in an ipsilateral flap. Also, the final positioning of an ipsilateral flap leaves the area with the least reliable blood supply on the lateral aspect of the reconstructed breast and not medially, therefore if there is any flap loss it will most likely be laterally as preferred. Suturing of an ipsilateral flap at the previous umbilical excision site will cone the breast at the desired lateral position.

In certain instances in which the caliber of the SIEA is questionable, we will examine the SIEV diameter before making the final call between the SIEA and DIEP flaps. If a substantial SIEV is present, we can presume superficial draining system dominance and we will strongly consider using the SIEA flap, rather than the DIEP flap, in spite of the unimpressive SIEA caliber.

After the SIEA flap has been selected and all aspects of the algorithm are met, the pertinent vessels are dissected and then we proceed with the rest of the flap elevation. The upper incision begins at the lateral termination of the upper incision line marked earlier (generally the ASIS) and continues to approximately 1 cm superior to the umbilicus. This incision is now continued deeply, through the adipose tissue to the loose areolar tissue plane just superficial to the muscular fascia of the abdominal wall. Next, careful elevation of the flap takes place from lateral to medial, using Bovie cautery to ensure that hemostasis is obtained. Complete hemostasis will provide an uncompromised view of the correct surgical planes and help to prevent any unwanted fascial incision. After that, the umbilicus is dissected away from the adjacent flap tissue. Avoid skeletonization of the umbilical stalk to ensure that enough blood supply is maintained with the umbilical stalk.

For bilateral reconstruction, we will complete the anastomosis of the first flap, before addressing the superficial inferior epigastric artery and vein of the second hemi-abdomen. The caliber of the vessels is evaluated, as earlier, and the algorithm is used once again to decide if the SIEA is the appropriate flap.

When the flap elevation is complete but the pedicle is still attached, we mark the superficial aspect of the pedicle for future use. Next, the flap edges are brought back together and stapled, and finally the mastectomy defects are addressed.

In almost all of our reconstructive cases the internal mammary vessels are the recipient vessels of choice. The dissection site will be either the second or third intercostal space, chosen based on the palpated width of the intercostal space. We may occasionally widen the intercostal space by resecting part of the rib costochondrium using a rongeur, although this is rarely necessary. After that, a small window is excised from the pectoralis muscle, and the intercostal muscles are then carefully resected for access to the internal mammary artery and vein. Next, the artery and vein are prepared for microanastomosis using Loupe magnification. We now compare the diameter of the recipient vessel, the IMA to the SIEA. If there is an arterial size discrepancy greater than 0.5mm between the recipient vessel and the SIEA, we will most likely consider reverting to a DIEP flap. For optimal exposure of the internal mammary vessels for anastomosis, the mastectomy skin should be carefully retracted. Next, the internal mammary vessels are prepared for anastomosis under the microscopic.

When the internal mammary vessels are ready, the SIEA, its venae commitantes, and the SIEV are ligated from the donor site. As mentioned earlier, the flap is rotated 180 degrees to properly position the pedicle for anastomosis. The coupler device is usually used for the venous anastomosis and 9-0 suture for the arterial anastomosis.

We prefer to use the venae commitantes (proximal to where they unite) instead of the SIEV that actually exits the flap separately. The similar caliber as well as the desirable proximity of the venae commitantes, which course alongside the SIEA, make these vessels more favorable and in our experience have shown lower risk of complication from vessel kinking when compared to utilization of the SIEV. As a result, we only tend to use the SIEV for cases in which the venae comitantes are insufficient or if a second venous anastomosis is needed.

Before closure of the donor site skin, we address any diastasis recti found intra-operatively by plicating the rectus fascia. The umbilicus is delivered, and sutured in place using 3-0 and 4-0 interrupted Monocryl sutures. Two 15F Blake drains placed in the lateral edge of the donor site defect before the abdomen closed in layers. The Scarpa's fascia is closed with interrupted 2-0 Monocryl sutures, followed by deep subcutaneous interrupted 3-0 Monocryl sutures, and finally a running subcuticular 4-0 Monocryl. The approximated edges of the skin are now sealed with liquid skin adhesive, and a dry dressing is placed on top.

7. Pitfalls

7.1 Crossing the midline in SIEA flaps

Tissue harvest across the midline involves resecting all of zone IV, as well as any inadequately perfused zone III tissue. The amount of remaining tissue across the midline that is satisfactorily perfused varies from patient to patient.

Visually delineate the zone of inadequate perfusion and mark the line of proposed resection on the flap skin. Most of the time, an obvious line of demarcation will appear on the flap skin. A more accurate estimate of flap perfusion can be achieved while the flap is still attached to the vessels at the abdominal site, compared to evaluating a reperfused flap following anastomosis, as it takes time for the true line of demarcation to appear on a recently reperfused flap. After the anastomosis is complete and the planned resection markings are reevaluated, some excess flap tissue will be excised.

7.2 Flap inset and the SIEA pedicle

The orientation is key when handling the final inset of the SIEA flap. The anatomy of the SIEA pedicle is very distinctive. In perforator based abdominal flaps the pedicle enters the flap from beneath, however the SIEA pedicle enters horizontally from the flap's inferior edge at the superficial subcutaneous tissue. The primary recipient vessels are the internal mammary vessels, found within the intercostal space. The recipient vessels are better positioned for abdominal perforator flaps. With pedicles on the underside of the flap, the vessels are less likely to kink along their course to the anastomosis. The pedicle of the SIEA flap travels from a more superficial plane to a deeper one, making it more vulnerable to vascular compromise from kinking, compression or malrotation.

7.3 Persistent donor site seromas after flap harvest

Abdominal drains usually remain in place longer in SIEA patients than with perforator flaps. This is most likely due to the more extensive dissection into the groin area and possible disruption of additional lymphatic channels. We remove the drains only when drainage is less than 25cc per day.

8. References

Arnez, Z. M., Khan, U., Pogorelec, D., and Planinsek, F. Breast reconstruction using the free superficial inferior epigastric artery (SIEA) flap. *Br. J. Plast. Surg.* 1999;52: 276-79.

Antia NH, Buch VI. Transfer of an abdominal dermo-fat graft by direct anastomosis of blood vessels. Br. J.Plast. Surg. 1971;24: 15- 9.

Chevray PM. Breast reconstruction with superficial inferior epigastric artery flaps: a prospective comparison with TRAM and DIEP flaps. Plast. Reconstr. Surg. 2004;114:1077-83.

Granzow JW, Levine JL, Chiu ES, Allen RJ. Breast reconstruction using perforator flaps. J Surg Oncol. 2006;94:441-54.

Grotting JC. The free abdominoplasty flap for immediate breast reconstruction. Ann. Plast. Surg. 1991;27: 351-4.

Hester TR Jr, Nahai F, Beegle PE, Bostwick J. Blood supply of the abdomen revisited, with emphasis on the superficial inferior epigastric artery. Plast. Reconstr. Surg. 1984;4:657-70.

Holm C, Mayr M, Ho¨fter E, Ninkovic M. The versatility of the SIEA flap: a clinical assessment of the vascular territory of the superficial epigastric inferior artery. J Plast Reconstr Aesthet Surg. 2007;60:946-51.

Holmström H. The free abdominoplasty flap and its use in breast reconstruction. An experimental study and clinical case report. Scand J Plast Reconstr Surg. 1979;13:423-27.

Reardon CM, O'Ceallaigh S, O'Sullivan ST. An anatomical study of the superficial inferior epigastric vessels in humans. Br J Plast Surg. 2004;57:515-19.

Schaverien M, Saint-Cyr M, Arbique G, Brown SA. Arterial and venous anatomies of the deep inferior epigastric perforator and superficial inferior epigastric artery flaps. Plast Reconstr Surg. 2008;121:1909-19.

Spiegel AJ, Khan FN. An Intraoperative algorithm for use of the SIEA flap for breast reconstruction. Plast Reconstr Surg. 2007;120:1450-9.

Stern HS, Nahai F. The versatile superficial inferior epigastric artery free flap. Br J Plast Surg. 1992;45:270-74.

Taylor GI, Daniel RK. The anatomy of several free flap donor sites. Plast Reconstr Surg. 1975;56:243-53.

Ulusal BG, Cheng MH, Wei FC, Ho-Asjoe M, Song D. Breast reconstruction using the entire transverse abdominal adipocutaneous flap based on unilateral superficial or deep inferior epigastric vessels. Plast Reconstr Surg. 2006;117:1395-403.

Volpe AG, Rothkopf DM, Walton RL. The versatile superficial inferior epigastric flap for breast reconstruction. Ann Plast Surg. 1994;32:113-17.

9

Double-Pedicle DIEP and SIEA Flaps and Their Application in Breast Reconstruction

Marzia Salgarello, Liliana Barone-Adesi and Giuseppe Visconti
University Hospital "Agostino Gemelli", Catholic University of "Sacro Cuore", Rome, Italy

1. Introduction

Autologous breast reconstruction with deep inferior epigastric artery perforator (DIEP) and superficial inferior epigastric artery (SIEA) flaps is nowadays considered the gold standard in post-mastectomy reconstruction. Excellent results could be achieved in term of softness and natural appealing breast, making these lower abdominal flaps very popular.

Nevertheless, large breast reconstruction still remains a challenge for the surgeons because the amount of fat that could be safely transferred with the DIEP and SIEA flaps in the conventional way could be insufficient to achieve a good symmetry with the contralateral breast. A contralateral reduction mammaplasty may solve some of these cases, but in other clinical situations a flap larger than standard is needed. This fact gains importance especially in patients with scant abdominal tissue or infraumbilical vertical scars, and in delayed reconstructions after previous modified radical mastectomy (MRM) where there is a severe lack of skin and subcutaneous tissue. Moreover, patients who previously had mastectomy plus expander breast reconstruction often show a depression of the cartilage rib cage which could need larger flap to be corrected.

2. Relevant applied microvascular anatomy of the DIEP and SIEA flaps

DIEP and SIEA flap relevant anatomy has been extensively explained in the relative chapters. In this paragraph we will focus on the microvascular anatomy of the abdominal flaps as its comprehension is key-point when choosing a double-pedicle instead of an unipedicle flap. A three- and four-dimensional computed tomographic angiography (CTA) study by Wong C. et al. on injected medial and lateral row DIE perforators demonstrates that the area of perfusion of a medial row DIE perforator is larger (around 300 cm^2) and more centralized when compared to the lateral row DIE perforator ones, that results smaller (around 200 cm^2) and more lateralized, encompassing almost only the ipsilateral hemiabdomen.

2.1 Arterial microvascular anatomy

When selecting a perforator for DIEP flap reconstruction, the largest perforator should be selected (i.e. the dominant perforator). The medial row perforators have been shown to often have dominance over the lateral row perforators. Furthermore, the "clinical" angiosome sustained by a medial row perforator is normally larger than the one sustained by a lateral row perforator.

The perfusion of the transverse lower abdominal flap was first described by Scheflan and Dinner on the unipedicle transverse rectus abdominis musculocutaneous (TRAM) flap. These authors divided the lower abdominal ellipse into four equal parts and named them with numbers according to their clinical impression of perfusion. However, the zoning system became known after Hartrampf's paper on the TRAM flap for breast reconstruction and took his name (Hartrampf zone of perfusion). As already described by Scheflan and Dinner, the flap is ideally divided in four zones, as follows. The abdomen midline divides the lower abdominal flap in two hemiabdominal flaps. These are ideally divided in two halves, thus resulting four zones, which are numbered from I to IV based on their perfusion and viability. Zone I is the most perfused zone being the one corresponding to the selected perforator. Zone IV is the most distant one and usually bad perfused and not viable. (figure 1)

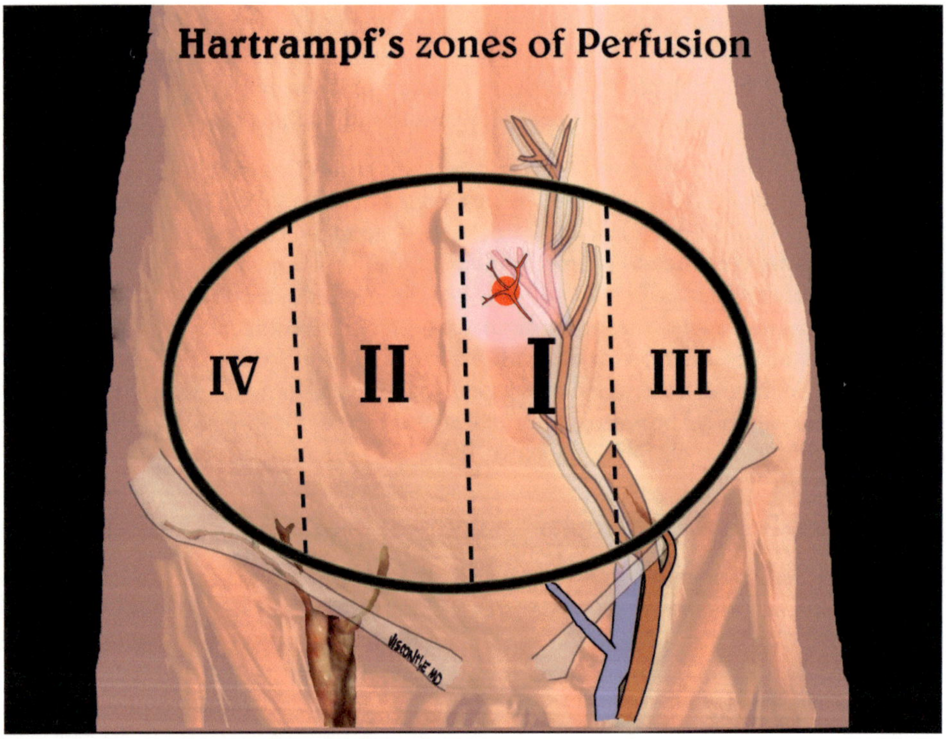

Fig. 1. The figure shows the dominant medial peforator and the corrisponding zoning system. This follows the Hartrampf's classification.

One year later Hartrampf's paper, Dinner's further investigation casted a shadow on the strictness of this zoning system as zone II and III should have to be switched. Twenty-three years later, Holm et al. confirmed Dinner's observation by decreeing that Hartrampf zone of perfusion II and III are reversed according to their fluorescent perfusion techniques. (figure 2).

It was only after the 3D and 4D CTA studies by Saint-Cyr et al., that the DIEP flap zones of perfusion were clarified. According to this study, zones of perfusion depend on the row position of the perforator harvested, as follows:

- Flap based on a single *medial row perforator* shows a more centralized perfusion thus following the Hartrampf's classification of perfusion zones. (figure 1)
- Flap based on a single *lateral row perforator* shows a more lateralized perfusion thus following the Holm's classification of perfusion zones. (figure 2)

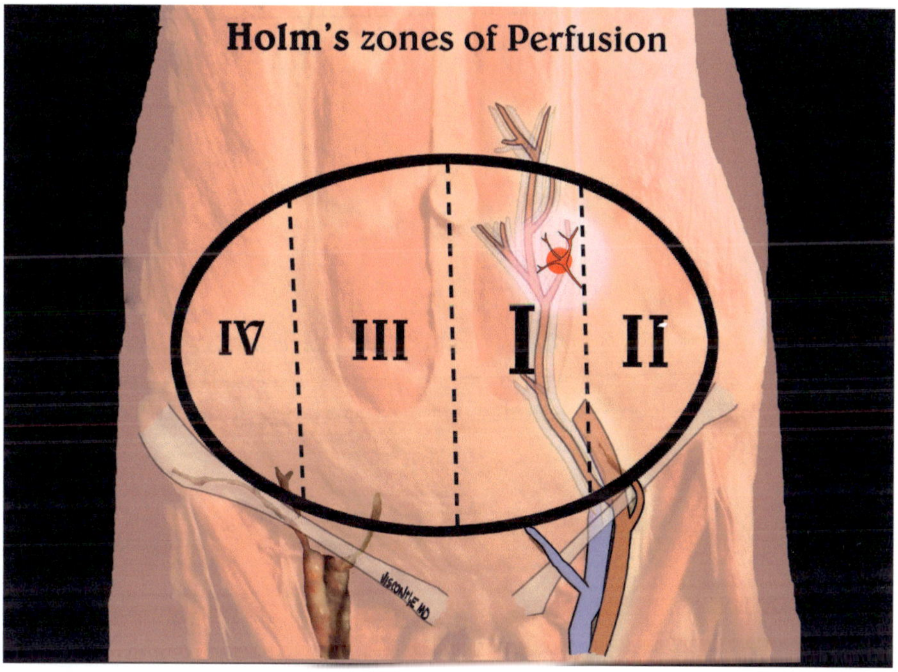

Fig. 2. The figure shows the dominant lateral peforator and the corresponding zoning system. This follows the Holm's classification.

However, both these theories are applied for a single dominant perforator. Depending on the perforator size and location, it is not uncommon that more than 1 perforator is harvested to improve DIEP flap perfusion.

Since Saint-Cyr et al. introduced the perforasome concept, nowadays the perforasome zone of perfusion (ZoP) theory is applied to the DIEP flap surgery (figures 3,4), as follows:

- *ZoP I:* it corresponds to the selected perforator, both medial or lateral row perforator;
- *ZoP II:* perforasomes just adjacent to the selected perforasome.
- *ZoP III.* next group of perforasomes, further distal to the selected perforasome.
- *ZoP IV and so on:* further distal perforasomes.

The perforasome concept is based on the fact that each perforator has its own vascular territory. It represents the "perforator" evolution of the Taylor's "anatomic angiosome".

Each perforasome is able to capture a variable number of adjacent perforasomes via direct and indirect linking vessels. This is what Taylor defines "clinical angiosome". Direct linking

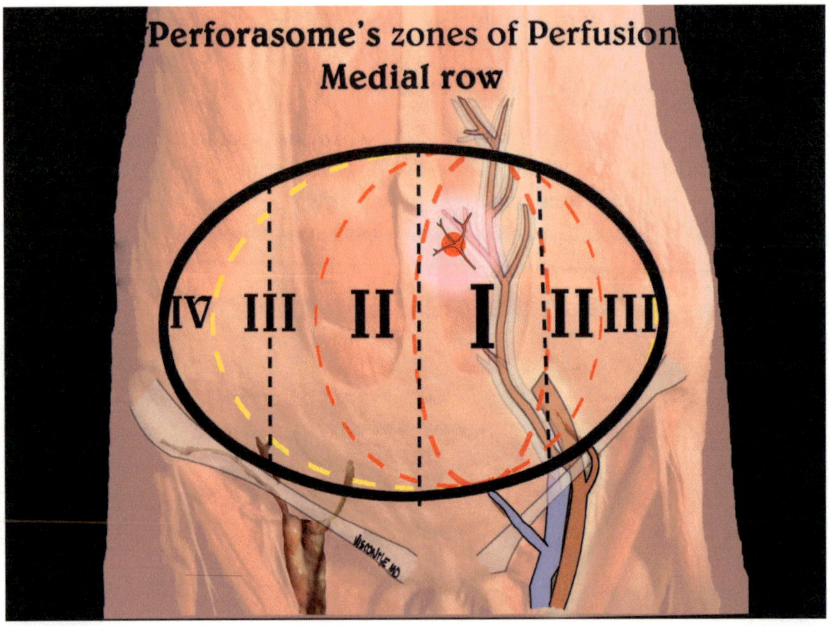

Fig. 3. The perforasome's zone of perfusion when selecting a medial row dominant perforator. The viable flap is more centralized and have a larger surface when compared to a lateral row perforator.

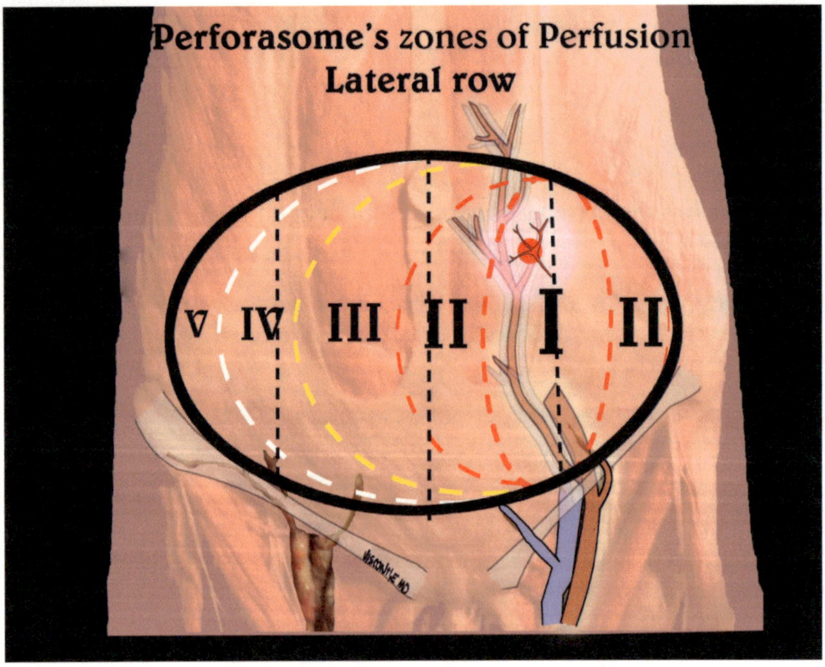

Fig. 4. The perforasome's zone of perfusion when selecting a lateral row dominant perforator. The viable flap is more lateralized and have a smaller surface when compared to a medial row perforator.

vessels have large calibre and allow to capture adjacent perforasomes through an interperforasome flow mechanism. Indirect linking vessels are small calibre vessels , similar to the Taylor's choke vessels, allowing to capture adjacent perforasome through a recurrent flow mechanism. This normally takes place in the subdermal plexus.

In DIEP flap, Saint Cyr et al. observed that:

- perforators of the same row of the selected perforator are connected via direct linking vessels.
- perforators of the other row than the selected perforator are connected via direct and indirect linking vessels.
- Perforators of the opposite hemiabdomen than the selected perforators are connected only via indirect linking vessels because the vascular connections at linea alba between the two hemiabdomens take place only via indirect vessels.

So far, in DIEP flap surgery, the dimension of the viable flap based on a selected perforator relies on the clinical angiosome of the selected perforator. In other word, it depends on the number of perforasomes that are perfused by the selected perforator.

What Hartrampf, Holm and the perforasome zones of perfusion have in common is:

- the distal contralateral area then the selected perforator hemiabdomen (zone IV) is usually not viable and reliable. However, Wong C. et al reported that around 20% of the medial row perforators DIEP flap vascular territories encroach zone IV, whereas none of the lateral row perforators do.
- the clinical angiosome of an unipedicle DIEP flap extends within the same perforator hemiabdomen and partially in the contralateral hemiabdomen.
- the unipedicle DIEAP flap based on a medial row perforators is more centralized thus extending more its viable area in the contralateral hemiabdomen.
- the unipedicle DIEAP flap based on a lateral row perforators is more lateralized and the viable area on the controlateral hemiabdomen is minimal.

Regarding the SIEA microvascular anatomy, Schaverien et al. demonstrated that the perfusion pattern mostly overlaps the lateral row DIEP perforator pattern being the controlateral hemiabdomen never interested. However, in literature larger SIEA pattern has been described. (figure 5)

The vascular connection between the superficial vessels and both the medial and lateral row perforators of the same hemiabdomen are via indirect linking vessels in the subdermal plexus (recurrent flow).

In conclusion, when facing with the need of a large DIEP flap, a medial row perforator DIEP flap should be the choice. However, if the need is to transfer the whole lower abdominal skin and soft tissues (four zone DIEP flap) a double-pedicle (i.e perforator of the contralateral DIE or the SIEA/SIEV pedicle) is usually needed to increase the flap viable area.

2.2 Venous microvascular anatomy

The arterial anatomy of the lower abdominal skin and soft tissue has been widely described, and advances have been made with the modern concept of perforasome zones of perfusion. On the other side, the venous microanatomy of the abdominal wall did not receive the same appraisal. In modern era of DIEP flap, the main vascular issues encountered are the venous drainage problems that can drive the flap from partial to complete necrosis.

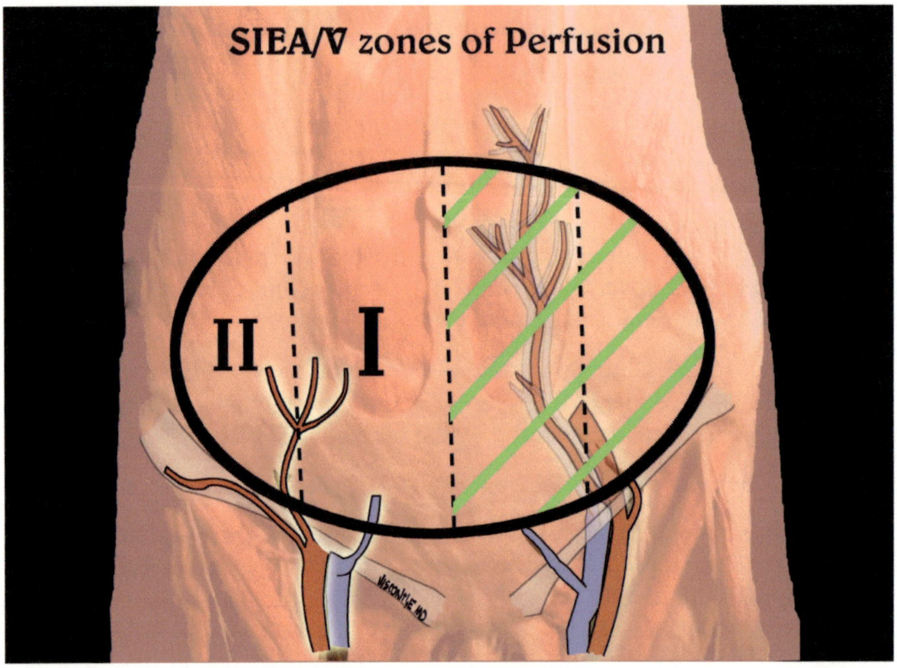

Fig. 5. The perfusion pattern of a SIEA/V flap. It is generally described as a hemiabdominal flap or I-II zones flap, being the contralateral hemiabdomen not perfused.

The venous drainage of the lower abdomen is provided by the superficial system belonging to SIEVs and the deep venous system belonging to DIEVs. Cadaver and in-vivo studies by Shaverien M et al. and Rozen WM et al. demonstrated the presence of small connecting veins (also called oscillating veins) between the superficial and the deep venous systems that usually diverts the subcutaneous venous flow from the superficial (SIEVs) to the deep veins (DIEVs) through the DIE perforator comitantes veins. In this case, the dominant perforator comitantes veins are often 1mm or bigger. On the other side, there could be also cases with prevalent venous drainage towards the superficial venous system, via SIEVs. A SIEV bigger than 1.5 mm at the inferior skin incision can be a pointer of this situation.

So far, the calibre of the selected perforator vein can be a limiting factor in DIEP flap drainage.

However, additional factors may be responsible for the lower abdomen soft tissue venous congestion:

- *The degree of communications between the superficial and deep system.* The links between the superficial and the perforating system are not uniform and frequently via small calibre vessels, also called *oscillating veins.* These may limit the efficiency of the venous drainage.
- *Midline cross-over connections by the SIEVs.* Each SIEV has been found to be a single trunk in the majority of the cases but sometimes can show a bifurcating or very rarely a trifurcating trunk below the umbilicus.

SIEV often supplies a medial branch that crosses the midline routinely at the arcuate line. Sometimes, there are additional cross-over just above and below the umbilicus. However, these midline cross-over connections can also be weak or even absent. These factors may also contribute to venous congestion.

In our centre, we usually study and evaluate the mid-line cross-over SIEV connections according to a grading scale where Grade I stands for absent connections at the midline, Grade II for weak connections, Grade III for good midline connection and Grade IV for good connections with at least one big size midline connection. (figure 6)

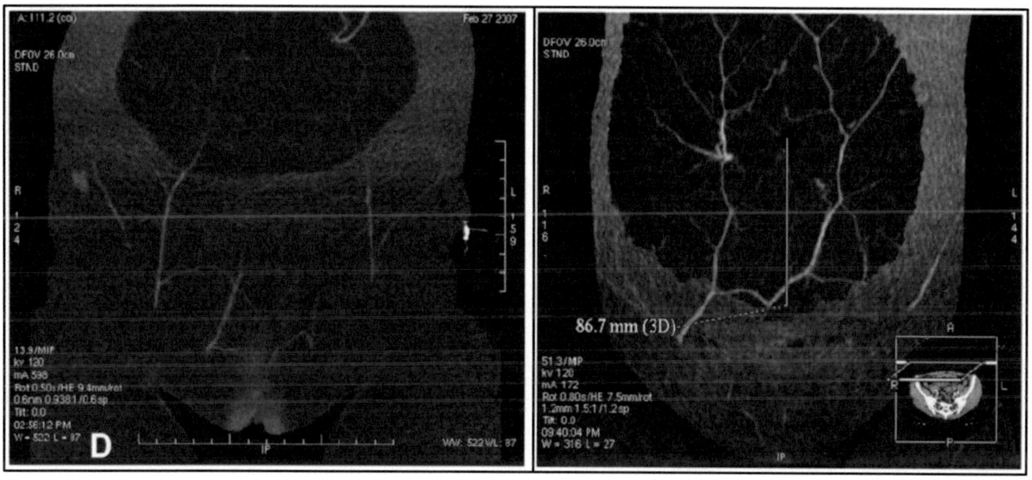

Fig. 6. (left) C-T coronal subvolume MIP (Maximum Intensity Projection) reconstruction of the subcutaneous fat of the lower abdomen shows multiple small connections among the superficial venous systems of both sides. Grade II connections.
(right) C-T coronal subvolume MIP (Maximum Intensity Projection) reconstruction of the subcutaneous fat of the lower abdomen shows a large venous connection between the superficial epigastric veins of both sides. Grade IV connections.

In conclusion, when planning a four zone DIEP flap is paramount to predict and to evaluate that the flap has adequate arterial input and venous discharge. In four zone DIEP flap, a double-pedicle flap is what is normally needed to assure both good perfusion to all the four zones as well as efficient venous discharge. With reliable SIEA/SIEV, it is possible to raise a four zone lower abdominal flap on DIEP on one side and contralateral SIEA/SIEV or even based on bilateral SIEA/SIEV. In the latter, it is more appropriate to talk about a double I -II zone flap as each SIEA/SIEV flap sustains the corresponding hemiabdomen only.

There are few situations where an unipedicle DIEP flap with an additional venous anastomosis (one of the SIEVs) can be enough.

All this will be better explained in the next paragraphs.

3. Relevant applied vascular anatomy of the internal mammary vessels

The internal mammary vessels are widely used as recipient vessels in autologous tissue breast reconstruction. Their central location, reliability in terms of size and constancy, freedom of flap insetting and the relatively resistance to atherosclerosis, preservation following radiation therapy and axillary surgery make them a natural choice as recipient vessel in breast reconstruction. Moreover, avoiding the use of thoracodorsal vessels as recipients, the latissumus dorsi (LD) flap is preserved as salvage option.

The internal mammary vessels are bilateral. On each side we can distinguish the internal mammary artery (IMA) and at least one internal mammary vein (IMV).

3.1 IMA

The internal mammary artery originates from the subclavian artery. Occasionally, it can have a common origin with the thyreocervical trunk, scapular artery, dorsal scapular artery, thyroid artery or costocervical trunk. It courses downward and medially joining the posterior surface of the first cartilaginous rib. It continues downward, ventral to the parietal pleura and on the posterior surfaces of the first six cartilaginous ribs being at the lateral sternal border. The distances between the IMA and the lateral sternal border is on average 15 mm, ranging from 6 to 24 mm. Starting from the third intercostal space, the IMA is found superficial to the trasversus thoracis muscle which separates the artery from the parietal pleura, making the dissection safer.

The IMA diameter varies at each intercostal space, being normally bigger proximally. Arnez et al. measures the IMA at the third, fourth and fifth intercostal spaces finding out an average diameter of 2.8, 2.6 and 2.6 mm, respectively. IMA tends to be larger on the right than the left side.

At the sixth intercostal space IMA normally splits in two trunks: the musculo-phrenic artery and the superior epigastric artery.

A combined radiologic and clinical study on 120 patients by Murray ACA et al. pointed out that in all patients both left and right IMA were always present and detectable both at ultrasound (US) and CTA. This study found out that in 99 % of the cases the IMA is a single trunk and in 1% of the case two trunks can be found. At the third intercostal space, where the IMV is normally split in two venous trunks, the IMA was found medial to the vein(s) in 22.5% of the cases, lateral to vein(s) in 6% of the cases and central positioned in 71.5% of the cases.

IMA shows anastomosis with the intercostal arteries of each space and gives off perforating branches at each intercostal space. However, a great variability has been described about IMA perforator calibre. The biggest IMA perforator is usually the one located at the second intercostal space followed by the ones at the third and first intercostal spaces with an average diameter of 1 mm, ranging from 0.5 to 2 mm. This makes the IMA perforator potential recipient vessels instead of the IMA itself, when the perforator has an acceptable calibre (more than 1 mm).

Besides all the positive aspects that makes the IMA the most favourite recipient vessel in breast reconstruction, there are rare cases where congenital anatomical variations, pathologic and iatrogenic phenomena can make the IMA not suitable as recipient vessel. This makes useful a preoperative radiologic assessment of IMA features by US or CTA. In our centre, we normally study the IMA preoperatively with color-doppler ultrasound (CDS).

3.2 IMV

Internal mammary veins originated from the confluence of the superior epigastric veins and the musculophrenic veins. This normally takes place at the sixth intercostal space. These veins are comitantes of the homonymous artery.

Generally, two IMVs accompany the IMA till the second/third intercostal spaces where the two venous trunks converge in an unique IMV. An anatomic study from Clark CP III et al showed that in 90 % of the cases, the IMV bifurcation takes place at the third rib on the left side and in 40% on the right side (in 60%of cases bifurcate downwards). This means that at the second intercostal spaces almost always a unique venous trunk is found on both right and left side. This place is the one we now prefer for the preparation of recipient vessels.

In literature, many authors choose the third intercostal space for recipient vessel preparation.

The IMV calibre varies at each intercostal space as the IMA calibre does. At the second intercostal space a vein about 3 mm is generally found. The same calibre is found only in 50 % of the cases at the third intercostal space, being generally not less than 2 mm till the fourth intercostal space. However, by progressing lower than the fourth intercostal space the vein calibre diminishes progressively till 1 mm or less, making the veins not consistent for a reliable anastomosis.

The physiologic IMV venous flow is toward the anonymous vein. The IMV is connected with intercostal and sternal veins at each intercostal space and gives off perforating vein at each intercostal space. A recent anatomic study by Mackey SP et al showed that IMV can contain a variable number of valves, mostly one and sometimes more (till 3). According to their cadaveric study on 32 human bodies, they found valves in 42% of male specimens and in 44% of female specimens. The valves has been found to be caudal to the second intercostal space in about 22 % of the cadavers and caudal to the third space in about 11 %. From a rheologic point of view, this means that once the IMV is divided to be anastomosed to the flap pedicle, the proximal vein should be use because an anterograde flow is present but the distal vein may be not reliable because of valves that would limit the establishment of a retrograde flow.

The successful use of the distal limb of IMV as recipient vein in autologous breast reconstruction makes this logic assertion incorrect. Despite the presence of valve in the IMV, clinical experiences show that a retrograde flow takes place in the IMV distal limb, making it an important further recipient vein in breast reconstruction. This is especially useful when a second venous anastomosis is needed in autologous tissue reconstruction. Many theories has been advanced to explain the presence of a retrograde flow in the IMV despite the valves. Essentially, valves may be:

- Not present at all.
- Not present caudal to the venous anastomotic site.
- *incompetent:* the venous pressure proximal to the valve is higher than distally. This can force the valves making them incompetent.
- *bypassed by collaterals:* the rich connections between IMV and intercostals and sternal veins as well as the perforating branches of the IMV at each intercostal space can allow a bypass of the valvular system by these collaterals.

- Both incompetent and bypassed by collaterals.

The retrograde flow in the distal limb of the IMV can be explained as follows:

- The IMV flow has been interrupted by the venous split and the corresponding decreased venous pressure gradient through the anonymous vein does not directly exist anymore for the IMV distal limb.
- the corresponding deep superior epigastric vein has been ligated if a double-pedicle DIEP flap has been harvested, because the DIE has been harvested. This reduces the venous flow and pressure through the IMV distal limb.
- The arterial input into the flap is responsible for the flap venous outflow and pressure.
- The higher venous pressure gradient of the flap output on the remaining IMV distal limb venous afferents makes the direction of the venous flow reversed, thus a retrograde flow takes place.

4. Indications

Lower abdominal tissue nowadays represents the gold standard in breast autologous tissue reconstruction.

The four zones DIEAP flap identifies the case when the whole lower abdominal skin and soft tissue is harvested.

Regarding the recipient site in single breast reconstruction, the four zone DIEP flap has these general indications:

- Need to *reconstruct a large breast* in patients with large contralateral breast that does not wish to reduce their breast size.
- Need to *reconstruct the breast mound and extramammary skin*, as in patients undergoing radical mastectomy o MRM with added skin resection. (figure 7)
- Patients with *rib cage congenital or acquired depressions* (i.e. Radiated mastectomy patients with expander). In these cases there is the need to fill the depression besides the breast mound reconstruction. (figure 8)

Regarding the donor site, the four zone lower abdominal tissue is required in single breast reconstruction in:

- Patients with scant abdominal tissue;
- Patients with *infraumbilical vertical scar* (in this case a double-pedicle flap is mandatory if more than a hemiabdominal flap is required).

Contraindications applied for standard DIEP and SIEA flaps are applied also to the four zone lower abdominal flap.

5. Flap markings

In the preoperative setting, abdominal mutidetector row computer tomography (MDCT) is very helpful to study the vascular architecture of the lower abdominal soft tissues in order to plan a reliable flap.

At our institution, all patients scheduled for lower abdominal flap breast reconstruction, undergo abdominal MDCT to investigate, localize and select "dominant" perforators. Care is taken on: diameters of perforators and their branching into the subcutaneous layer, perforator's localization, intramuscular course, connection to the superficial epigastric veins (SIEV), DIEA branching pattern and superficial venous architecture.

Indications for the four zone lower abdominal flap

Relative to the recipient site features:

- Patient with large native breasts who does not wish to reduce the contralateral breast.
- Patient with wide skin resection besides the mastectomy
- Patients with rib cage costitutional or acquired deformities.
- Patients with both the needing of reconstruct large breast and rib cage deformities.

Relative to the donor site features:

- Patients with scant abdominal tissue.

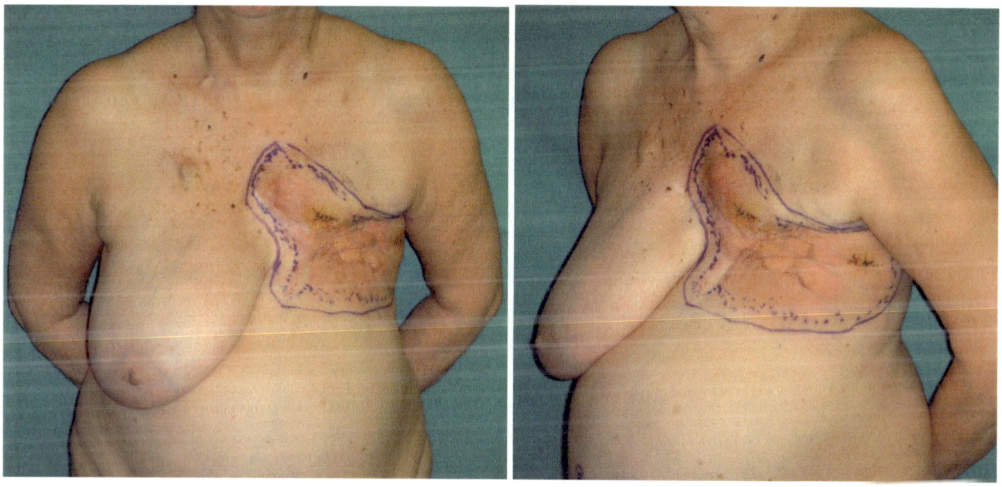

Fig. 7. Patient with a history of modified radical mastectomy, left axillary clearance and adjuvant radiation therapy. The patient developed a chest wall angiosarcoma. The skin resection needed is wider than the classic mastectomy pattern.

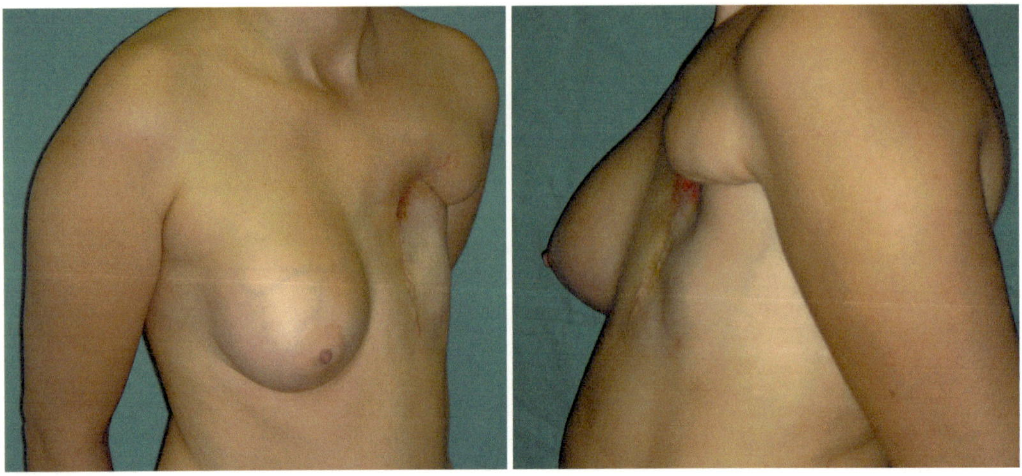

Fig. 8. Patient with a history of modified radical mastectomy, immediate tissue-expander placement and adjuvant radiation therapy. She developed a breast carcinoma recurrence. Note the left side chest wall depression as sequelae of the tissue-expander contracture.

When a four zone DIEP flap is needed for unilateral breast reconstruction, a double-pedicle DIEP flap is usually planned, as follows:

- when "true dominant" perforators are found on each hemiabdomen, the four zone flap will be raised based on these two perforators. The presence of a "dominant" lateral row perforator would be preferable in the double-pedicle four zone DIEP flap as better perfusion of the lateralmost part of the flap is expected. Moreover, dissection will be easier and faster than with the medial row perforators.
- when one or multiple medium caliber perforators are found without the presence of a "true dominant" perforator, the best perforators are selected on each hemiabdomen. In this cases, more than one perforator for each hemiabdomen can be included in the flap, preferring to include perforators of the same row.

A four zone lower abdominal flap can be also raised on one DIE pedicle and one SIE pedicle. As a premise of the followings, it has to be remarked that we prefer to inset the flap after 180 degree rotation, in order to place the fattiest portion of the flap (i.e. the periumbelical one) to reconstruct the inferior quadrants. In the case of a flap raised on one DIE pedicle and one SIE pedicle, due to short pedicle of the superficial system (range 5 to 8 cm), it would be preferable to have the superficial pedicle on the ipsilateral side of the breast to reconstruct in order to avoid the need of further recipient vessel dissection than the internal mammary vessels (i.e. thoracodorsal vessels) and/or to use an artery and vein graft to allow anastomosis to the internal mammary vessels. Another option is to use the contralateral SIE pedicle anastomosed to the ipsilateral DIE pedicle (distal DIE stump or other row stump) with an intraflap anastomosis.

There are rare cases, when a four zone DIEP flap can be safely raised based on only one pedicle with additional SIEV supercharging in patients without mid-line abdominal scar. This is possible when a "true dominant" medial row perforator is present, a large caliber SIEV (more than 1.5 mm) is found along with good midline cross-over SIEV connections (grade III to IV).

The perforators identified by MDCT are then reported on the abdominal site, possibly with aid of CDS that further analyzes the caliber of perforators and flow velocity.

Markings begin on the abdominal area while the patient is in a supine position. The markings follows those of the standard abdominoplasty.

6. Surgical technique

6.1 Double-pedicle DIEP flap harvest

The patient is placed in supine position with the arm of the side of affected breast elevated in order to expose the axilla (in immediate reconstruction) or the arms lying along the sides (in delayed reconstruction). The harvest of the flap begins by the dissection of the SIEV bilaterally. If a suitable SIEA is encountered on the ipsilateral side of the affected breast with a diameter of 1,5 mm at the level of the inferior skin incision, it can be dissected as well. The decision if the ipsilateral flap has to be raised on the SIE pedicle or on the DIEP pedicle depends on the characteristics of the dominant perforator/s. In case the dominant perforator/s caliber is bigger than 1,5mm at the preoperative MDCT, the choice shift toward the DIEP flap.

Harvesting the flap is done in standardized approach using perforators from both sides (or SIEA on one side). The DIE pedicle has to be dissected up to its entry into external iliac vessels to keep it as long as possible. The distal extent of DIE pedicle and the stump of the second row, when present, have to be dissected 1-2 centimeters futher to be ready for possible additional anastomoses.

6.2 Vascular construct

After dissection of both vascular systems on each side, consideration has to be given to the location and the dissection of the recipient vessels. Recipient vessels selection is highly influenced by the configuration that could provide the best orientation for flap positioning and inset.

Over the last thirty years the internal mammary vessels has become the gold-standard as recipients in autologous tissue breast reconstruction. Moreover, their diameter is favorable as it normally matches the one of the deep inferior epigastric artery and veins allowing an easier end-to-end anastomosis. However, other recipients site can be used. The most frequent alternative recipients to the internal mammary vessels are the thoracodorsal vessels. However, these vessels are laterally located and more prone to damage from previous axillary surgery and from radiation therapy. Furthermore, their use may preclude the possibility to rely on the LD flap as salvage option.

When raising the double-pedicle lower abdominal flap entails the need of simultaneous restoration of the blood supply of both pedicles. Various methods of reconstructing the blood supply of double pedicle flaps have been reported.

The most common technique is to combine two different recipient vessels. Many anatomical solutions exist, the most popular one being internal mammary vessels, or its perforators when possible, and thoracodorsal vessels. In case they could not be both available, such as in some delayed reconstruction, other options are still possible:

- Circumflex scapular vessels.

- Serratus branches
- Thoracoacromial vessels.
- Contralateral internal mammary vessels, with the drawback of an additional visible scar.

However, the split internal mammary vessels can be used to reconstruct both the arterial and venous flow of the double-pedicle flap. Since its first description almost ten years ago, we routinely use the inferior limb of the internal mammary artery and vein when an arterial and/or venous supercharging is needed.

Thus, there are two possibilities to reconstruct the vascular connection of the double-pedicle flap by using a single set of internal mammary vessels, as follows:

- *Double anastomoses to a single set of internal mammary vessels.* DIE double anastomoses to both the superior and inferior limbs of the split internal mammary vessels, being with antegrade flow the superior limb anastomosis and with retrograde flow the inferior limb one (figure 9), as already described by Li S et al. and Xu H et al. This is also our preferred choice.

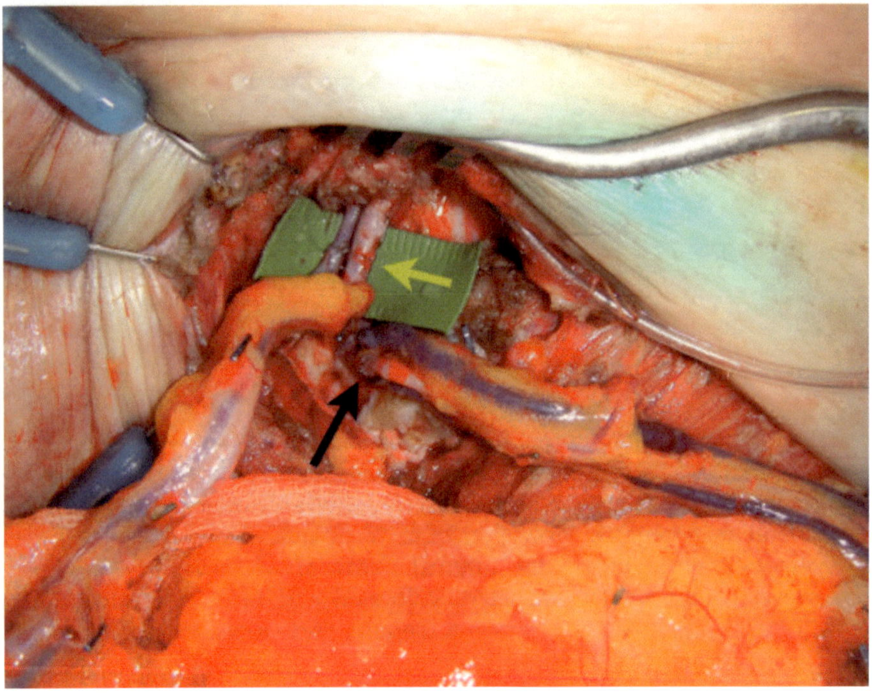

Fig. 9. The two DIEP pedicle are anastomosed to a single set of internal mammary vessels. The black arrow points the contralateral DIEP pedicle anastomosed to the inferior limb of the internal mammary vessel. The blood flow is retrograde. The yellow arrow points the homolateral DIEP pedicle anastomosed to the superior limb of the internal mammary vessel. The blood flow is antegrade.

- *The "serial" intraflap anastomosis.* Premising that the flap is 180 degree rotated, the contralateral DIE pedicle is anastomosed to the ipsilateral pedicle. The intraflap anastomosis may be performed on the abdomen while the flap is still perfused by the ipsilateral DIE pedicle, in order to reduce the ischaemia time. Moreover, this allows to check the patency of the intraflap anastomosis before completely dividing the DIE pedicle from the abdomen. This can be accomplished in an end-to-end fashion to the distal end of the ipsilateral DIE pedicle or to the other row stump of the DIE (if present).

One key point in harvesting double pedicle lower abdominal flaps is keeping the pedicles as long as possible to easily perform the additional anastomoses and to accommodate the pedicles according to these spatial configurations, thus avoiding subsequent stretching of the pedicles.

6.3 Cases images

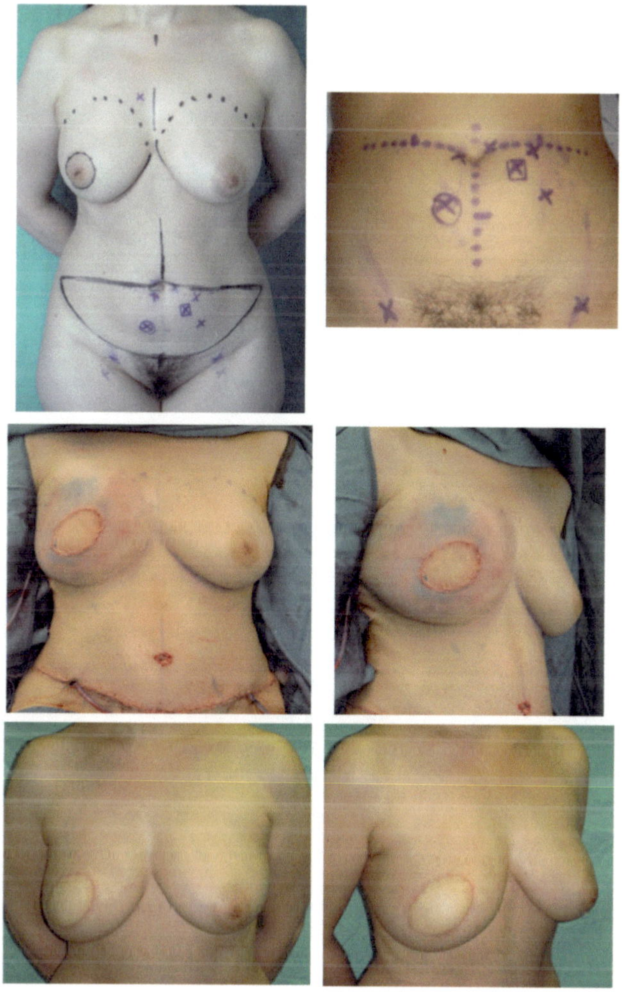

Fig. 10. (Above, left and right) Preoperative planning of a double pedicle DIEP flap. The patient was planned for a Type I skin-sparing mastectomy. She did opt for the autologous tissue reconstruction and did not wish to reduce contralateral breast size. A four zone flap is needed to reconstruct a similar size right breast. The abdominal wall perforators have been

marked after the MDCT scan and CDS. The dominant perforators have been circled. (center, left and right) Intraoperative pictures after flap inset. (Below, left and right) Six month postoperative pictures.

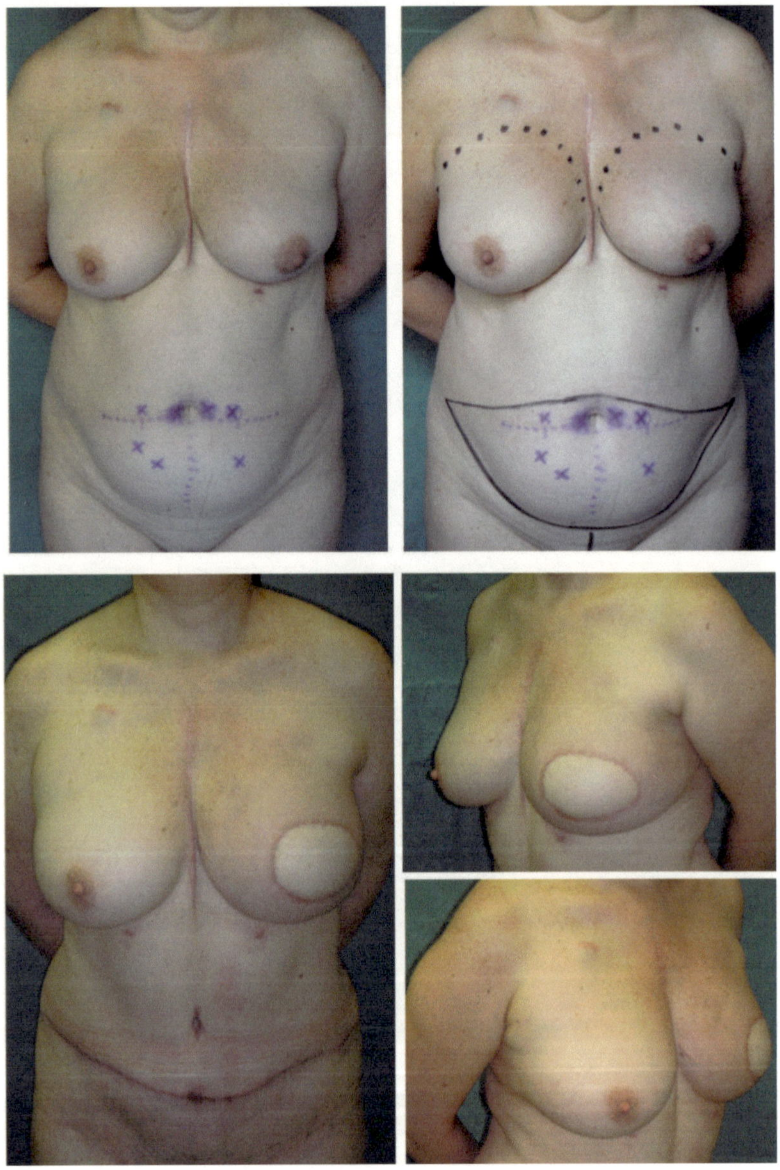

Fig. 11. (Above, left and right) Preoperative planning of a double pedicle DIEP flap. The patient had history of timoma extirpartion and mantle irradiation. She was planned for a Type I skin-sparing mastectomy and autologous tissue reconstruction. She did not wish to reduce contralateral breast size. A four zone flap is needed to reconstruct a similar size left breast. The abdominal wall perforators have been marked after the MDCT scan and CDS. The dominant perforators have been circled. (Below, left and right) Three month postoperative pictures

6.4 Flap inset

The flap is usually *folded* on one or both ends to create the most projecting point of the breast mound according with the contra lateral volume and shape of the breast.

Special attention has to be payed before the anastomoses to the spatial configuration of the pedicles in order to avoid kinking, twisting or their stretching. This is particularly true when the double DIE pedicle is anastomosed to both the superior and inferior limb of the internal mammary vessels.

DellaCroce FJ et al. extensively described another option for a full lower abdominal flap inset in single breast reconstruction with "stacked" DIEP flap. This is a layered combination in the recipient site of a two hemiabdominal free DIEP/SIEA flaps. Firstly, one hemiabdominal DIEP flap is deepithelialized and inset into the breast pocket, orienting its vascular pedicle for the anastomosis with the internal mammary vessels. Then, the second flap is inserted after performing the intraflap to the distal stump or other row stump of the first flap pedicle (DIEP or SIEA flaps).

7. Postoperative care and complications

Postoperative management of a four zone DIEP/SIEA flap are identical to that of a standard DIEP flap as well as the complications that could be experienced. Compared to a unipedicle DIEP flap, the likelihood of venous congestion are rarely experienced as we should think to double-pedicle flap as two I-II zones flaps. Consequentially, the rate of liponecrosis experienced in double-pedicle flaps is also faraway smaller than a unipedicle flap.

8. Acknowledgment

Thanks to Emiliano Visconti, M.D., Resident in-training, Department of Bioimages and Radiologic Sciences, University Hospital "A. Gemelli", Rome - Italy for its contribution in digital artworks

9. References

Arnez ZM, Valdatta L, Tyler MP et al (1995) Anatomy of the IM veins and their use in free TRAM flap breast reconstruction. Br J Plast Surg 48:540.

Bailey SH, Saint-Cyr M, Wong C, Mojallal A, Zhang K, Ouyang D, Arbique G, Trussler A, Rohrich RJ. The single dominant medial row perforator DIEP flap in breast reconstruction: three-dimensional perforasome and clinical results. Plast Reconstr Surg. 2010 Sep;126(3):739-51.

Beahm EK, Walton RL. The efficacy of bilateral lower abdominal free flaps for unilateral breast reconstruction.Plast Reconstr Surg. 2007 Jul;120(1):41-54

Clark CP 3rd, Rohrich RJ, Copit S, Pittman CE, Robinson J. An anatomic study of the internal mammary veins: clinical implications for free-tissue-transfer breast reconstruction. Plast Reconstr Surg. 1997 Feb;99(2):400-4.

DellaCroce F J, Sullivan SK, Trahan C. Stacked deep inferior epigastric perforator flap breast reconstruction: a review of 110flaps in 55 cases over 3 years. Plast Reconstr Surg 2011 Mar;127(3):1093-9

Dinner MI, Dowden RV, Scheflan M. Refinements in the use of the transverseabdominal island flap for postmastectomy reconstruction. Ann Plast Surg. 1983 Nov;11(5):362-72.

Hartrampf CR. Breast reconstruction with living tissue. Norfolk: Raven Press Ltd. Hampton Press Publishing Company; 1991

Holm C, Mayer M, Hofter E, Ninkovic M. Perfusion zones of the DIEP flap revisted: a clinical study. Plast Reconstr Surg 2006; 117:37-43.

Kerr-Valentic MA, Gottlieb LJ, Agarwal JP. The retrograde limb of the internal mammary vein: an additional outflow option in DIEP flap breast reconstruction. Plast Reconstr Surg. 2009 Sep;124(3):717-21.

Li S, Mu L, Li Y, xu J, Yang M, Zhao Z, Liu Y, Li J, Ling Y. Breast reconstruction with the free bipedicled inferior TRAM flap by anastomosis to the proximal and distal ends of internal mammary vessels. J Reconstr Microsurg 2002;18:161-168

Li S, Mu L, Li Y, xu J, Yang M, Zhao Z, Liu Y, Li J, Ling Y. Clinical study of the hemodynamics of both ends (proximal and distal) of the internal mammary artery and its following-up. Chin J Plast Surg 2002;18:140-142

Mackey SP, Ramsey KW. Exploring the myth of the valveless internal mammary vein--a cadaveric study. J Plast Reconstr Aesthet Surg.2011 Sep;64(9):1174-9.

Murray AC, Rozen WM, Alonso-Burgos A, Ashton MW, Garcia-Tutor E, Whitaker IS. The anatomy and variations of the internal thoracic (internal mammary) artery and implications in autologous breast reconstruction: clinical anatomical study and literature review. Surg Radiol Anat. 2011 Oct 11. [Epub ahead of print]

Rahmanian-Schwarz A, Rothenberger J, Hirt B, Luz O, Schaller HE. A combined anatomical and clinical study for quantitative analysis of the microcirculation in the classic perfusion zones of the deep inferior epigastric artery perforator flap. Plast Reconstr Surg. 2011 Feb;127(2):505-13.

Rozen WM, Pan WR, Le Roux CM, Taylor GI, Ashton MW. The venous anatomy of the anterior abdominal wall: an anatomical and clinical study. Plast Reconstr Surg. 2009 Sep;124(3):848-53.

Saint-Cyr M. Assessing perforator architecture. Clin Plast Surg. 2011 Apr;38(2):175-202.

Salgarello M, Barone-Adesi L, Sturla M, Masetti R, Mu L. Needing a large DIEAP flap for unilateral breast reconstruction: double-pedicle flap and unipedicle flap with additional venous discharge. Microsurgery 2010;30(2):111-7

Salgarello M, Cervelli D, Barone-Adesi L, Finocchi V. Anterograde and retrograde flow anastomoses to the internal mammary vessels in the third intercostal space. J Reconstr Microsurg. 2010 Nov;26(9):637-8

Schaverien M, Saint-Cyr M, Arbique G, Brown SA. Arterial and venous anatomy of the deep inferior epigastric perforator and superficial inferior epigastric artery flaps. Plast Reconstr Surg. 2008 Jun;121(6):1909-19.

Scheflan M, Dinner MI. The transverse abdominal island flap: part I. Indications, contraindications, results, and complications. Ann Plast Surg. 1983 Jan;10(1):24-35.

Scheflan M, Dinner MI. The transverse abdominal island flap: Part II. Surgical technique. Ann Plast Surg. 1983 Feb;10(2):120-9.

Wong C, Saint-Cyr M, Mojallal A, Schaub T, Bailey SH, Myers S, Brown S, Rohrich RJ. Perforasome of the DIEP flap: vascular anatomy of the lateral versus medial row perforators and clinical implications. Plast Reconstr Surg. 2010 Mar;125(3):772-82.

Xu H, Dong J, Wang T. Bipedicle deep inferior epigastric perforator flap for unilateral breast reconstruction: seven years' experience. Plast Reconstr Surg 2009 Dec;124(6):1797-807

Zeltzer AA, Andrades P, Hamdi M, Blondeel PN, Van Landuyt K. The use of a single set of internal mammary recipient vessels in bilateral free flap breast reconstruction. Plast Reconstr Surg. 2011 Jun;127(6):153e-4e. No abstract available.

10

The Omentum Flap

Sirlei dos Santos Costa and Rosa Maria Blotta
Reconstructive Surgery Center of Porto Alegre,
Universidade Federal do Rio Grande do Sul,
Brazil

1. Introduction

The omentum flap with its well known characteristics has been used in the last two centuries to recover the most different purposes. Nowadays, its most recently observed attributes permits new applications with superb results, mainly in breast surgery.

In 1888, Senn employed it to protect an intestinal anastomosis (Irons et al,1983) and in 1963, Kiricuta described the use of the great omentum as a flap in cases of breast cancer surgery (Kiricuta, 1963).

McLean and Buncke in 1972, described the omentum free flap (McLean & Buncke, 1972). Laparoscopic harvesting of the omentum was carried out for the first time by Saltz in 1993 in order to repair soft tissue defects in the knee (Saltz et al, 1993).

Costa presented a totally closed video laparoscopic procedure in 1996, where the flap was dissected in the abdominal cavity and transposed through a subcutaneous tunnel to the thoracic wall, used to treat breast cancer patients. In 1998, for the first time, Costa utilized the omentum flap to treat Poland's syndrome deformities (Costa, 1998).

Various options have been proposed to reconstruct the breast's volume, including local flaps, expanders and implants, transposition of the latissimus dorsi, gluteus or the rectus abdominis muscle flaps. Although these techniques may achieve excellent results, depending on the degree of deformity, satisfaction with aesthetic reconstruction of the more detailed deformities, have been disappointing. Moreover, an additional scar is left in the patient's donor region of those muscular flaps.

In an attempt to solve these problems, the laparoscopically harvested omentum flap can be considered an excellent reconstructive option that offers a very interesting aesthetic result. The advantages of the omentum flap are numerous and significant: it is extremely malleable, adapts easily to irregular surfaces, and has a long and reliable vascular pedicle. The omentum is composed of highly vascularized fatty connective tissue and is attached to the greater curvature of the stomach. It adheres to the transverse colon forming the gastrocolic ligament. It continues separating the transverse colon and folds of the small intestine from the anterior abdominal wall. Left and right gastroepiploic arteries supply blood and this vascular net is anatomically constant enough so as to enable systematic dissection. The flap measures approximately 25x35 cm and its volume varies according to patient size (Arnold et al, 1976; Das, 1976).

In the first six months after the procedure the omentum flap presents a variable growth that needs to be considered when planning repair of the deformity (Costa et al, 2010; Costa et al, 2011).

The omentum (Fig.1) has several advantages including the flap's large absorption capacity, which reduces the postoperative time period during which drains are needed, since the flap helps absorb the lymphatic fluid resulting from lymph node dissection. The use of laparoscopy to harvest the flap offers minimal insult to the abdominal wall (Fig. 2), ensuring a short and comfortable postoperative recovery period (Cothier-Savey et al, 2001; Ferron et al, 2007; Zaha et al, 2006). A review of all available literature about laparoscopically harvested omentum flaps indicates that there are no severe postoperative complications.

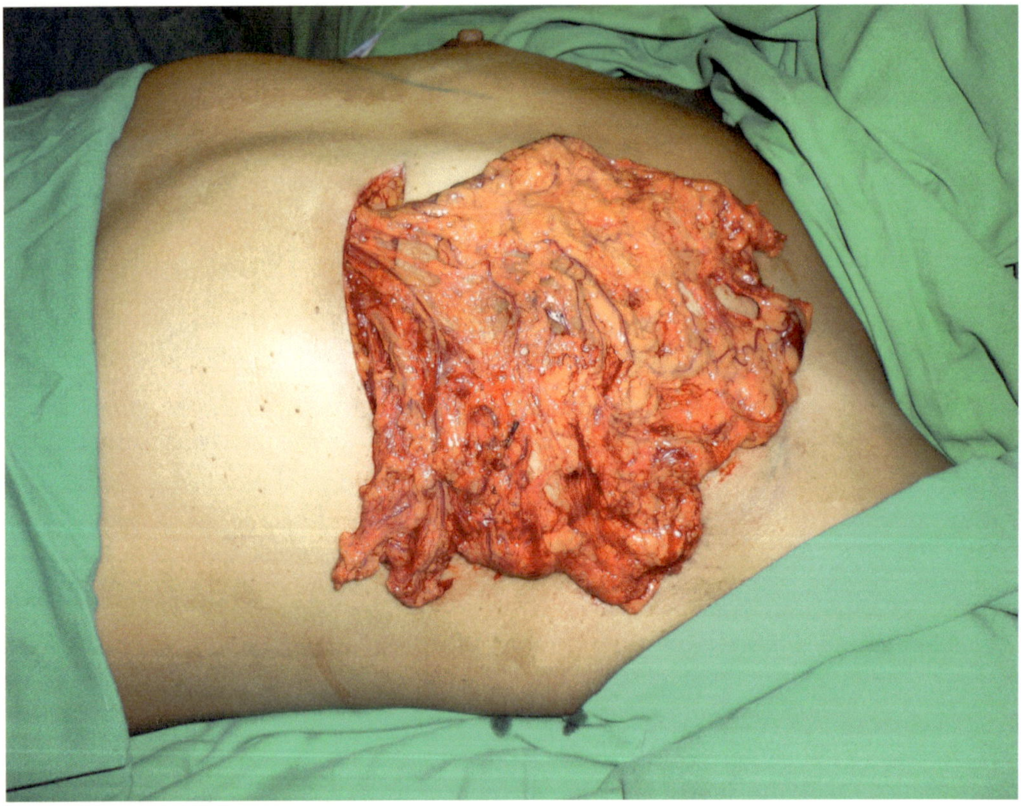

Fig. 1. The omentum flap over the thorax wall.

A difficulty of this technique is that it is not possible to precisely define the final omentum volume available in order to plan the reconstruction. The complementation of the volume and equalization with the contra-lateral breast may be done during the same surgical time or, even better, at another time, four to six months later; when it is possible to take into consideration the spontaneous growth of the flap that always occurs after its transposition.

Finally, the resulting consistency is very similar to the contra-lateral breast, enabling more satisfactory reparation of the anterior axillary pillar than any other reconstructive option.

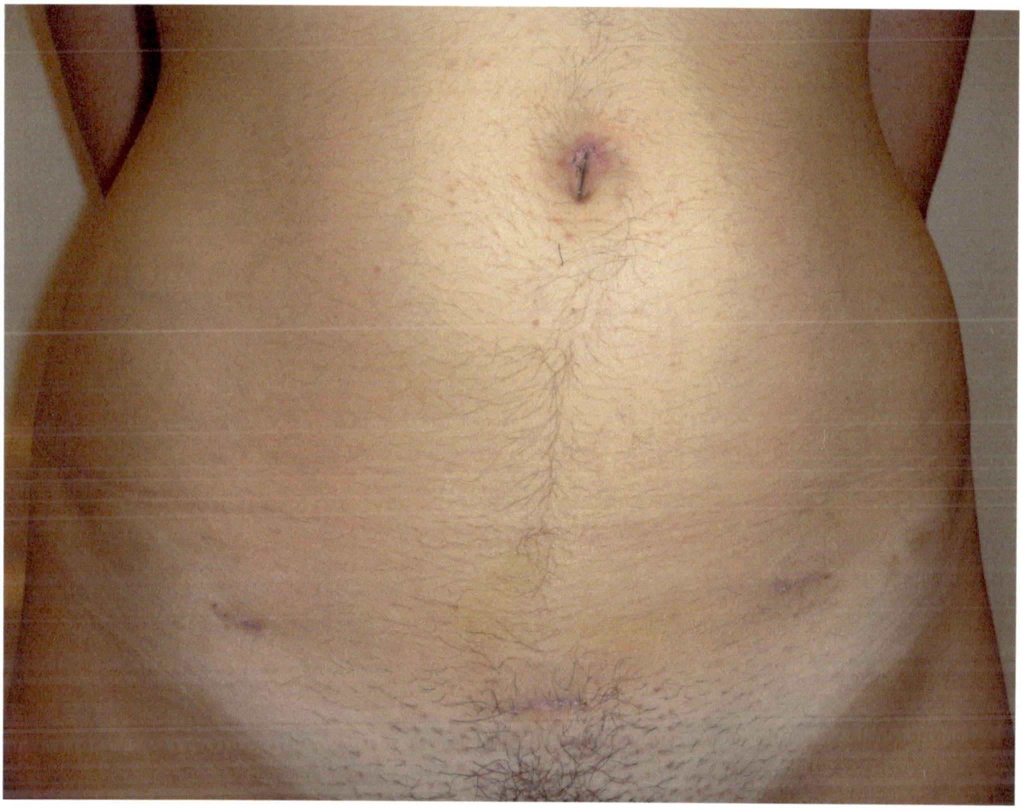

Fig. 2. Scars in the abdominal wall.

2. Indications

The omentum flap may be used in many different situations.

In breast reconstruction it can be used to treat congenital malformations and the principal utilization of the omentum flap is in the Poland's syndrome that is characterized by abnormalities in thorax wall, vertebrae and superior member. It is possible to treat the transverse sulcus in the anterior axillary's pillar, the infraclavicular depression and the anomalous breast contour with thin cover, unable to hide an implant (Fig. 3)

Benign diseases sequels, such as after a giant fibro adenoma resection (Fig. 4) or in visible wrinklings through the thin breast skin covering an implant that shows the visible muscle contraction, can be treated with the omentum flap (Fig. 5).

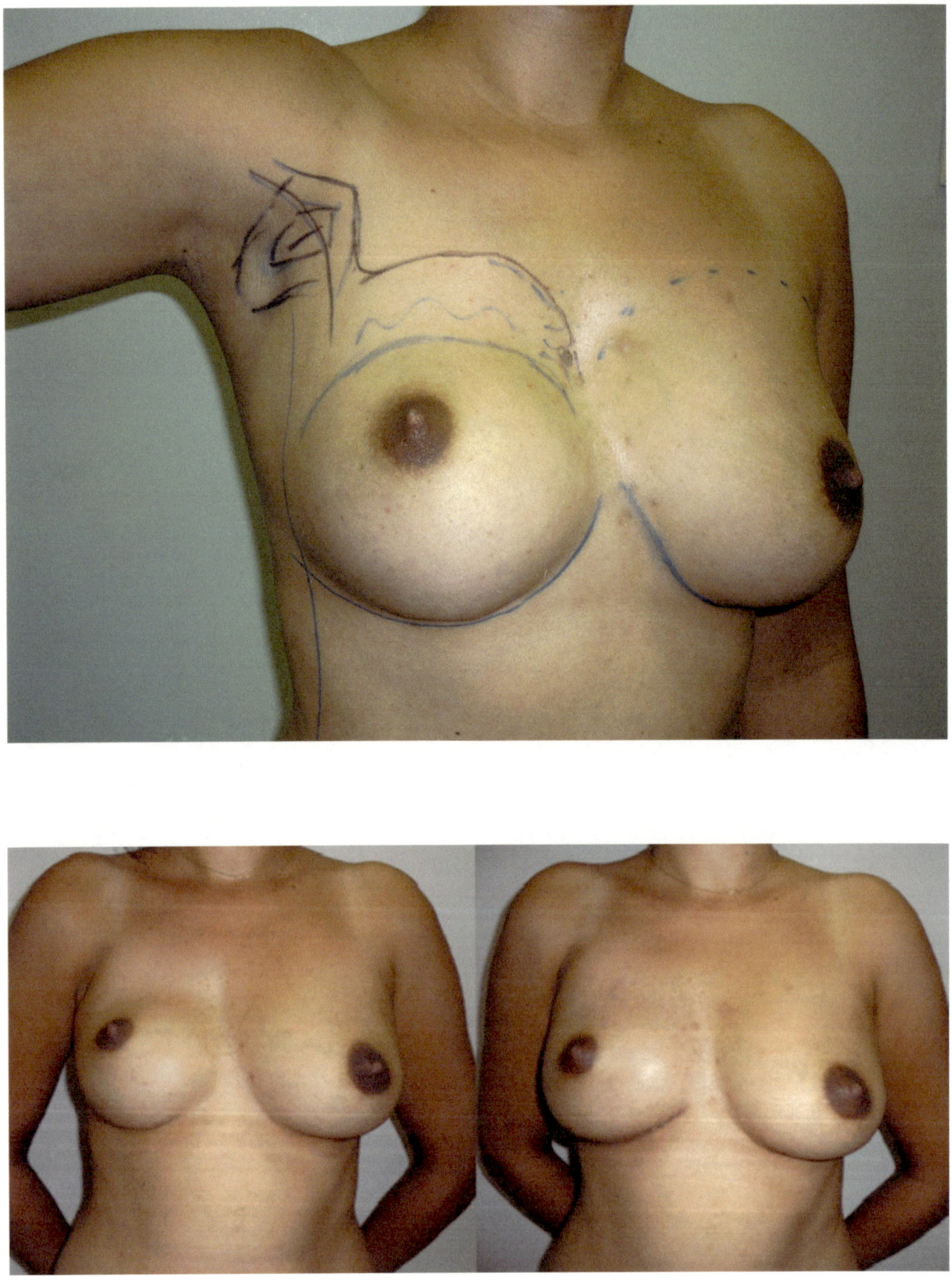

Fig. 3. Patient with Poland's syndrome treated with omentum flap.

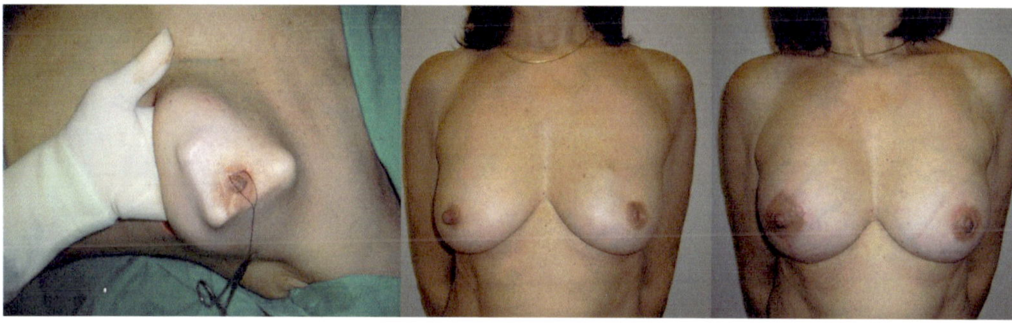

Fig. 4. Sequel of a giant fibro adenoma resection of the left breast treated with omentum flap.

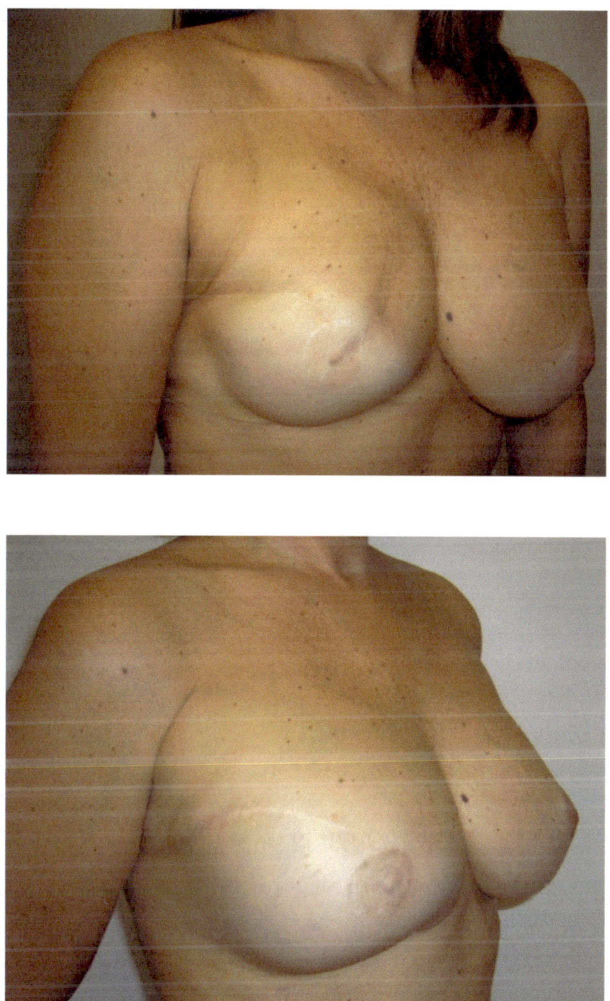

Fig. 5. The thin breast skin covering an implant and showing the visible muscle contraction treated with the omentum flap.

After breast cancer treatment, it can be used in partial or total resection of the breast, with or without prosthesis to complete the final volume.

The omentum is particularly interesting in radiotherapy sequels where its use may repair the ischemic condition of the skin, decreasing the local fibrosis and giving a soft appearance to the breast (Fig. 6).

There are many advantages to use the omentum flap: when dissected by video laparoscopy the abdominal wall is preserved with minimal scars. It is extremely malleable and adapts to the surface irregularities. It has a long pedicle with big caliber and the procedure presents minimal blood loss with short hospitalization time and fast recovery. The omentum flap has big absorption capability and stimulates new angiogenesis.

Other flaps like latissimus dorsi, gluteus or the rectus abdominis muscle flaps are preserved for another situation and the new breast consistency is similar to a natural one.

There are limitations for omentum use as the necessity of skin enough to cover the new breast, previous diseases in abdominal cavity that may damage the integrity of the omentum (inflammatory or surgical sequel), the variability of its volume and size and the necessity of the use of implants in some cases to complete the final volume desired.

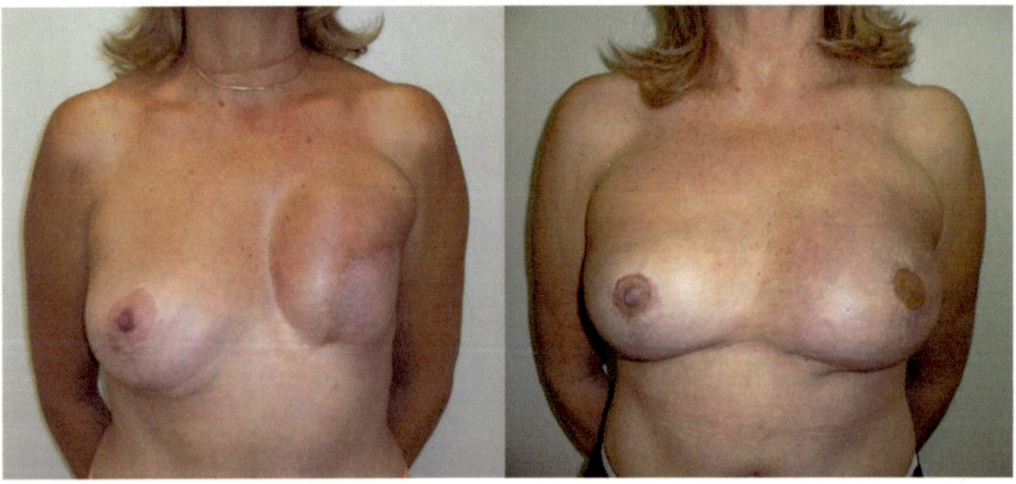

Fig. 6. Radiotherapy sequels treated with Omentum flap.

2.1 Omentum in breast cancer

The first breast reconstructions were carried out in surgical fields left by mastologists with great skin loss, which left the aesthetic result of the reconstruction difficult and poor. The advances in diagnosis and treatment of breast carcinoma over the last years have permitted greater preservation of the skin.

The omentum flap can be used in patients with sufficient skin to reconstruct a neo-breast, small than the first, but with a normal shape. In case of breast ptosis, where the removal of the entire breast is necessary, but part of the skin can be preserved, the omentum can be a good option.

Even in small breasts, in case of small tumors, where it is possible to conserve sufficient skin to reconstruct a neo-breast, the omentum flap can be an alternative to add volume (Fig. 7).

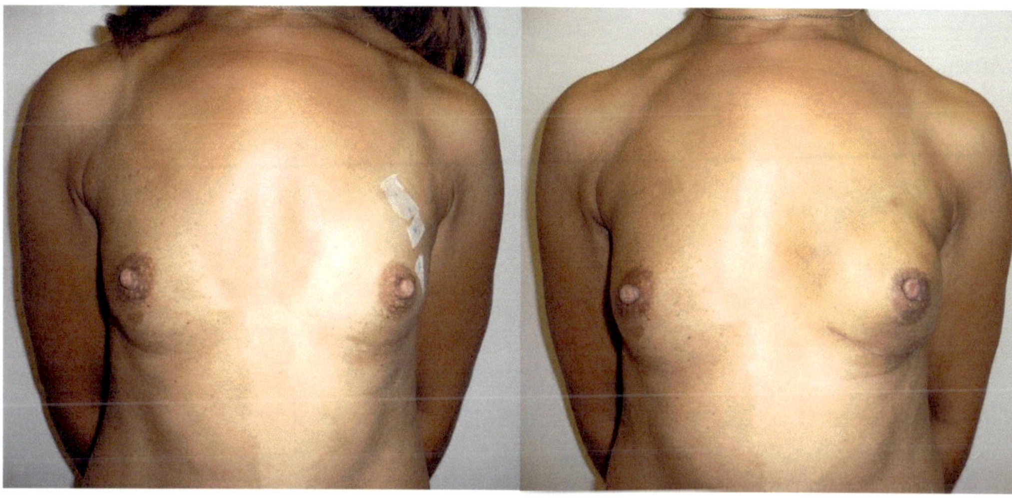

Fig. 7. Left breast reconstruction with omentum flap after left mastectomy.

The complementary post-operative treatment in patients with breast cancer using radiotherapy may cause fibrosis and vascular alterations resulting in a fragile skin which is inadequate to receive a prosthesis.

In these cases, the omentum can be transposed and offers a considerable improvement in vascularization and malleability of the skin flaps, enabling a breast reconstruction with expansor and prosthesis (Fig. 6).

2.2 Omentum in breast malformations

The main congenital malformation of breast is the Poland's syndrome (Fig.8). Patients with Poland's syndrome may present with numerous ailments such as absence of the sternal-costal portion of the *pectoralis* major muscle, upper extremity hypoplasia, brachysyndactyly, and syndactyly. Various other muscles may also be affected: *pectoralis* minor, latissimus dorsi, serratus anterior, external oblique, and deltoid. Skeletal deformities such as partial agenesis of the ribs, *sternum*, and spine (sometimes with *scoliosis*) may occur. Breast hypoplasia or aplasia, nipple abnormalities, skin atrophy, and absence of the sweat glands and surrounding structures are other features (Cobben et al, 1989; Bainbridge et al, 1991; Perez et al, 1996).

In Poland's syndrome, thoracic wall deformities are not as obvious at birth as hand deformities. However, when female patients reach adolescence, the thoracic deformity seems to become more evident as absence or asymmetry of the developing breasts occurs. To minimize this, a tissue expander may be placed in the developing breast to accompany contra-lateral breast growth. Unfortunately, however, surgical treatment of the breast deformities cannot be accomplished before 17-19 years of age, when development of the body is complete.

The most uncomfortable physical alterations are the transversal skin fold in the anterior axillary pillar (caused by the absence or hypoplasia of the pectoral muscles), the infra-clavicular depression, and an anomalous breast contour (Seyfer et al, 1988). The resulting aesthetic derangement is difficult to hide, leads to thoracic asymmetry, and imposes significant psychological trauma and social withdrawal in both men and women.

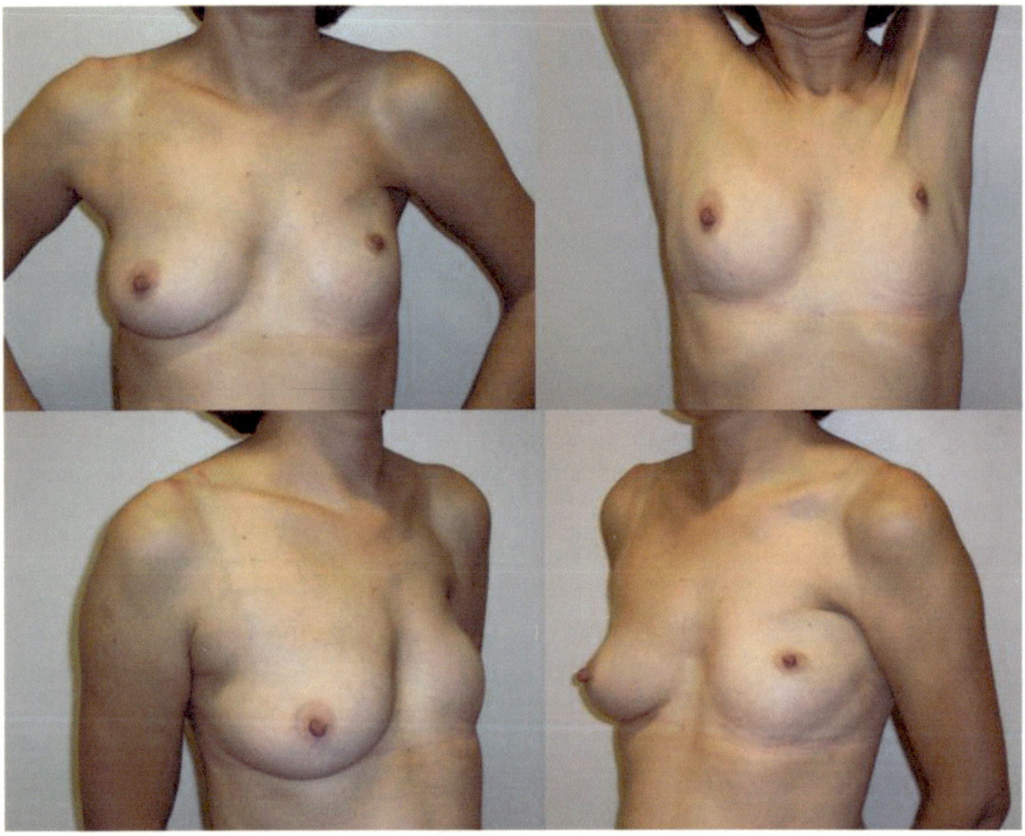

Fig. 8. Patient with Poland's syndrome in the left side.

Patients with Poland's syndrome treated with omentum flap achieved a final aesthetic result better than those patients who were treated with other techniques, as shown in figures 9 to 11. With the omentum flap, it is possible to correct particular details of breast contour due to flap tissue malleability, an outcome impossible to achieve with all other techniques. Utilization of the omentum flap improves breast contouring, filling in the infra-clavicular depression and reconstructing the anterior axillary pillar. When implants are employed below the flap, it provides appropriate concealment and a better quality coverage system that results in improved symmetry with the opposite hemi-thorax. The palpation of the flap in the new site is similar in consistency to a normal breast. This flap is the only one that gives the patient this possibility. All other flaps do not achieve such a perfectly similar consistency of the breast-like omentum.

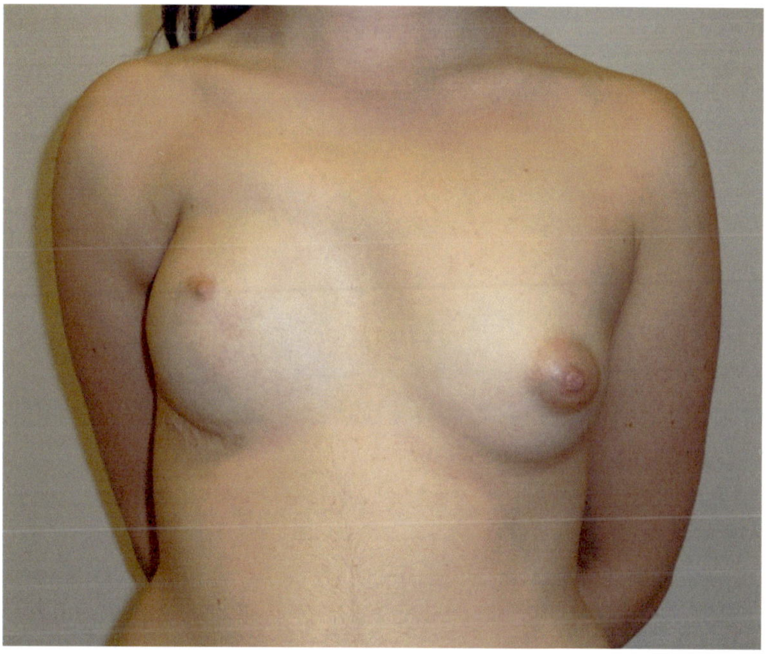

Fig. 9. Patient with Poland's syndrome in the right side first treated only with a prosthesis with a poor aesthetic result.

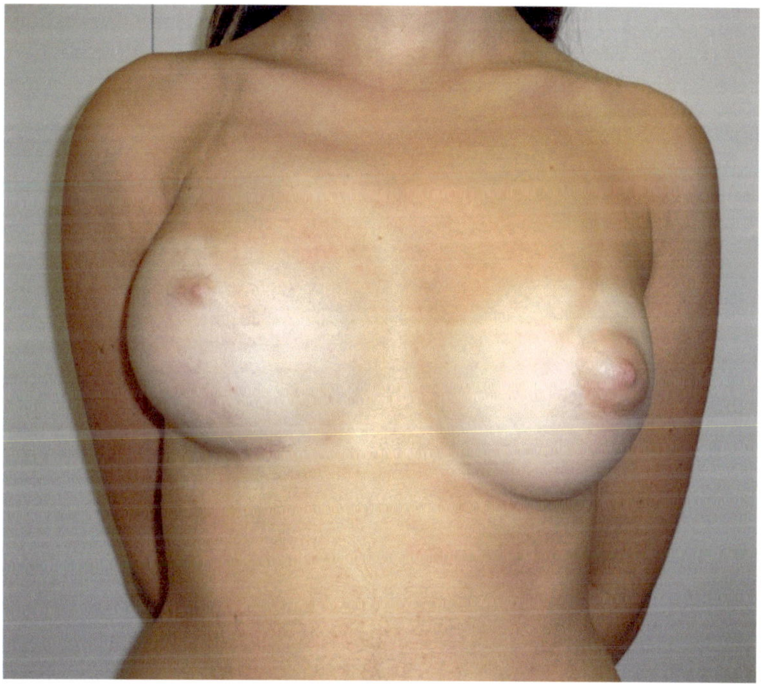

Fig. 10. Patient after omentum flap transposition to the right breast and bilateral breast augmentation with prosthesis.

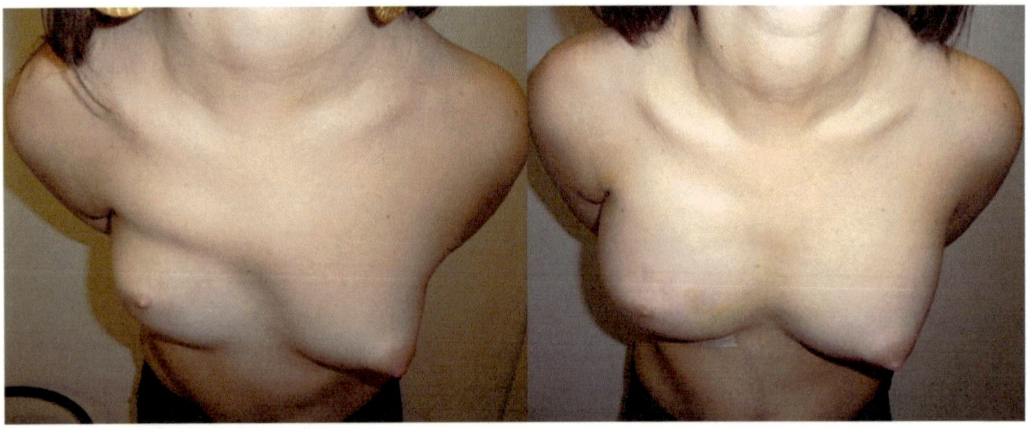

Fig. 11. A comparative view of the breasts.

3. Surgical techinique

Harvesting of the omentum flap is performed using standard laparoscopic surgery techniques. Four ports are usually placed; CO_2 pneumoperitoneum of 8-10 mmHg is maintained during the procedure. Dissection of the flap is initiated by clamping and elevation of the gastric wall (Fig. 12). The right gastro-epiploic artery (RGEA) is isolated and preserved; ligations of the short gastric arteries along the greater curvature are then performed until the left gastro-epiploic artery (LGEA) is reached (Fig. 13). The omentum should be disconnected from the transverse colon by a carefully dissection in order to preserve the mesocolon vascularity (Fig. 14). The flap will be totally liberated when ligations of the LGEA are accomplished adjacent to the left colic flexure (Fig. 15).

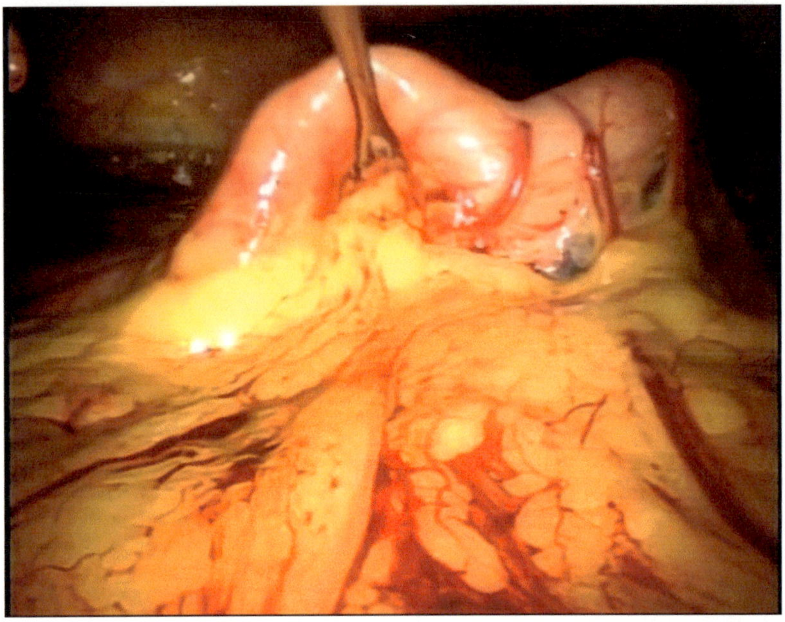

Fig. 12. Elevation of gastric wall.

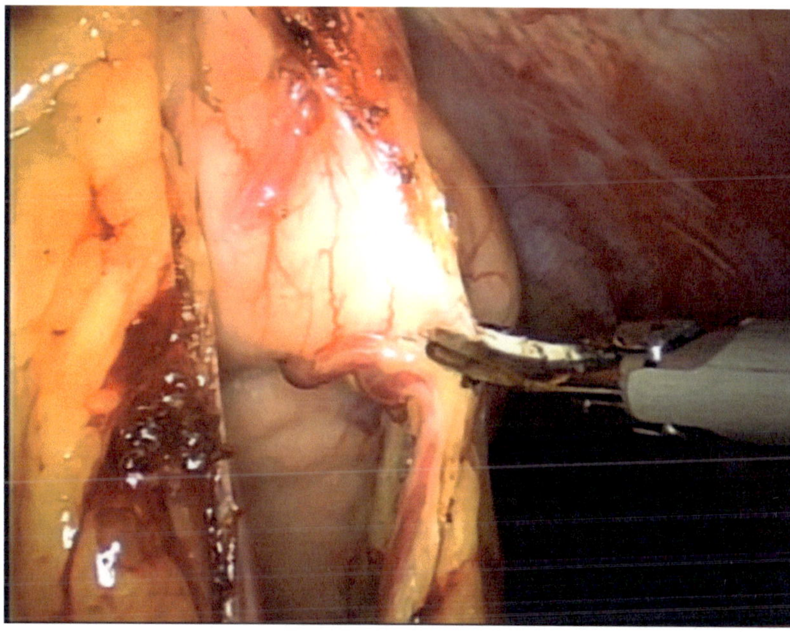

Fig. 13. Ligations of the short gastric arteries along the great gastric curvature showing the RGEA preserved.

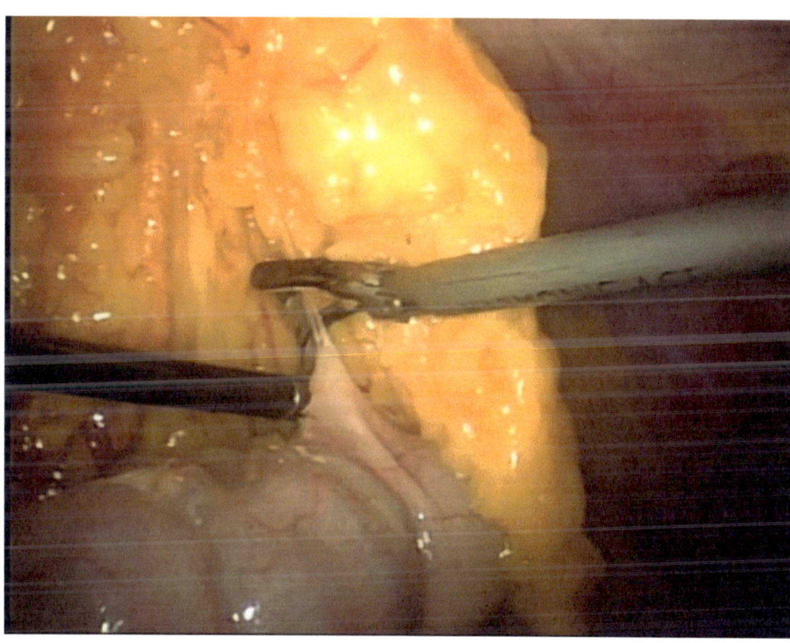

Fig. 14. Liberation of the colon segment of omentum attachment.

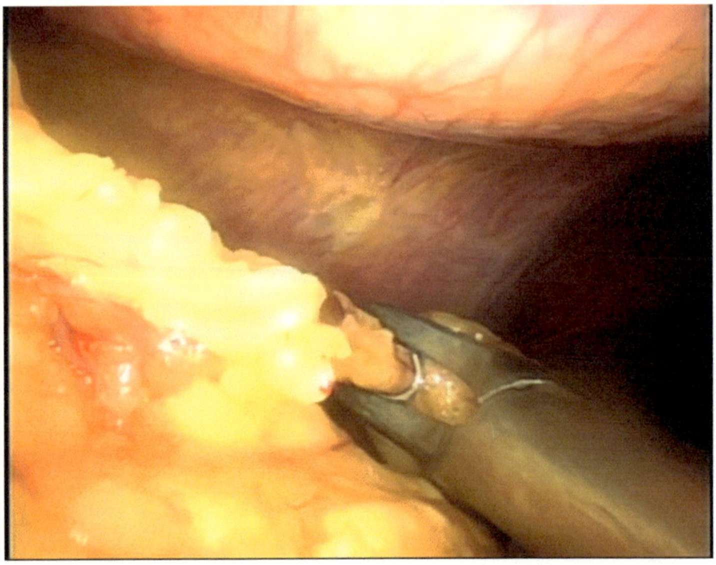

Fig. 15. Ligation of the LGEA.

Finally, through a small incision in the infra-mammary fold a subcutaneous tunnel is dissected until the costal border to open the aponeurose in the medial line, in the direction to the abdominal cavity (Fig. 16). With a digital maneuver the omentum is pulled from the abdominal cavity to the breast region to permit passage and placement of the flap over the specific thoracic wall region (Figs. 17-19). This tunnel is placed to the left or right side of the round ligament depending on the site that needs reconstruction. The location of the deformity is then dissected and filled in with the omentum flap, which is fixed into place. Both procedures are performed under video-assisted guidance.

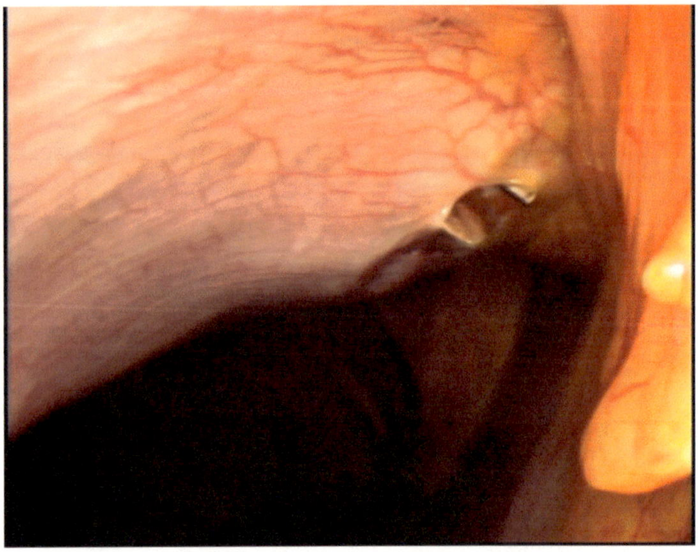

Fig. 16. Incision in the peritoneum to communicate the abdominal cavity with the breast region through a subcutaneous tunnel.

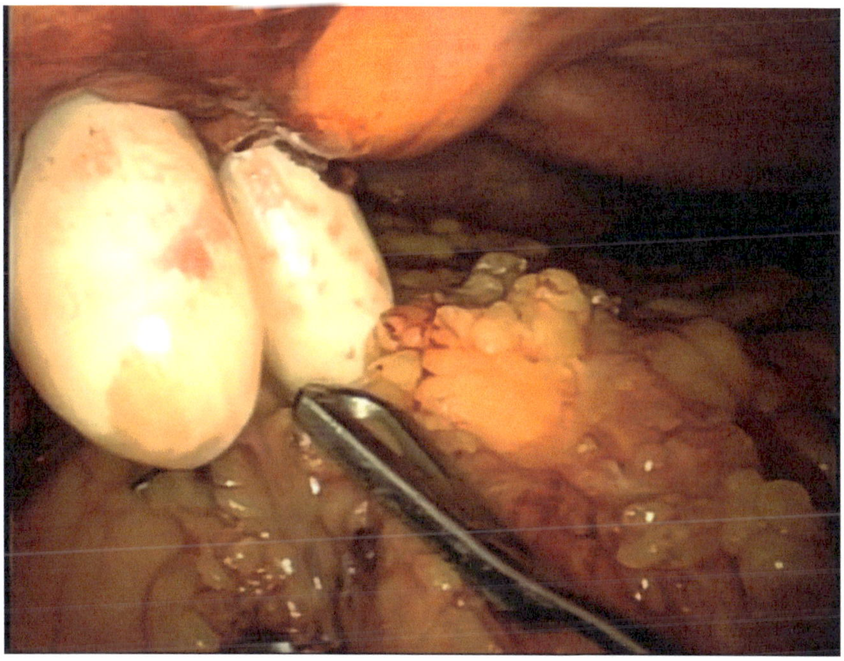

Fig. 17. Taking the omentum flap with finger maneuver to pull it from abdominal cavity to breast region.

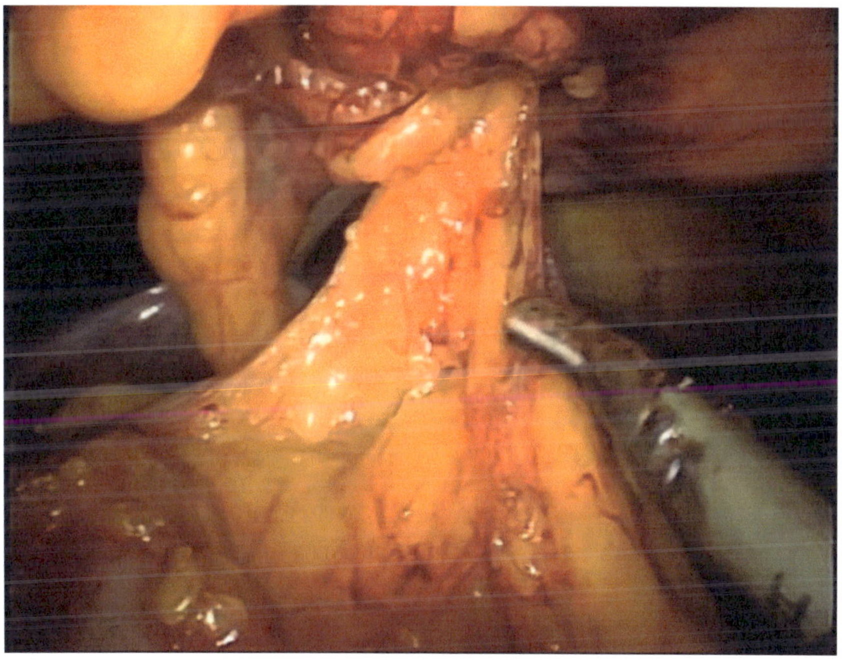

Fig. 18. Final position of the pedicle flap into the abdominal cavity.

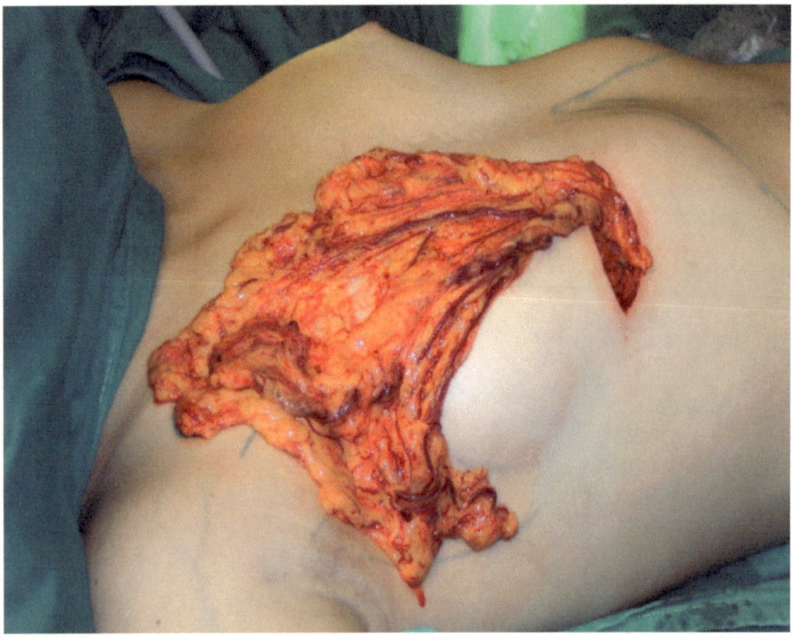

Fig. 19. Omentum flap upon thoracic wall.

4. Changes in the omentum flap after transposition

When laparoscopically harvested omentum flap was used to treat breast deformities, a significant volume increase of the omentum was noticed in the first months following its transposition in all the patients (Fig. 20 and 21).

The omentum is composed, predominantly, of mature adipocytes that do not have the capacity to multiply and that represent an important share of visceral fat in the human body. The omentum also has adult stem cells and progenitor cells or preadipocytes, which are smaller and able to differentiate (Fonseca-Alaniz et al, 2006).

The growth of the adipose tissue can be controlled by local vascularization. The degree of development of the adipocytes and of the vascular morphology is dependent on the volume of deposit of triglycerides whereas the size of the adipocytes does not depend on this volume of storage (Hausman & Richardson, 2004). When the supply of triglycerides for storage increases very much, preadipocytes may become mature adipocytes because the tissue needs storage room; thus, there will be hypertrophy and, then, hyperplasia. The increase in the bulk of adipocytes is accompanied by an increase in the microvascular net (Zhong et al, 2009) and, conversely, there is the need for an increase in neovascularization during the growth of adipose tissue. Evidence suggests that the O_2-sensitive signaling mechanism regulates adipogenesis (Lolmede et al, 2003). However, the differentiation of the preadipocyte is inhibited under hypoxic conditions, and, therefore, there would be only hypertrophy of the adipocytes and not hyperplasia (Frye et al, 2005).

The transposed omentum suffers hypoxia caused by a transitory ischemia. It causes a growth stimulation of VEGF (vascular endothelial growth factor) in the endothelial receptors that promotes neo-angiogenesis (Ignjatovic et al, 2001).

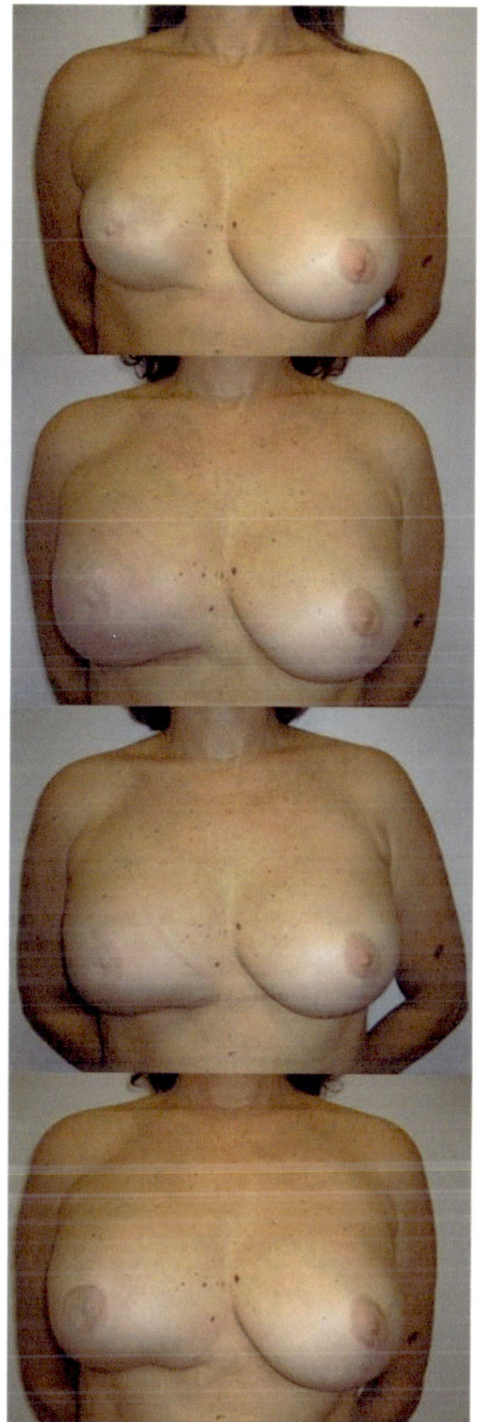

Fig. 20. Volume increase of the omentum in the first months following its transposition. Pre-operative and after 30, 60 and 100 days.

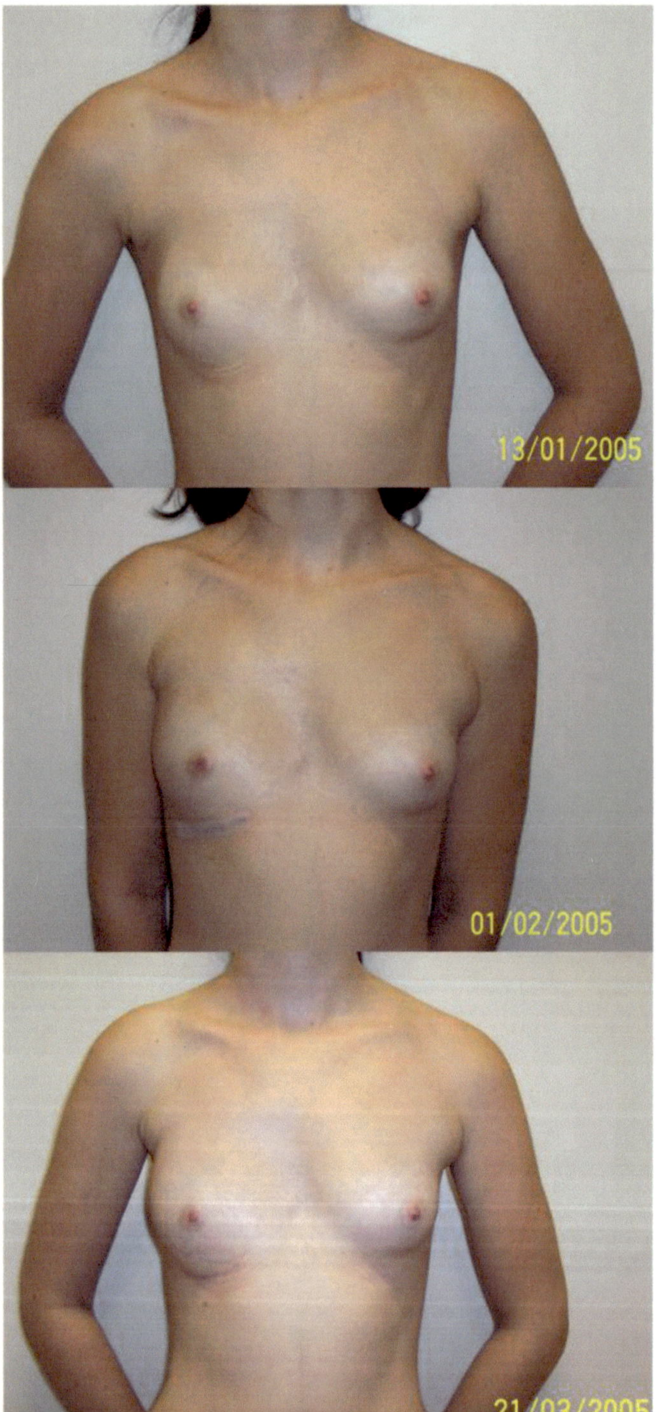

Fig. 21. Patient with Poland's syndrome in the right side showing the increase in volume of the omentum flap transposed to the right breast.

A high level of consistency is found in the literature so that we can safely use the measurement of VEGF, neoangiogenesis by the CD31(cluster of differentiation molecule) or PECAM-1 (Platelet Endothelial Cell Adhesion Molecule) and morphometric measurements of the adipocyte to investigate, clarify, and document the increase in postoperative volume of the omentum flap (Jernas et al, 2006; Fox & Harris, 2004).

In order to assess the nature of the apparent volume increase of the omentum when transposed to the breast, Costa et al studied patients that were treated with omentum flap. There was used the CD31 marker to do the measurement of angiogenesis as we do in cancer. The increase in the number of vessels in the second sample (Fig. 22) suggests neoangiogenesis stimulated by the initial increase in VEGF values documented in the first sample The histological study of Costa, comparing the adipocyte size; before and after the omentum transposition, presented a significant statistical difference (p <0,001) (Fig. 23). This difference ranged from a big to a very big effect. The confidence intervals of these effect sizes were always above moderate (Costa et al, 2011).

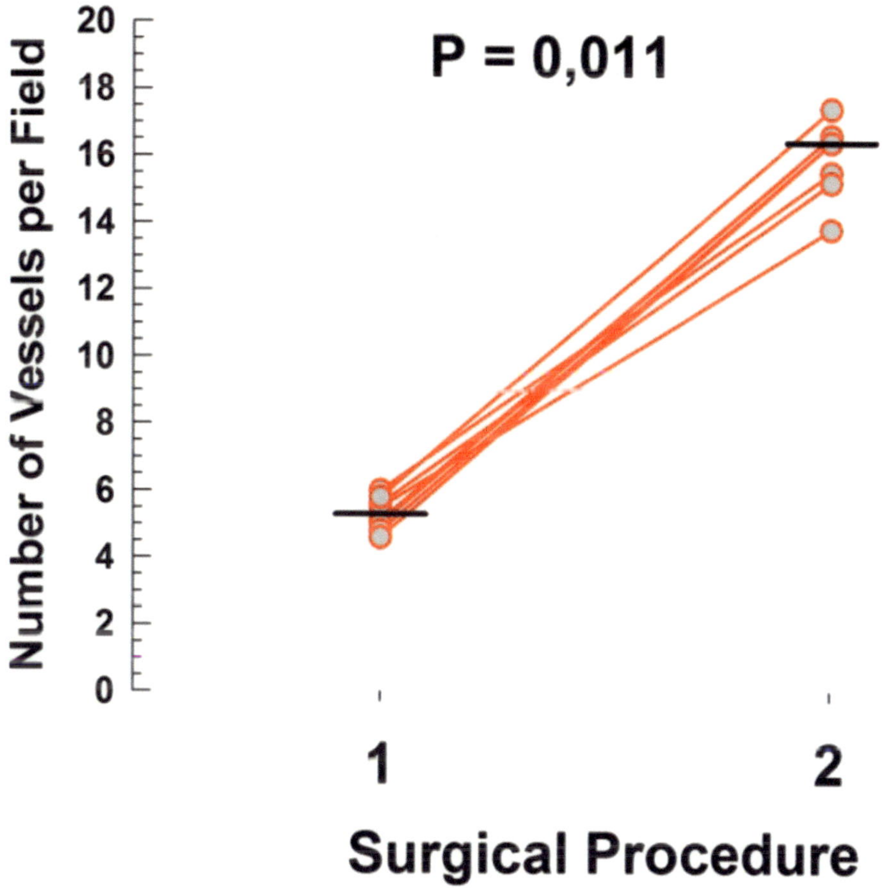

Fig. 22. Scoter plot with lines showing the variation of the number of vessels per field between surgical procedure 1 and 2. Short thick lines represent the series median values.

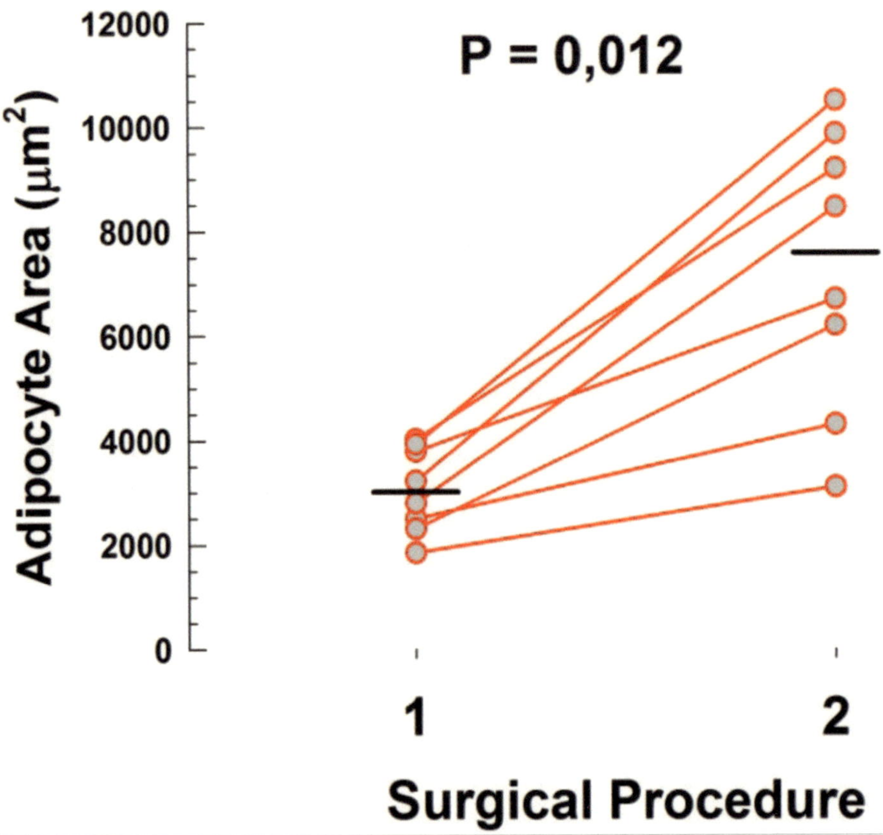

Fig. 23. Scoter plot with lines showing the variation of the adipocyte area between surgical procedure 1 and 2. Short thick lines represent the series median values.

5. Omentum flap versus adipocyte cells graft

Nowadays the use of adipocyte cells grafts can offers a possibility to treat small defects with good results, although it needs more than one surgical procedure even in small deformities. On the other hand, the omentum flap offers the possibility to restore a deformity in a single procedure without reabsortion of part of the volume transferred and even with a gain in the final volume after three or four months.

6. Conclusion

In conclusion, the employment of the omentum flap in the treatment of breast deformities enables reconstruction of the anterior axillary pillar as well as filling in of the infra-clavicular depression and provides volume and a soft coverage system that is thick enough to conceal silicone implants, a feature that no other technique seems able to achieve with so good aesthetic result.

7. Perspectives for the future

With the current knowledge regarding the new attributions and functions of the adipocytes and especially of the omentum cells, innumerous other indications of use of this tissue may arise in a near future. The omentum flap has great chances of becoming a rich source of material to correct and reconstruct segments or human organs unthinkable even today, but already exhaustively searched for by experimental medicine.

8. References

Arnold, P.G.; Hartrampf, C.R. & Jurkiewicz, M.J. (1976). *One-stage reconstruction of the breast, using the transposed greater omentum. Case report.* Plast Reconstr Surg.; 57(4):520-2.

Bainbridge, L.C.; Wright, A.R. & Kanthan, R. (1991). *Computed tomography in the preoperative assessment of Poland's syndrome.* Br J Plast Surg; 44(8):604-7.

Cobben, J.M.; Robinson, P.H.; Van Essen, A.J.; Van der Wiel, H.L. & Ten Kate, L.P. (1989). *Poland anomaly in mother and daughter.* Am J Med Genet; 33(4):519-21

Costa, S.S.; Pedrini, J.L.; Recamonde, A. & Penczek, F. (1998). *Tratamento cirúrgico da síndrome de Poland com omento transposto por Videolaparoscopia.* In:, editors. XI Congresso Brasileiro de Mastologia. Foz do Iguaçu-Paraná: XI Congresso Brasileiro de Mastologia;. p. 186.

Costa, S.S.; Blotta, R.M.; Mariano, M.B.; Meurer, L. & Edelweiss, M.I.A. (2010) *Aesthetic Improvements in Poland's Syndrome Treatment with Omentum Flap.* Aesth Plast Surg:1-6, April 24.

Costa, S.S.; Blotta, R.M.; Mariano, M.B.; Meurer, L. & Edelweiss, M.I.A. (2010). *Laparoscopic treatment of Poland's syndrome using the omentum flap technique.* Clinics; vol.65 no.4 São Paulo.

Costa, S.S.; Blotta, R.M.; Meurer, L. & Edelweiss, M.I.A (2011). *Adipocyte morphometric evaluation and angiogenesis in the omentum transposed to the breast: a preliminary study.* Clinics (Sao Paulo). February; 66(2): 307–312.

Cothier-Savey, I.; Tamtawi, B.; Dohnt, F.; Raulo, Y. & Baruch, J. (2001) *Immediate breast reconstruction using a laparoscopically harvested omental flap.* Plast Reconstr Surg;15;107(5):1156-63; discussion 64-5.

Das, S.K. (1976). *The size of the human omentum and methods of lengthening it for transplantation.* Br J Plast Surg; 29(2):170-44.

Ferron, G.; Garrido, I.; Martel, P.; Gesson-Paute, A.; Classe, J.M. & Letourneur, B. (2007). *Combined laparoscopically harvested omental flap with meshed skin grafts and vacuum-assisted closure for reconstruction of complex chest wall defects.* Ann Plast Surg; 58(2):150-5.

Fonseca-Alaniz, M.H.; Takada, J.; Alonso-Vale, M.I. & Lima, F.B. (2006). *[The adipose tissue as a regulatory center of the metabolism].* Arq Bras Endocrinol Metabol;50:216-29.

Fox, S.B. & Harris, A.L. (2004). *Histological quantitation of tumour angiogenesis.* APMIS;112:413-30.

Frye, C.A.; Wu, X. & Patrick, C.W. (2005). *Microvascular endothelial cells sustain preadipocyte viability under hypoxic conditions.* In Vitro Cell Dev Biol Anim;41:160-4.

Hausman, G.J. & Richardson, R.L. (2004) *Adipose tissue angiogenesis.* J Anim Sci;82:925-34.

Ignjatovic, M.; Pervulov, S.; Cuk, V.; Kostic, Z. & Minic, L. (2001) *Early angiogenic capabilities of the transposed omental flap after omentomyelopexy.* Acta Chirf Iugosl;48(2):41-3.

Irons, G.B.; Witzke, D.J.; Arnold, P.G. & Wood, M.B. (1983). *Use of the omental free flap for soft-tissue reconstruction*. Ann Plast Surg;11(6):501-7.

Jernas, M.; Palming, J. & Sjoholm, K. (2006). *Separation of human adipocytes by size: hypertrophic fat cells display distinct gene expression*. FASEB J;20:1540-2.

Kiricuta, I. (1963). *[The use of the great omentum in the surgery of breast cancer.]*. Presse Med; 5;71:15-7.

Lolmede, K.; Durand de Saint Front, V.; Galitzky, J.; Lafontan, M. & Bouloumie, A. (2003) *Effects of hypoxia on the expression of proangiogenic factors in differentiated 3T3-F442A adipocytes*. Int J Obes Relat Metab Disord;27:1187-95.

McLean, D.H. & Buncke, H.J. (1972). *Autotransplant of omentum to a large scalp defect, with microsurgical revascularization*. Plast Reconstr Surg; 49(3):268-74.

Perez Aznar, J.M.; Urbano, J.; Garcia Laborda, E.; Quevedo Moreno, P. & Ferrer Vergara, L. (1996) *Breast and pectoralis muscle hypoplasia. A mild degree of Poland's syndrome*. Acta Radiol; 37(5):759-62.

Saltz, R.; Stowers, R.; Smith, M. & Gadacz, T.R. (1993). *Laparoscopically harvested omental free flap to cover a large soft tissue defect*. Ann Surg;217(5):542-6; discussion 6-7.

Seyfer, A.E.; Icochea, R. & Graeber GM. (1988). *Poland's anomaly. Natural history and long-term results of chest wall reconstruction in 33 patients*. Ann Surg.; 208(6):776-82.

Zaha, H.; Inamine, S.; Naito, T. & Nomura, H. (2006). *Laparoscopically harvested omental flap for immediate breast reconstruction*. Am J Surg;192(4):556-8.

Zhong, X.; Yan, W.; He, X. & Ni, Y. (2009). *Improved fat graft viability by delayed fat flap with ischaemic pretreatment*. J Plast Reconstr Aesthet Surg;62:526-31.

Part 4

Fat Graft in Breast Reconstruction

11

Autologous Fat Transplantation – A Paradigm Shift in Breast Reconstruction

Daniel Del Vecchio[1] and Hetal Fichadia[2]
[1]*Back Bay Plastic Surgery and Massachusetts General Hospital, Boston MA,*
[2]*St. Elizabeth's Medical Center, Tufts University, Boston MA,*
USA

1. Introduction

Fat grafting to the breast is not a new concept. It has been under consideration since the 19th century when pioneers attempted inserting bulk volumes of fat (Neuber, 1893, Czerny 1895). Interest in fat grafting was rekindled with the introduction of liposuction, which provided an easy and reliable source of fat. After a brief pause in evolution of breast fat grafting due to concerns over confounding radiologic findings, and risk of carcinogenesis, fat grafting is once again at the forefront of cosmetic and reconstructive breast surgery as these concerns are have become more manageable. The plastic surgery community has re-assessed its position and has called for further clinical and basic science research in this versatile technique. As discussed below, fat grafting is becoming an invaluable tool for breast reconstruction both for core reconstruction and as an ancillary technique after various procedures for breast reconstruction.

2. History

Given the aesthetic importance of preservation of the breast mound and easy availability of adipose tissue, it is only natural that the early beginnings of breast reconstruction and fat grafting are interlinked. Vincent Czerny, a German physician first described breast reconstruction by fat transfer (Czerny, 1895). This was not only a first breast reconstruction, but also one of the initial few attempts at autologous fat transfer (Neuber, 1893). Describing the case of a 41-year-old singer who required unilateral mastectomy for chronic interstitial mastitis and fibroadenoma, Czerny wrote:

" Since both breasts were very well developed, an unpleasant asymmetry, which would have resulted after removal of one breast, would have been a particular hindrance to her stage activity. Luckily the lady had a lipoma, larger than a fist in the right lumbar region. I decided, therefore, to use this for a reconstruction of the extirpated breast " (Goldwyn, 1978)

2.1 History of breast reconstruction

The history of breast reconstruction must follow the history of breast cancer surgery. As the various techniques for extirpative cancer cure evolved over the past century, the reconstructive strategies had to likewise evolve. Halsted, who was a pioneer in breast cancer surgery, discouraged initial attempts at breast reconstruction. His teachings kept breast reconstruction from emerging as an option because he believed it could conceal local recurrence. (Halsted 1894, 1907, McGraw 1980, Losken and Jurkiewicz 2002). Therefore, many of the initial attempts at breast reconstruction took place in Europe. Ombredanne in France is credited with using the first muscle flap (a reflected pectoralis minor) to create a breast mound, whereas Tansini is credited with using a latissimus dorsi myocutaneous flap (Losken and Jurkiewicz, 2002). In the pre-antibiotic era, the use of prosthetic materials like polyvinyl sponges resulted in high complication rates (DeCholnoky, 1963).

In the post antibiotic era following World War II, the introduction of prosthetic materials like silicone implants ushered in a new era in breast reconstruction (Cronin and Gerow, 1963), and these received a wider acceptance after use of tissue expansion as an initial step after mastectomy (Radovan, 1982). Around the same time, with a better understanding of the vascular supply to the skin, microvascular techniques were developed and this resulted in re-introduction of the latissimus dorsi muscle flap for breast reconstruction (Schneider et al, 1977). This became a workhorse flap for a brief period of time, but had shortcomings like inadequate bulk of the muscle, often necessitating an underlying implant to fully reconstruct the breast volume. In addition, the donor site scar left on the back was significant. In 1982, Carl Hartrampf introduced the transverse rectus myocutaneous flap "TRAM" flap (Hartrampf, 1982). The TRAM flap with its many modifications is one of the most popular methods of autologous breast reconstruction today. Its donor site has an abdominoplasty scar, and there is often adequate soft tissue in the flap to reconstruct most defects. A major disadvantage of this flap is the sacrifice of the rectus muscle, which often results in donor site deformities such as muscle weakness, and abdominal wall hernias.

With further development of microsurgical techniques, perforator flaps became popular in the 1990s with development of DIEP and SGAP. Such flaps use the subcutaneous fat and skin of the TRAM flap, but obviate the need for the rectus to be harvested as the vascular pedicle. This procedure demands expertise in microsurgical techniques and is time consuming, requiring meticulous dissection of the donor vessels, and still leaves a donor site scar.

2.2 History of breast fat grafting

With the advent of liposuction in the 1980s, large amounts of unwanted fat could be removed from different body areas using small access incisions and a suction cannula. In this setting, fat grafting was re-introduced in the early '80s, pioneered by Mel Bircoll, who first described a series of fat transplantation for breast augmentation and reconstruction (Bircoll, 1987). Bircoll's contribution to fat grafting, albeit impressive, was met with a considerable amount of criticism from the plastic surgery leadership, with the American Society of Plastic Surgeons ("ASPS") releasing a position statement about the procedure in 1987. Plastic surgeons were essentially banned from attempting this technique (Snyderman, 1987). With all the concerns regarding the unknown risks of carcinogenesis and radiologic changes with fat grafting, the procedure was never adopted and fell into obscurity.

Some Europeans, undeterred by the American position, persisted and continued to push for the technique, though not for cosmetic augmentation. Emmanuel Delay in Lyon, France had begun using fat grafting to the breast for reconstruction as early as 2000 (Delay, 2009) and

Gino Rigotti in Verona, Italy also had a large series that he presented at the European of Aesthetic Plastic Surgeons in 2007 (Rigotti, 2007).

At the 2006 meeting of the American Society for Aesthetic Plastic Surgery (ASAPS), Baker et al., presented a series of 20 patients augmented with a combination of external expansion and fat grafting (Baker, 2006). Using serial breast MRI and 3D volumetric analysis Baker documented a 180 ml augmentation with documented volumetric survival of the grafts. None of the women had difficult-to-interpret findings on the mammogram. At the latest update of this prospective clinical trial, with over 40 women followed up for at least 6 months and for an average of 30 months, there were still no issues with breast imaging or difficult to interpret masses.

In 2007, Coleman published his landmark review of 17 breast augmentation and reconstruction patients who were treated using autologous fat and were followed up with serial photography (Coleman and Saboeiro, 2007). The results were overall successful with maintenance of volume over 7-12 years of follow up. Coleman used serial grafting sessions instead of injecting large volumes in a single session in a pre-expanded recipient breast like Baker et al.

With the growing realization that with optimal technique, fat grafts to the breast have potential to survive long term and that the radiographic arguments behind the ASPS-imposed ban were no longer valid many surgeons across the world have started publishing their previously unpublished work (Khouri and Baker, 2002, Rigotti and Marchi, 2007, Gosset et al 2008)

3. Physiology of volume maintenance in fat transplantation

The physiology of fat grafting was initially studied scientifically in 1950 by Peer (Peer, 1950), who observed that isogenous fat grafts have a 100% resorption rate whereas autogenous fat grafts have a 45% resorption rate. It should be noted that Peer's work preceded liposuction and he was using blocks of adipose tissue that were excised using open surgical techniques. Peer observed that the larger the graft transplanted, up to a point, the better the survival seemed to be. He postulated that there may be a critical element of micro-angiogenesis that occurs and once it does, perfusion could be re-established to the entire block of tissue. Tissue therefore needed to survive prior to this angiogenesis event, or the entire block would undergo necrosis. Peer postulated this 'cell-survival theory' to explain his findings, but this work was largely overlooked as the trends in plastic surgery at the time focused on skin and fascial flaps for soft tissue reconstruction.

Based partly on the initial work by Peer, there are two main theories explaining maintenance of volume after adipocytes are transplanted into recipient tissue. The "Diffusion/Angiogenesis" theory postulates that adipocytes survive by oxygen diffusion in the recipient site during the first 7-14 days following grafting, with eventual micro angiogenesis and the formation of a viable blood supply to the grafted cells. In this scenario, the transplanted adipocytes are envisioned as surviving the transplantation event in whole or in part, and constitute the volume maintenance that is observed clinically. Overcrowding or excessive interstitial pressure in the recipient site is thought to interfere with diffusion, which leads to cellular death, apoptosis and loss of graft volume. This accounts for the use of successful small graft volume (18 to 34 cc) that has been reported in breast reconstruction where ancillary fat grafting has been used successfully for breast reconstruction of border-zone contour irregularities (Kanchwala, 2008). Smaller volumes of graft compared with the recipient-site volume capacity potentially result in maintenance of a physiologic interstitial pressure environment and a favorable surface-to-volume ratio of graft to recipient, improving oxygen diffusion in the early days after grafting. Just like in a skin graft, early trauma or shearing of the graft-recipient interface is thought to damage micro-angiogenesis and decrease graft survival.

A competing theory of graft volume maintenance is based on the experimental work of Morrison who demonstrated adipocyte proliferation and angiogenesis in a perforated hollow tube filled with a non-viable poly (D, L-lactic-co-glycolic acid) ("PLGA") sponge matrix which was implanted in the groin of rats (Dolderer et al, 2007). In the so-called "Morrison" (or better described as the "Scaffold") theory of volume maintenance post fat transplantation, all or most of the transplanted adult adipocytes are destined to die. Rather than survive to maintain volume, these dead cellular elements act as a non-viable matrix or scaffold, through which macrophages penetrate and through which recipient-site stem cell-mediated angiogenesis and adipogenesis occurs. Interestingly, Peer's original 1950 "cell survival theory" postulated that human fat grafts disappeared completely a short time after transplantation and noted that "small autogenous multiple grafts had surviving portions that one year after transplantation appeared like normal fat tissue."

Rather than choose between mutually exclusive theories, it is our belief that a third theory exists to explain volume maintenance after fat transplantation. According to the "Tandem" theory, some transplanted adipocytes survive by diffusion and receive a blood supply by eventual micro-angiogenesis, while others do not and act as a scaffold for recipient site cells to enter and remodel. Thus, both mechanisms are working in tandem in any given system.

4. Not all fat grafting is the same – Definition of mega-volume fat grafting

Early applications of fat grafting in breast reconstruction involved injection of small amounts of fat for contour correction or filling defects left after breast conservation therapy (Losken et al 2011, Rietjens et al 2011). However, there have been reports of complete breast reconstruction after mastectomy being accomplished by fat grafting with good results (Serra-Renom et al, 2011, Babovic, 2010, Fitoussi et al 2009, Delay et al 2010). The technique of fat grafting used in the face for nasolabial folds is different from the technique of fat grafting used to treat chronic wounds, or to reconstruct radiated mastectomy sites. What is apparent is that not all fat grafting can be lumped into one technique, as not all fat grafting is the same. Sometimes fat is required to only provide volume, whereas in other cases its use is more to supply a regenerative effect, as in the case of a chronic wound (Cervelli et. al, 2009). Therefore, we propose there are at least four separate categories of fat transplantation: high volume vs. low volume, and regenerative vs. non-regenerative, as depicted in Figure 1, below:

We define mega-volume fat grafting as transplantation of over 100 cc of processed fat for core volume projection replacement. In so doing, our technical strategies will cater to the demands of this large volume, mainly non-regenerative case.

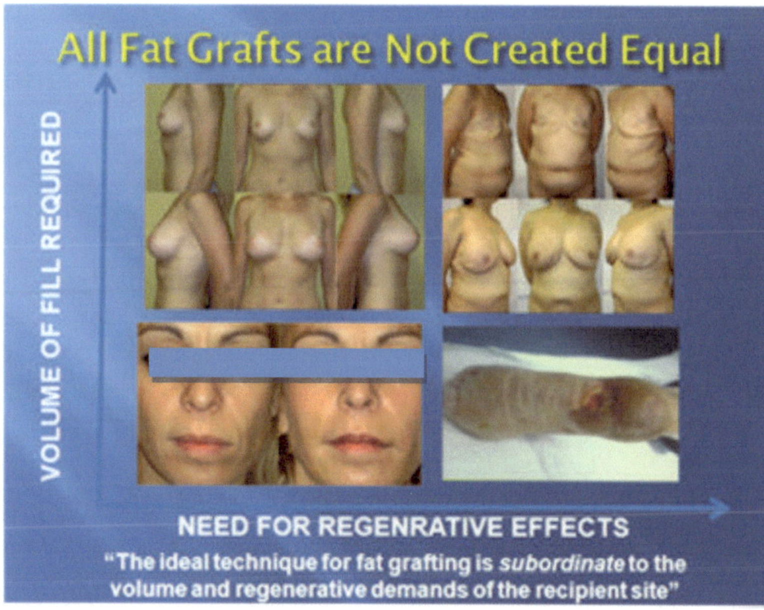

Fig. 1. A Matrix Classification of Fat Grafting. The correct strategy for fat grafting must take into consideration the relative volume capacity and regenerative demands of the recipient site. (Reconstruction case courtesy of Roger Khouri, MD)

5. From science to the operating room – Surgical variables in fat transplantation

Four clinical factors appear to have a significant effect on the survival of grafted fat cells:

1. Fat Harvesting
2. Fat Processing
3. Fat Grafting
4. Role of the Recipient Site

5.1 Fat harvesting

Cannulas: Diameter and Hole Size: Although it has been reported in a histological study that larger cannula sizes (6mm) harvest fat with better viability than with smaller cannulas (Erdim et al, 2009), viability in this report was measured using cell isolation and counting adipocytes with a haemocytometer. Such an experimental endpoint only represents the first step of a multi-stage procedure that must consider all stages, with the clinical endpoint being long-term (six months or greater) volume retention after transplantation into an animal host.

Smaller cannula sizes theoretically create less donor site trauma and allow for removal of smaller sized lobules of fat, which may improve flow characteristics and reduce trauma during re-injection. An important consideration besides cannula size is *cannula hole size* and *number of holes*. A 12-gauge cannula with 6-8 side holes 2x1 mm in size can extract a significant amount of fat despite its small caliber.

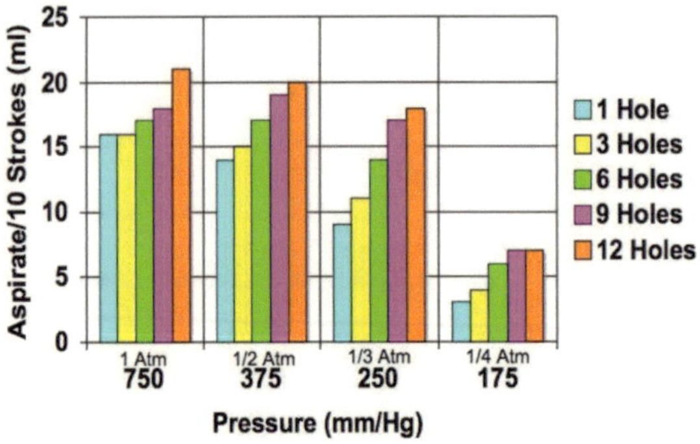

Fig. 2. Varying negative pressure and hole size, the volume of fat flowing through cannulas (measured in cc of fat per 10 strokes) is efficient at 6-12 holes, even at lower negative pressures. (Data: courtesy of Roger Khouri, MD)

The summation of the surface area of the individual openings on a 12 gauge, 12-hole cannula approaches or exceeds the surface area of the opening of a classic 10 mm one-hole cannula, once used in the 1980s. The result is better tissue flow with less donor area trauma. Further, each hole selects for lobules of uniform small size, which are more likely to flow easily through the injection cannula during the grafting phase of the procedure, without the need for further processing or syringe transfers. The hole sizes on the aspiration cannula approach the size of the hole on the injection cannula, providing "equalization" of hole sizes for more efficient fat flow (see below under fat injecting).

Negative Pressure: The literature regarding the isolated effects of negative pressure suggests that adipocytes can be suctioned below 700 mm Hg without undue trauma (Shiffman, et al, 2001). Any claims of syringe suctioning being safer than machine suctioning should be carefully examined. While a standard liposuction machine can generate up to one atmosphere (760 mm Hg) of negative pressure, a 60 cc syringe connected to an in-line manometer can also generate nearly one atmosphere of negative pressure (Fig. 3). With regards to the effect of negative pressure on adipocyte viability, it is likely that absolute pressure and not the source of this pressure is the key variable in adipocyte trauma.

Location of Donor Fat: Animal studies have not demonstrated superior donor site fat based on anatomic location (Ullman et al, 2005), and clinically we have not observed anatomic location of the donor fat to be of significance in terms of volume retention. Although reports in the literature (Padoin et al, 2008) suggest the lower abdomen and inner thighs to be richer in the source of stem cells, this study used C-Kit expression as a proxy measurement for stem cells. C-Kit expression also measures lymphocytes and on this basis the conclusions of this paper are in question. In reality, what is more important to consider is the relative abundance and requirements of donor graft in each individual case, and the surgical plan should aim to avoid or minimize donor site deformities. It may turn out that that adipocyte cellular size, which varies in different body regions and also among different patients may be a more important variable than location per se. Larger cells have a higher likelihood of mechanical cell membrane damage during extraction, and it may be this variable of cell size relative to cannula hole-size that is more important than the specific area on the body used for harvest per se.

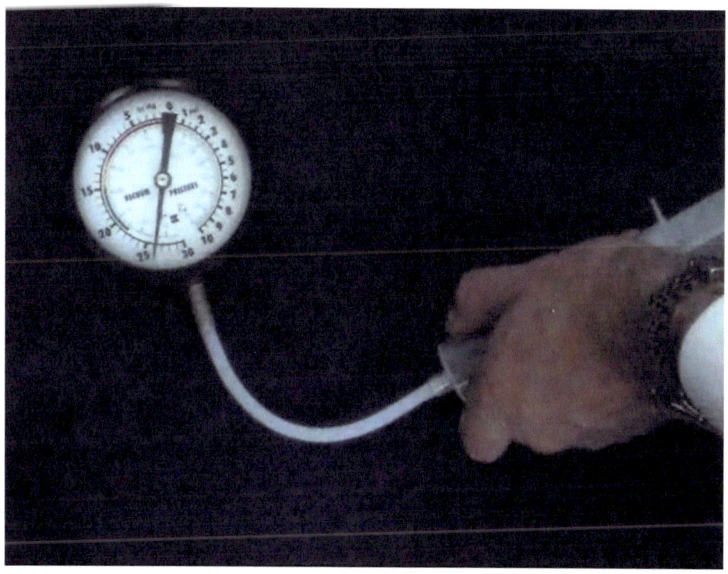

Fig. 3. A 60cc syringe can generate close to one atmosphere (30 in = 760 mm Hg) of negative pressure, dispelling the myth that syringe suction is "safer" than machine suction.

Another variable of unknown importance in fat harvesting remains the negative impact of air exposure (Kaufman et al, 2007). Despite its widespread mention, there is a paucity of scientific data quantifying the effect of air exposure on adipocyte viability (Aboudib et al, 1992). Techniques of fat processing range from drying fat on Telfa Rolls (high air exposure), to completely closed systems employing intravenous tubing, three way stopcocks and IV bags for collection.

5.2 Fat processing

Peer's cell survival theory of grafted *en bloc* fat dates back over 50 years and suggests that the number of calls transplanted at the time of transplantation may correlate with the ultimate fat graft survival volume (Peer, 1950). After Ilouz's breakthrough application of liposuction (Ilouz, 1983), fat became available in a fragmented form. The cell survival theory of solid fat transplantation may have influenced the use of high-speed centrifugation as a potential strategy for effective fat grafting. Historically, the penchant for centrifugation may have arisen from the need to graft as much adipocyte biomass as possible into a limited space. Although centrifugation can process highly concentrated fat, there are potential problems associated with it when this technique is employed in megavolume fat grafting:

- The cells may be damaged due high G-forces (Kurita et al, 2008)
- It is a time and labor-consuming process
- High fat concentrations may cause clumping and more difficult flow during re-injection

One of the most confusing metrics in fat grafting is a lack of standardization when one discusses "percent yields". Once fat is lipo-aspirated as donor graft there are an infinite number of different concentrations of adipocyte volume relative to non-adipocyte volume (blood, serum, crystalloid) that can be reached prior to grafting the recipient site. Unless the concentration of adipocytes in the grafted material can be accurately measured and unless the process of fat concentration is standardized, one cannot reliably measure the percent of adipocyte volume that survived grafting. In an effort to move toward an acceptable technical standard and to allow for better comparison of volumetric data in clinical series, careful documentation of the following data should be performed in mega-volume fat grafting patients:

- Obtain a baseline mammogram of the breast
- Prior to expansion, objectively document breast volume (MRI, 3D imaging, or both)
- Document the process used for crystalloid separation (decanting, low speed centrifugation, high speed centrifugation)
- Document the volume of processed material grafted in cc
- Objectively document the post graft volume of the breast at 6 months or more (MRI, 3D imaging, or both)

Our strategy in mega-volume fat grafting is based on the concept of minimizing extracorporeal adipocyte time ("EAT"). Whichever theory of fat volume maintenance one believes is true, all should agree that excess time is detrimental for patient safety, cells, and lastly, surgeons. Therefore, we employ the large syringe technique to process 480 cc of fat in 2 minutes, which is the most efficient method of fat dehydration currently available.

5.3 Fat injecting and shape-modifying techniques

The selection of an injection cannula used in mega-volume fat grafting follows similar principles to those of harvesting. Small gauge cannulas theoretically reduce trauma to the breast recipient site, which potentially reduces the risks of bleeding, hematoma, and resultant poor graft oxygen diffusion. The hole size of the injection cannula should match closely with the hole sizes of the aspiration cannula. By matching hole sizes, the selected size of the harvested lobules of fat are more likely to flow easily through the injection cannula without blockage or undue resistance (Fig 4).

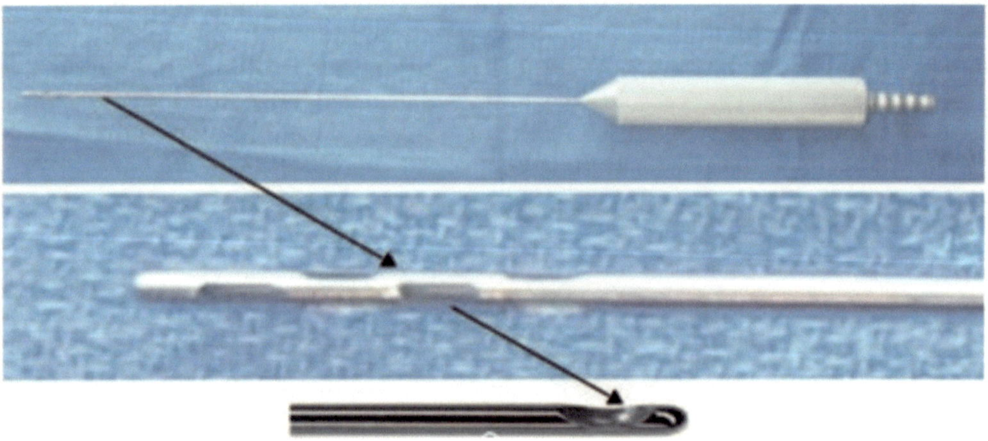

Fig. 4. Equalization of Hole Size. The opening in the 3 mm, 9-hole aspiration cannula (*top, center*) is nearly equal in size to the hole opening in the 16-gauge blunt tipped side hole injection cannula (*bottom*), improving tissue flow on injection.

There are currently two methods of injecting fat in a manner that seeks to increase dispersion and surface to volume contact with the recipient site - the "Mapping" technique and the "Reverse Liposuction" technique. Despite using these different techniques, the authors' independent long-term volume maintenance is essentially the same, each demonstrating an average increase in breast volume of 250 cc on average at six months by quantitative volumetric MRI imaging.

The Mapping Technique: Donor cells have the highest chance of survival with the technique that best ensures an even, three-dimensional dispersion of the fat. The mapping technique involves the use of small (3 cc-5 cc) syringes handheld and connected directly to a 16 Gauge blunt curved side-hole cannula. Markings are made in the recipient areas to aid in a systematic, diffuse and even injection of the entire recipient area. 8-10 circum-mammary and 4 circum-areolar entry points are usually made with a 14G hypodermic needle (Fig. 5). Through each entry point the 15-20 cm long cannula makes multiple tunnels that fan out radially and injects 1-2 cc of fat only upon axial withdrawal. The cannula is then inserted into another adjacent entry point and the fanning process is repeated to yield a 3-D weave that evenly crisscross and covers the recipient space.

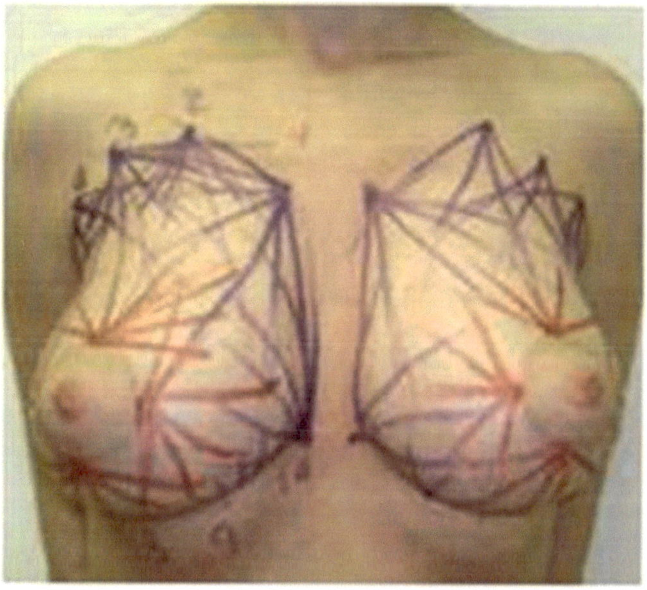

Fig. 5. Markings for the Mapping Technique of Fat Injection. On the breasts, 8-10 circum-mammary and 4 circum-areolar needle puncture entry sites with radially fanning tunnels from each site provide a well- diversified insertion of the grafts

Multiple levels of graft are deposited, deep from the base of the breast just above the pectoralis fascia, to the subcutaneous space immediately subjacent to the dermis. Direct injection of fat into the dense parenchyma of the breast is never performed. This technique is deliberate and exact but does take time. In addition, it requires the operator to deploy the plunger and withdraw the needle at the same time. Overall, the Mapping technique may be more suitable for surgeons beginning mega-volume fat grafting for breast augmentation because it is more exact and deliberate. For breast reconstruction, it is clearly beneficial, especially in scarred areas caused by mastectomy and/or irradiation where a careful and deliberate graft placement is necessary.

The "Reverse Liposuction" Technique: The reverse liposuction technique seeks to evenly disperse the fat into the subcutaneous and non-breast parenchyma in as efficient a manner as is possible. 6-8 needle insertions are made using a 14-gauge needle on the breast, along the infra-mammary fold ("IMF") and spaced 4-5 cm laterally toward the axilla. Using a straight, 15 cm blunt side- hole, 16 gauge needle loaded directly onto 60 cc syringes, the fat is injected using a controlled "to and fro" liposuction movement with constant light depression on the plunger. With every pass of the needle the direction is changed slightly to create a fanning pattern of vectors. This is repeated in each different insertion site and at multiple planar levels from the base of the breast. The axillary insertion is also used to place graft in the sub-muscular position and this approach is felt to be the safest method of navigating the sub pectoral space. The rate of graft insertion in this technique should be 1-2 seconds per cc, which results in a 1-2-minute/60 cc of fat rate, or a 300 cc per breast grafting session performed in 10-15 minutes on each breast. The Reverse Liposuction Technique is more time efficient and can be utilized in cases where there is no internal breast scarring, no dense adherence of skin to the chest wall, and where the breast is adequately expanded. Hence, this technique might not be the best technique for breast reconstruction in an irradiated breast. Another potential benefit of the reverse liposuction technique is that 60 cc syringes generate lower maximum pressures than do 5 cc syringes, which generate higher pressure. Therefore, if there is a blockage of flow along the insertion needle due to clumping, this will occur at a lower pressure using a 60 cc syringe, with less potential damage to the grafted cells and less likelihood of pushing the blockage through, creating a bolus.

5.3.1 Breast shape modification using 3 dimensional ligamentous band release

Once the fat is grafted, the internal parenchyma is under higher pressure. Contour irregularities due to internal ligamentous tethering can be manifest, especially seen at the interface between the natural infra-mammary fold and the newly augmented breast mound. A technique first described by Rigotti, who employed a pickle fork to release heavily scarred recipient site radiated tissue, is used to release subcutaneous ligaments and scars in breast augmentation and reconstruction with fat grafting. This technique is called three dimensional ligamentous band release, or "Rigottomy". 3D Ligamentous band release is a powerful technique that can change breast shape. This technique, like meshing a two-dimensional skin graft, releases contour deformities of the breast parenchyma in three dimensions. Grafted fat immediately fills space created and the fat keeps distance between the transected scar or band, so the scar or band does not reform.

5.4 The role of the recipient site in fat transplantation

Negative pressure on the breast prior to fat transplantation creates internal expansion of the breast parenchyma by drawing in more fluid, creating an edema-like state, and by increasing the size and caliber of blood vessels. The authors postulate that non-surgical pre-operative expansion of the breast recipient site enhances fat grafting results by five main effects:

Bigger potential spaces available for overall volume of graft;

Reduces the demand on adipocytes to act as internal expanders, resulting in undue pressure;

Augments tension on internal constrictions and scars, so breast *shape* can be addressed;

Variables that are time consuming (e.g. centrifugation) become less demanding;

Angiogenesis effect may increase recipient site oxygen tension and lead to better graft take.

The VAC® device has markedly improved outcomes in many types of difficult open wounds by clearance of bacteria and reduction in fluid volume (Saxena et al, 2007). In open wounds, micromechanical forces such as negative pressure elicit tissue deformation forces that stretch individual cells, thereby promoting proliferation in the wound microenvironment. The application of micromechanical forces on cells has been demonstrated as a useful method with which to stimulate wound healing through the promotion of cell division, angiogenesis, and local elaboration of growth factors (Saxena et al, 2004, 2007). The deformational forces of the VAC® device are consistent with this mechanism of action and are similar to the negative pressure exerted on the breast when BRAVA pre-expansion is used. Pre-expansion to the breast may therefore be more than just "increasing space". Negative pressure therapy to the breast may demonstrate similar effects of angiogenesis, cell division, and up-regulation of growth factors in the breast recipient site.

For small graft volumes (100 ml or less), pre-expansion is not a pre-requisite as much as it is for breast augmentation, as it does not result in high interstitial pressures, as the capacity of the recipient site can receive such a small volume with relative ease.

6. Surgical technique

Fat grafting for breast augmentation or reconstruction does not begin with surgery. Proper patient selection and motivation for use of the external expansion device, and finally education as to the unknown potential risks of fat grafting and the need for staged procedures is essential to success. A breast reconstruction from a mastectomy takes 3-4 sessions of fat grafting spaced 4 months apart; if the patient has had radiation the number of sessions is increased to 4-5. Patients must be counseled prior to initiating the process that tis is a long reconstructive effort in which the patient plays and active (pre-expansion) role.

Following proper patient selection, patients undergo three weeks of pre-operative external expansion using the BRAVA device. The device is worn during awake hours, usually in the evenings after work, as night-time use proves ineffective because the device detaches during sleep. Patients are encouraged to expand 6-8 hours a day and are checked regularly in the office to monitor their progress. The use of 3-D imaging aids in the qualitative measurement of progress or the lack thereof. A 2-3 fold increase in volume of the breast mound or breast is sought prior to grafting (Fig. 6 & 7).

Preoperatively, the patient is initially marked for areas to be suctioned, and the breasts are marked circumferentially for areas of proposed needle insertions. Any constricted areas are outlined for planned release using a percutaneous needle. Markings are placed at 8-10 proposed sites, circumferentially around the breast.

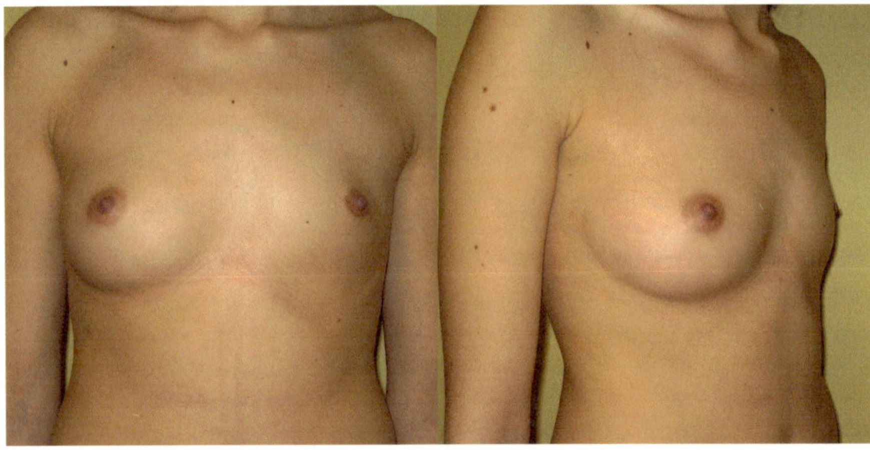

Fig. 6. 18-year-old patient with absence of left breast following tumor excision as an infant. This patient would be a poor candidate for prosthesis, as a breast implant could never match the natural breast on the right. A complex flap like a TRAM would leave a significant donor site deformity, and the patient does not have excess abdominal fat. In addition, she may be considering child bearing making an abdominal muscle closure less attractive. Note the lack of left breast parenchyma and skin, with decreased clavicle to nipple-areolar distance.

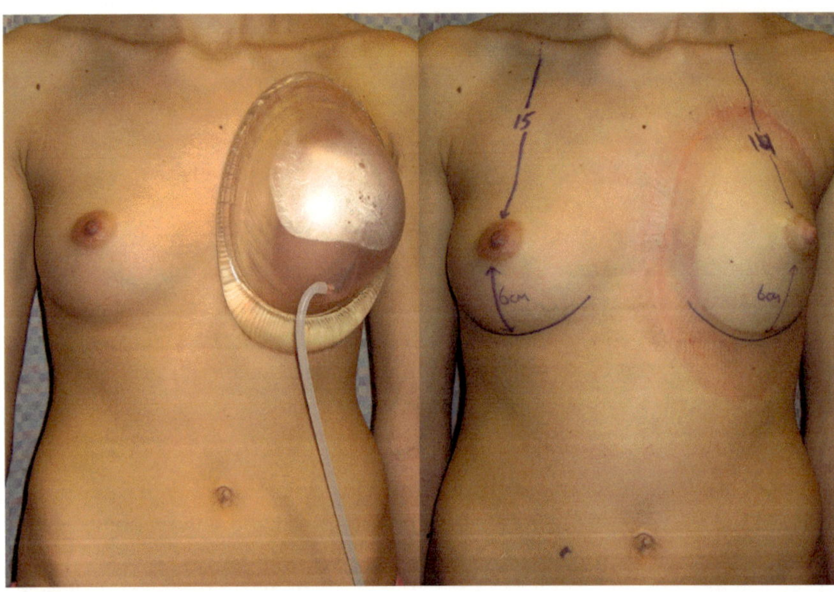

Fig. 7. Preoperative external pre-expansion for reconstruction of the left breast. The patient wore the BRAVA device 6-8 hours a day for three weeks. Note the increased volume, and the increased skin as the left nipple areola complex is almost even with the right.

Liposuction is performed using a 12-gauge multi-hole (9-12 hole) cannula. Smaller cannula sizes lead to less subcutaneous tissue trauma, faster recovery, and smaller fat lobules, which result in better fat flow and less clumping. Multiple holes lead to more efficient and faster fat removal. Our collection technique is as follows:

Using a sterile "in-line" container, fat is aspirated at 2/3 to 3/4 of an atmosphere (500-600 mm Hg) suction by attaching a sterile clear collection canister to a standard vacuum machine off the sterile field. A 3 mm 9 hole cannula with a wide handle and ribbed connector end is used to attach to the liposuction tubing. Maximal negative machine pressures are avoided when using this technique and vaporization of the fat ("boiling" appearance) in the collection canister is to be avoided at all costs. This technique initially collects the fat into 1200 cc canisters and can be performed with existing equipment used in an operating room (Figure 8).

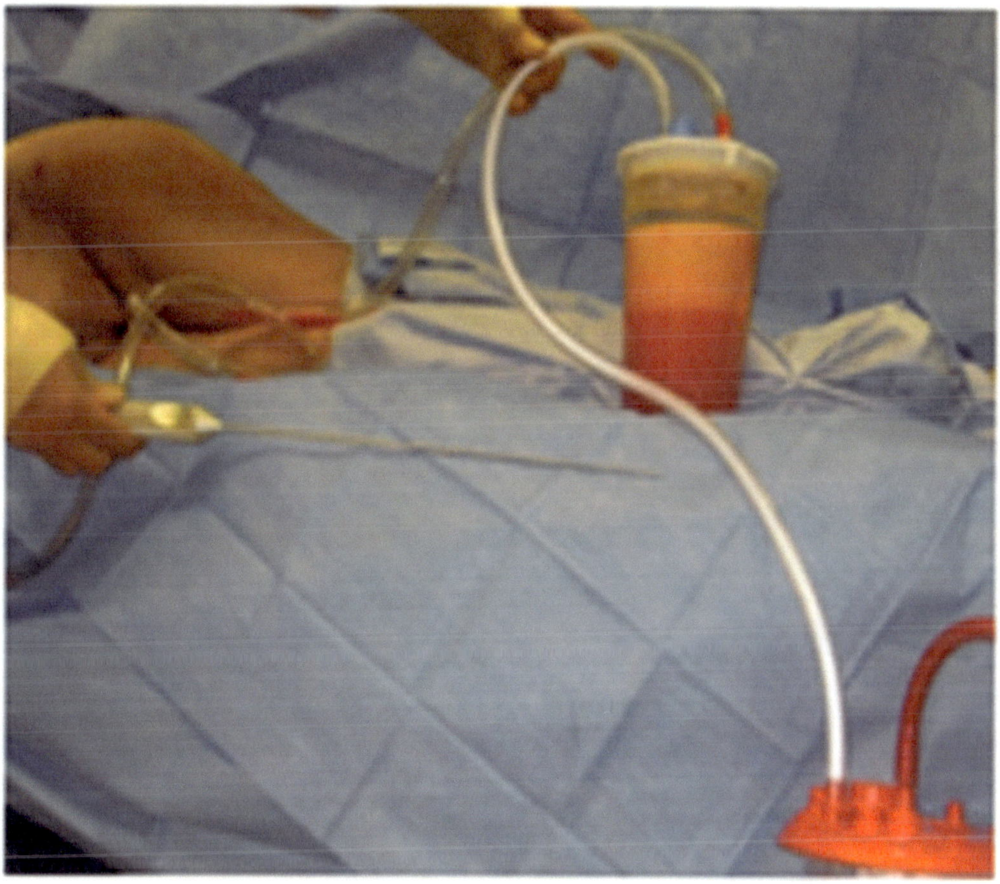

Fig. 8. "In line method" of fat collection in mega volume fat transplantation. A sterile plastic canister on the field collects the fat and is in line with the liposuction machine canister (shown in red). No fat should be lost to the non-sterile canister.

Ideally, fat should be processed so as to separate blood, infiltration fluid, and cell debris from healthy adipocytes with minimal trauma. Once the fat is collected, we use the following method for removing unwanted crystalloid:

"Large Syringe" Method: Several in-line collection canisters are used during the machine liposuction. (Figure 9, a-e). Every time a canister is full, a new canister replaces it. The canisters containing the lipoaspirate (a) are then allowed to stand for 10 minutes allowing fat to separate from crystalloid. This fat is then drawn up into 60 cc syringes (b) directly from the collection canister, and placed in a mega volume centrifuge (c). Additional low-G force centrifugation of these 60 cc syringes then removes an additional 20% crystalloid (d,e).

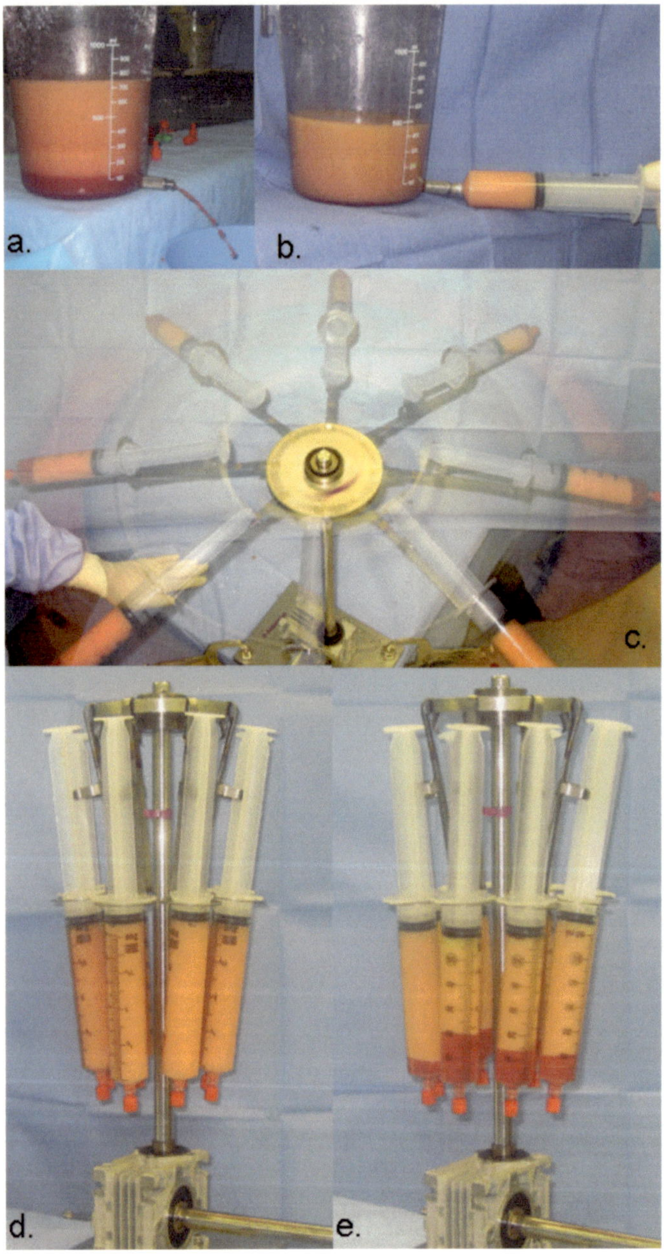

Fig. 9. "Large Syringe" method of fat processing. Fat that appears to be pure fat after decanting at 1G (a,b) actually still has considerable (20%) amounts of crystalloid, that can be efficiently removed in minutes using a low-G force hand cranked sterile centrifuge (c). Before (d) and after (e) centrifugation, demonstrating the extraction of unwanted fluid and blood.

If the recipient site has been pre-expanded for complete breast reconstruction, then the emphasis on hyper-concentrated fat, separated at 1300G is unnecessary. This is because over- expansion of the recipient site affords is the opportunity to inject less concentrated fat. This less concentrated fat is theoretically less traumatized, flows better, disperses better because it is less concentrated, and finally takes less operative time and manpower to process. These are the essential elements of the large syringe technique. We have focused on effective expansion of the recipient site and an efficient timely procedure, and have shifted our focus away from hyper concentrated fat and from "over-correction", because of resultant overcrowding, interstitial hypertension, and volume capacity limitations leading to subsequent fat necrosis.

Once the fat is separated from unwanted crystalloid, injection into the breast begins. Injections are performed using 15 cm "Coleman" (Mentor Incorporated, Santa Barbara, California) side hole needle. We employ the so-called "Reverse Liposuction" technique (Fig 10). If fat has been harvested and collected using the "In Line" machine and Large Syringe techniques, the fat is already in 60 cc syringes. These syringes are simply loaded onto the Coleman needle and injected into the breast. Multiple insertion holes are employed in a pattern around the breast periphery and in the areas that require volume for symmetry. Insertions along the medial upper quadrant are generally avoided to reduce the possibility of pigmented large needle scars, as this is the part of the breast often seen in low cut clothing. Transplanting fat for augmentation or reconstruction is an iterative process, with surgical artistry and judgment about how much fat and where to inject the fat being based on a continually changing breast as the procedure evolves. Knowing where to graft, when to stop, and how to release bands to effect shape change become the knowledge and skill of the fat grafting surgeon.

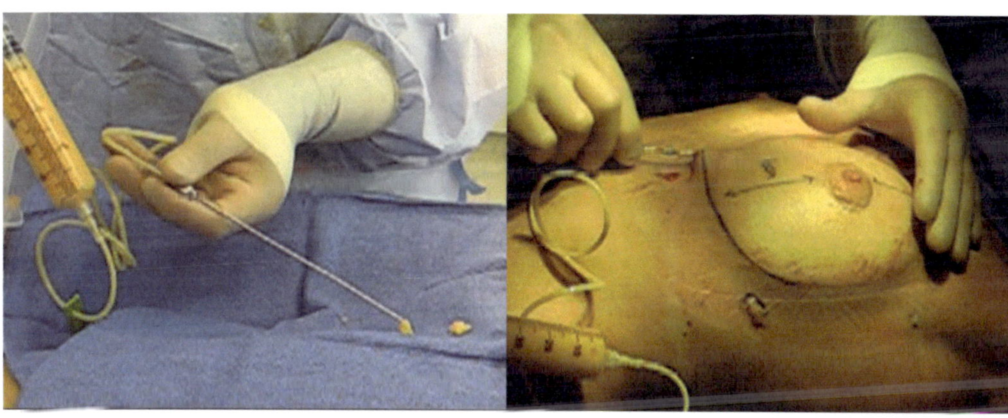

Fig. 10. Reverse liposuction technique used in breast fat transplantation. (Left) In this setup, an assistant applies syringe pressure via connected intravenous extension tubing. An alternative is for the surgeon to hold the syringe directly connected to the infusion cannula (Right) Grafting using the Reverse Liposuction Technique along needle sticks in the infra-mammary crease.

7. Post operative care

In the first 24 hours post grafting there is no external compression or negative pressure used. Patients are placed in standard girdles as for routine liposuction. Beginning at 24-48 hours after grafting, patients are placed into BRAVA domes, which are placed under low suction for a period of 14-21 days. The use if BRAVA in the postoperative period may act as a splint to protect the graft and may aid in volume maintenance by continued stimulation of the recipient site.

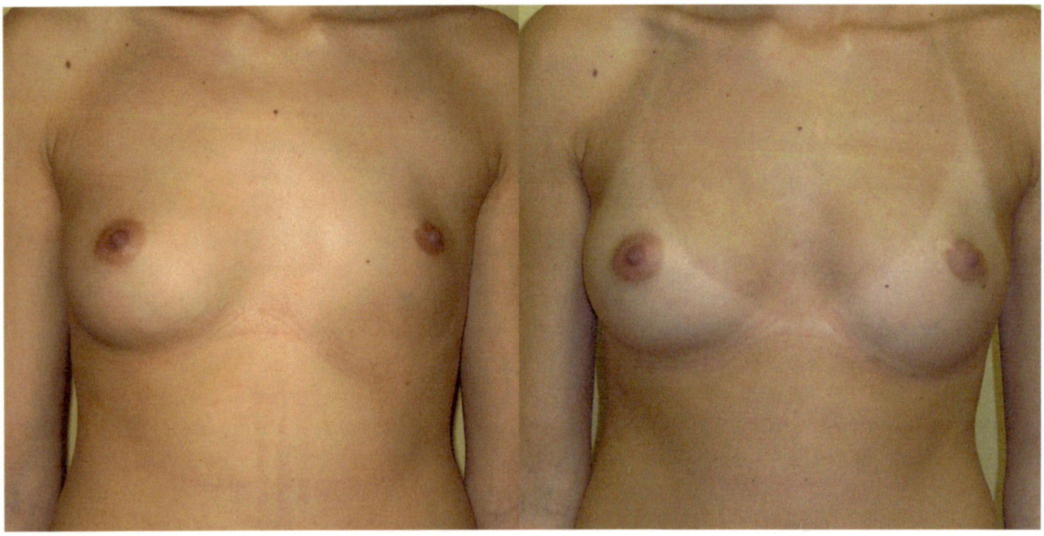

Fig. 11. Before (left) and after (right) reconstruction of the left breast. This patient received 300cc of transplanted fat. Her result is stable at 3 years postop.

8. The emerging role of fat grafting in breast reconstruction

Due to the wide availability of donor fat, ease of collection and minimal morbidity associated with liposuction, fat grafting has the potential to become a versatile tool in breast reconstruction. A review of the literature reveals there are a growing number of published reports on the use of fat grafting in breast reconstruction after surgery for breast cancer. While some of them are case reports (Del Vecchio 2009, Babovic 2010, Delay 2010, Panettiere 2011, Fitoussi 2009), a considerable number describe their experience with 40 or more patients (Spear 2005, Serra-Renom 2010, Sinna 2010, Rietjens 2011, Losken 2011, Missana 2007, Delay 2008, Panettiere 2009, Kanchwala 2009).

In 2005, Spear et al published one of the initial studies about the use of fat grafting in breast reconstruction. This study reported results of 37 small-volume cases (six patients bilateral) for small border zone cosmetic irregularities after reconstructive breast surgery (25 implant reconstructions, 17 transverse rectus abdominis muscle (TRAM) reconstructions, one TRAM and implant reconstruction). The average injected volume was relatively small (116 ml) and these cases were not intended for reconstruction of core volume. The complication rate of 8.5% (cellulitis and oil cysts) at a mean follow up of 15 months is manageable, with 85% of patients realizing some satisfactory result.

Similar findings were reported by Missana et al in 2007 when they published their experience with small volume non-core fat grafting in 69 patients (74 injections) for revision of border zone defects following flap reconstruction or for defects following lumpectomy.

The average volume injected was 67--77 ml for breast conservation therapy and between 140-300 ml for implant and autologous flap reconstruction revisions. These cases must be distinguished from core volume reconstructions. In addition, they did not use pre-expansion and therefore these cases required multiple injection sessions. 86.5% of patients were deemed to have good or very good results. The rate of fat necrosis was 7.4%

In addition to using fat simply as a filler, the regenerative work of Rigotti et al (2007) demonstrated a significant reversal in radiation damage after fat grafting in 20 patients. Fat, not acting simply as a filler, appeared to have a regenerative effect on the reversal of the radiation fibrosis and scarring. All the patients' LENT SOMA scores improved from 3-4 to 0-1. (LENT SOMA is a scale developed to have an objective assessment of post-radiation skin changes like degree of retraction or atrophy, edema, ulceration, telangiectasia, post-radiation fibrosis, arm lymphedema, skin sensation and pigmentation change). The number of procedures ranged from 1-6 with most patients needing 2-3 procedures. The volume injected varied between 60-80 cc in each injection. The mean follow up was 30 months and they reported no complications. This study used hyper concentrated fat for grafting and attributed the radiation damage reversal to the angiogenic potential of adipose derived stem cells (ADSC), which reside in natural fat.

Panettiere et al. reported similar improvement in radiation damage using fat grafting in 2009 (Panettiere et al, 2009). Their study population addressed 62 patients (20 active, 42 controls) who had undergone mastectomy, radiation and implant reconstruction. Fat grafting once again, was used as an ancillary technique to smooth border zone defects or to treat radiation damaged tissue. These patients did not undergo pre-expansion and had relatively tight, small-capacity recipient sites. The mean number of fat grafting sessions performed on each reconstructed breast was 3.4 with an average volume of 24.5 ml of autologous fat injected in each session. LENT SOMA scores improved in all patients in the intervention group and capsular contractures were downgraded as well. They reported no complications.

Delay et al (2008) reported extremely high patient satisfaction scores after using fat grafting to treat the sequelae of breast conservation therapy (lumpectomy and radiation) in 42 patients. Delaporte et al (2009) used fat grafting to reconstruct mastectomy defects in 15 patients. Average volume injected was 600 ml over 3 sessions. They reported good patient satisfaction scores as well.

The overwhelming theme in all of these studies is that small volume fat grafting for border zone defects and for radiation damage can be successfully performed in the absence of pre-expansion, especially when fat is hyper-concentrated, small volumes (less than 100cc) are used, and fat is transplanted in serial sessions. This is distinctly different from mega volume fat grafting for core volume replacement, which we employ as a first-line treatment for breast reconstruction. Such findings support our previously stated contention that not all fat grafting is the same, and must be stratified along a matrix of volume and regenerative demands at the recipient site.

Despite the large number of patient series of breast reconstruction patients receiving small amounts of fat as a final touch for achieving better aesthetic outcomes, there are few reports of "core volume" breast reconstruction being done exclusively by fat grafting (Del Vecchio,

2009, Babovic 2010, Delay et al 2010, Panettiere et al 2011, Fitoussi et al 2009). Because in all but one of these reports pre-expansion was not used and one begins with an absent breast mound or a thinned mastectomy skin flap, there are recipient site capacity issues in these cases and these operations often require more than 3 sessions.

9. Controversies and future directions

9.1 Sequelae of fat transplantation and cancer surveillance

As early as Lyndon Peer's work in fat grafting (Peer, 1950), it is a clinically accepted reality that not all that maintains volume following fat grafting represents viable adipocytes. Peer in fact stated his estimated 45% resorption rate was due to a combination of apoptosis and necrosis that subsequently lead to fibrosis, oil cysts and calcification. Legitimate concerns over these sequelae served as the cause for fat grafting's dismissal from the plastic surgery community through the ASPRS 1987 position paper on the subject. The paper stated:

"The committee is unanimous in deploring the use of autologous fat injection in breast augmentation. Much of the injected fat will not survive, and the known physiological response to necrosis of this tissue is scarring and calcification. As a result, detection of early breast carcinoma through xerography and mammography will become difficult and the presence of disease may go undiscovered."(ASPRS, 1987).

Breaking down the ASPRS statement into two parts, one can, in 2011, address each of them with a more evidence-based approach than was merely expert opinion in 1987:

We really still no not know how much of the injected fat survives, and there is no good accurate method to do so. Proponents of the scaffold theory do not believe any of the fat survives. In 2011, detection of early breast cancer can easily be distinguished from fat necrosis and oil cysts. In fact, the radiographic changes after fat grafting to the breast are no different than those after other conventional and well-accepted breast surgery (Pierrefeu-Lagrange et al, 2006, Coleman and Saboeiro, 2007, Gosset et al, 2008, Zheng et al, 2008, Veber et al, 2011).

The answer to addressing radiographic sequelae of fat grafting, perhaps, lies in a risk-adjusted approach to classifying radiographic findings after breast fat grafting (Del Vecchio, 2011). The ASPS revised their position on fat grafting and their new policy statement reads:

"Based on a limited number of studies with few cases, there appears to be no interference with breast cancer detection; however, more studies are needed to confirm these preliminary findings" (Level IV, V evidence) (Gutowski, 2009)

9.2 Neoplastic potential

The role of adipose-derived stem cells (ADSC) in wound healing has been described (Kim et al, 2007) and may have clinical use in treating radiation injury to irradiated breast tissue. Although this has been attributed to the secretion of angiogenic factors by human adipose stromal cells (Rehman et al, 2004), the naked truth is we really do not currently have a clear mechanism of action for this clinical observation. Some bone marrow derived stem cells, when placed into animal cancer models, appear to accelerate the growth of the underlying cancer (Liu et al, 2011). This observation cannot however, be translated to the risk of natural fat and their inherent concentration of adipocyte derived stem cells initiating breast cancer.

Women have a 1 in 8 risk of being affected by breast cancer in their lifetime. There is no evidence to date that this incidence is any greater in women who have had fat injected into all or part of their breasts. Although proxies for long-term carcinogenic effects on fat grafting and breast cancer have been reported in patients following breast cancer treatment with or without subsequent fat grafting (Delay et al, 2009), these are not prospective studies of a normal population of women with or without fat transplantation over many years, which is what will be necessary to fully answer the carcinogenesis question. To date, there appears to be no increased risk but it is too early to draw any conclusions. Therefore, in 2011, the use of fat grafting to the breast for reconstruction or for augmentation should include a thorough discussion of the *unknown risk* of fat causing breast cancer, and this discussion should be made clear with the patient and be well documented in the medical record.

10. Conclusion

Fat grafting to the breast has rapidly evolved as a safe technique with a wide range of applications in breast reconstructive surgery. There is still a lack of standardization in the techniques used, but trends towards time management and simplification of technique are appearing. Standardization in mammography imaging and reading in the fat-grafted breast is expected to improve and ease concerns over calcifications and oil cysts being misread as cancer, reducing the risk of unnecessary biopsies.

At this point of time, its technically simpler and lower-risk indication is for contour correction in conjunction with other reconstructive operations. However, it can be exclusively used for breast reconstruction for core volume projection, obviating the need for an initial core volume strategy that eventually requires fat transplantation for correction in the majority of cases.

11. References

Aboudib JHC, Cardoso de Castro C, Gradel J. Hand rejuvenescence by fat filling. Ann Plast Surg 1992 Jun; 28: 559-64

ASPRS Ad-Hoc Committee on new Procedures: Report on Autologous fat transplantation. Plast Surg Nurs 1987 Winter; 7(4):140–141

Babovic S. Complete breast reconstruction with autologous fat graft - a case report. J Plast Reconstr Aesthet Surg. 2010 Jul; 63(7): 561-3

Baker, T. BRAVA Non-Surgical Breast Expansion. Presentation at the American Society of Aesthetic Plastic Surgeons Annual Meeting, Orlando, Florida. April, 2006

Bernard RW, Beran SJ. Autologous fat graft in nipple reconstruction.Plast Reconstr Surg. 2003 Sep 15; 112(4): 964-8

Billings E Jr, May JW. Historical review and present status of free fat graft autotransplantation in plastic and reconstructive surgery. Plast Reconstr Surg 1989 Feb; 83(2):368–381

Bircoll M. Cosmetic breast augmentation utilizing autologous fat andliposuction techniques. Plast Reconstr Surg. 1987 Feb; 79(2): 267-71

Bircoll M, Novack BH. Autologous fat transplantation employing liposuction techniques. Ann Plast Surg. 1987 Apr; 18(4): 327-9

Cervelli V, Palla L, Pascali M, De Angelis B, Curcio BC, Gentile P. Autologous platelet-rich plasma mixed with purified fat graft in aesthetic plastic surgery. Aesthetic Plast Surg. 2009 Sep; 33(5): 716-21.

Chajchir A. Fat injection: long-term follow-up. Aesthetic Plast Surg 1996; 20: 291-6

Coleman, Sydney R. M.D.; Saboeiro, Alesia P. M.D. Fat Grafting to the Breast Revisted: Safety and Efficacy. Plast Reconstr Surg. 2007 Mar; 119(3): 775-85; discussion 786-7

Cronin T, Gerow F. Augmentation Mammaplasty: A new natural feel prosthesis. Transactions of the Third International Congress of Plastic Surgery, Amsterdam. Excerpta Medica Foundation. 1964; 41-49

Czerny V. DreiPlastischeOperationen.III. Plastischer Ersatz der Brustdrüsedurchein Lipom.Verhandlungen der DeutschenGesellscahftfürChirurgie 1895;II:216-217

De Cholnoky T. Late adverse results following breast reconstructions. Plast Reconstr Surg. 1963 May;31:445-52

Del Vecchio D. Breast reconstruction for breast asymmetry using recipient site pre-expansion and autologous fat grafting: a case report. Ann Plast Surg. 2009 May; 62(5): 523-7

Del Vecchio DA. Discussion: Clinical analyses of clustered microcalcifications after autologous fat injection for breast augmentation. Plast Reconstr Surg. 2011 Apr; 127(4): 1674-6

Delay E, Gosset J, Toussoun G, Delaporte T, Delbaere M. [Efficacy of lipo-modelling for the management of sequelae of breast cancer conservative treatment]. Ann Chir Plast Esthet. 2008 Apr;53(2):153-68

Delay E, Garson S, Tousson G, Sinna R. Fat injection to the breast: technique, results, and indications based on 880 procedures over 10 years. Aesthetic Surg J.2009 Sep-Oct;29(5):360-76

Delay E, Sinna R, Chekaroua K, Delaporte T, Garson S, Toussoun G. Lipomodelingof Poland's syndrome: a new treatment of the thoracic deformity. Aesthetic Plast Surg. 2010 Apr; 34(2): 218-25

Dolderer JH, Abberton KM, Thompson EW, Slavin JL, Stevens GW, Penington AJ, Morrison WA. Spontaneous large volume adipose tissue generation from avascularized pedicled fat flap inside a chamber space. Tissue Eng. 2007 Apr; 13 (4): 673-81

Erdim M, Tezel E, Numanoglu A, Sav A. The effects of the size of liposuctioncannula on adipocyte survival and the optimum temperature for fat graft storage: an experimental study. J Plast Reconstr Aesthet Surg. 2009 Sep; 62(9): 1210-4

Fitoussi A, Pollet AG, Couturaud B, Salmon RJ. Secondary breast reconstruction using exclusive lipofilling Ann Chir Plast Esthet. 2009 Aug; 54(4): 374-8

Goldwyn RM. Vincenz Czerny and the beginnings of breast reconstruction.Plast Reconstr Surg. 1978 May;61(5):673-81

Gosset J, Guerin N, Toussoun G, Delaporte T, Delay E. Radiological evaluation after lipomodelling for correction of breast conservative treatment sequelae. Ann Chir Plast Esthet. 2008 Apr; 53(2): 178-89.

Gumucio CA, Pin P, Young VL, Destouet J, Monsees B, Eichling J: The effect of breast implants on the radiographic detection of microcalcification and soft-tissue masses. Plast Reconstr Surg 1989 Nov; 84(5): 772-8; discussion 779-82

Gutowski KA; ASPS Fat Graft Task Force. Current applications and safety ofautologous fat grafts: a report of the ASPS fat graft task force. Plast Reconstr Surg. 2009 Jul; 124(1): 272-80

Halsted WS. I. The Results of Operations for the Cure of Cancer of the Breast Performed at the Johns Hopkins Hospital from June 1889 to January 1894. Ann Surg. 1894 Nov; 20(5): 497-555

Halsted WS. I. The Results of Radical Operations for the Cure of Carcinoma of the Breast. Ann Surg. 1907 Jul; 46 (1): 1-19

Hang-Fu L, Marmolya G, Feiglin DH. Liposuction fat-fillant implant for breast augmentation and reconstruction. Aesthetic Plast Surg. 1995 Sep-Oct; 19(5): 427-37

Hartrampf CR, Scheflan M, Black PW. Breast reconstruction with a transverse abdominal island flap. Plast Reconstr Surg. 1982 Feb; 69(2): 216-25

Hyakusoku H, Ogawa R, Ono S, Ishii N, Hirakawa K. Complications after autologous fat injection to the breast. Plast Reconstr Surg. 2009 Jan; 123(1): 360-70

Illouz YG. Body contouring by lipolysis: a five-year experience with over 3000 cases. Plast Reconstr Surg 1983; 72(5): 591-597

Illouz YG, Sterodimas A. Autologous fat transplantation to the breast: a personal technique with 25 years of experience. Aesthetic Plast Surg. 2009 Sep; 33(5): 706-15

Kanchwala SK, Glatt BS, Conant EF, Bucky LP. Autologous fat grafting to the reconstructed breast: the management of acquired contour deformities. Plast Reconstr Surg. 2009 Aug; 124(2): 409-18

Kaufman MR, Bradley JP, Dickinson B, Heller JB, Wasson K, O'Hara C, Huang C,Gabbay J, Ghadjar K, Miller TA. Autologous fat transfer national consensus survey: trends in techniques for harvest, preparation, and application, and perception of short- and long-term results. Plast Reconstr Surg. 2007 Jan; 119(1):323-31

Khouri RK, Baker TJ. Initial experience with the BRAVA nonsurgical system of breast enhancement. Plast Reconstr Surg. 2002 Nov; 110(6):1593-1595.

Kim WS, Park BS, Sung JH, Yang JM, Park SB, Kwak SJ, Park JS. Wound healing effect of adipose-derived stem cells: a critical role of secretory factors onhuman dermal fibroblasts. J Dermatol Sci. 2007 Oct; 48(1):15-24

Kononas TC, Bucky LP, Hurley C, May JW, Jr.: The fate of suctioned and surgically removed fat after reimplantation for soft-tissue augmentation: a volumetric and histologic study in the rabbit. Plast Reconstr Surg 1993 Apr; 91(5): 763-768

Kurita M, Matsumoto D, Shigeura T, Sato K, Gonda K, Harii K, Yoshimura K. Influences of centrifugation on cells and tissues in liposuction aspirates: optimized centrifugation for lipotransfer and cell isolation. Plast Reconstr Surg 2008 Mar;121(3):1033-41; discussion 1042-3

Lexer E. Fatty tissue transplantation. In: Die Transplantation, Part I. Stuttgart, Ferdinand Enke, 1919, pp. 265–302

Liu, S, Ginestier C, Sing, J et al. Breast Cancer Stem Cells Are Regulated by Mesenchymal Stem Cells through Cytokine Networks. Cancer Research 2011. 71(2); 614–24

Losken A, Jurkiewicz MJ. History of breast reconstruction. Breast Dis.2002;16:3-9

Losken A, Pinell XA, Sikoro K, Yezhelyev MV, Anderson E, Carlson GW.Autologous fat grafting in secondary breast reconstruction. Ann Plast Surg. 2011 May; 66(5):518-22

Manabe Y, Toda S, Miyazaki K, Sugihara H. Mature adipocytes, but not preadipocytes, promote the growth of breast carcinoma cells in collagen gel matrix culture through cancer-stromal cell interactions. J Pathol. 2003 Oct; 201 (2): 221-8

McCraw JB. The recent history of myocutaneous flaps. Clin Plast Surg. 1980 Jan; 7(1):3-7

Missana MC, Laurent I, Barreau L, Balleyguier C. Autologous fat transfer in reconstructive breast surgery: indications, technique and results. Eur J Surg Oncol. 2007 Aug; 33(6):685-90

Moseley, Timothy A. Ph.D.; Zhu, Min M.D.; Hedrick, Marc H. M.D. Adipose-Derived Stem and Progenitor Cells as Fillers in Plastic and Reconstructive Surgery. Plast Reconstr Surg: Volume 118(3S) Suppl1 September 2006 pp 121S-128S.

Neuber GA. Verhandlungen der Deutschen Gesellschaftfür Chirurgie 1893;1:66

Padoin AV, Braga-Silva J, Martins P, Rezende K, Rezende AR, Grechi B, Gehlen D, Machado DC. Sources of processed lipoaspirate cells: influence of donor site on cell concentration. Plast Reconstr Surg. 2008 Aug; 122(2):614-8

Panettiere P, Marchetti L, Accorsi D. The serial free fat transfer in irradiated prosthetic breast reconstructions. Aesthetic Plast Surg. 2009 Sep; 33(5):695-700

Panettiere P, Accorsi D, Marchetti L, Sgrò F, Sbarbati A. Large-Breast Reconstruction Using Fat Graft Only after Prosthetic Reconstruction Failure Aesthetic Plast Surg. 2011 Feb 27. [Epub ahead of print]

Peer LA. Loss of weight and volume in human fat grafts: With postulation of a "cell survival theory." Plast Reconstr Surg 1950; 5:217–230

Peer LA. Cell survival theory versus replacement theory. Plast Reconstr Surg 1955 Sep; 16(3): 161-8

Peer LA. The neglected free fat graft, its behavior and clinical use. Am J Surg. 1956 Jul; 92(1): 40-7

Pierrefeu-Lagrange AC, Delay E, Guerin N, Chekaroua K, Delaporte T.Radiological evaluation of breasts reconstructed with lipomodelling. Ann Chir Plast Esthet. 2006 Feb; 51(1):18-28

Pulagam SR, Poulton T, Mamounas EP. Long-term clinical and radiologic results with autologous fat transplantation for breast augmentation: case reports and review of the literature. Breast J. 2006 Jan-Feb; 12(1): 63-5

Radovan C. Breast reconstruction after mastectomy using the temporary expander.Plast Reconstr Surg. 1982 Feb; 69(2):195-208

Rehman J, Traktuev D, Li J, Merfeld-Clauss S, Temm-Grove CJ, Bovenkerk JE,Pell CL, Johnstone BH, Considine RV, March KL. Secretion of angiogenic and antiapoptotic factors by human adipose stromal cells. Circulation. 2004 Mar 16;109(10):1292-8

Rietjens M, De Lorenzi F, Rossetto F, Brenelli F, Manconi A, Martella S, IntraM, Venturino M, Lohsiriwat V, Ahmed Y, Petit JY. Safety of fat grafting in secondary breast reconstruction after cancer. J Plast Reconstr Aesthet Surg. 2011 Apr; 64(4):477-83

Rigotti, Gino M.D.; Marchi, Alessandra M.D et al. Clinical Treatment of Radiotherapy Tissue Damage by Lipo-aspirate Transplant: A Healing Process Mediated by Adipose-Derived Adult Stem Cells. Plast Reconstr Surg. 2007 April 119(5): 1409-1422

Rigotti G, Marchi A, Battistoni A. Bioengineering of the mammary region with adipocyte derived stem cells: a new concept in expander implant breast reconstruction in patients affected by radiation side effects, local fat deficiencies and/or important skin changes. Presented at the European Association of Plastic Surgeons Annual Meeting, Gent, 2007

Saxena V, Hwang CW, Huang S, Eichbaum Q, Ingber D, Orgill DP. Vacuum-assisted closure: micro-deformations of wounds and cell proliferation. Plast Reconstr Surg 2004 Oct; 114(5):1086-96; discussion 1097-8

Saxena V, Orgill D, Kohane I. A set of genes previously implicated in the hypoxia response might be an important modulator in the rat ear tissue response to mechanical stretch. BMC Genomics 2007 Nov 23;8:430

Schneider WJ, Hill HL Jr, Brown RG. Latissimus dorsi myocutaneous flap for breast reconstruction. Br J Plast Surg. 1977 Oct;30(4):277-81

Serra-Renom JM, Muñoz-Olmo JL, Serra-Mestre JM. Fat grafting in postmastectomy breast reconstruction with expanders and prostheses in patients who have received radiotherapy: formation of new subcutaneous tissue. Plast Reconstr Surg. 2010 Jan; 125(1):12-8

Serra-Renom JM, Muñoz-Olmo J, Serra-Mestre JM.Breast reconstruction with fat grafting alone. Ann Plast Surg. 2011 Jun; 66(6):598-601

Shiffman MA, Mirrafati S. Fat transfer techniques: the effect of harvest and transfer methods on adipocyte viability and review of the literature. Dermatol Surg. 2001 Sep; 27(9):819-26

Sinna R, Delay E, Garson S, Delaporte T, Toussoun G. Breast fat grafting (lipomodelling) after extended latissimus dorsi flap breast reconstruction: a preliminary report of 200 consecutive cases. J Plast Reconstr Aesthet Surg. 2010 Nov; 63(11): 1769-77

Snyderman RK. Breast cancer and fat transplants. Plast Reconstr Surg. 1988 Jun; 81(6):991

Spear SL, Wilson HB, Lockwood MD. Fat injection to correct contour deformities in the reconstructed breast. Plast Reconstr Surg. 2005 Oct;116(5):1300 5

Ullmann Y, Shoshani O, Fodor A, Ramon Y, Carmi N, Eldor L, Gilhar A. Searching for the favorable donor site for fat injection: in vivo study using the nude mice model. Dermatol Surg. 2005 Oct; 31(10): 1304-7

Veber M, Tourasse C, Toussoun G, Moutran M, Mojallal A, Delay E. Radiographic findings after breast augmentation by autologous fat transfer. Plast Reconstr Surg. 2011 Mar; 127 (3): 1289-99

Zheng DN, Li QF, Lei H, Zheng SW, Xie YZ, Xu QH, Yun X, Pu LL: Autologous fat grafting to the breast for cosmetic enhancement: experience in 66 patients with long-term follow up; J Plast Reconstr Aesthet Surg. 2008 Jul; 61(7): 792-8.

Zocchi ML, Zuliani F Bicompartmental breast lipostructuring. Aesthetic Plast Surg. 2008 Mar;32(2):313-28.

Part 5

Breast Reconstruction After Conservative Treatment

12

Breast Reconstruction Approach to Conservative Surgery

Egidio Riggio and Valentina Visintini Cividin
Unit of Plastic Reconstructive Surgery, Fondazione IRCCS Istituto Nazionale dei Tumori, Milano, Italy

1. Introduction

Breast conservative treatment (BCT) can be advantageous compared with skin-sparing (SSM) or nipple-sparing mastectomy for many patients affected by unicentric ductal carcinoma in situ (DCIS), Paget's disease, invasive lobular carcinoma (ILC) and invasive ductal carcinoma (IDC) up to 2-3 cm as diameter and without extension to skin (T1; part of T2 in larger breast), and more recently T2 up to 5 cm previously treated by neoadjuvant chemotherapy with positive effect on tumor size reduction. Partial or segmental mastectomy, i.e. quadrantectomy, should include 1.5–3cm excision of normal tissue around the tumour, including the ductal tree, and the removal of a portion of overlying skin and underlying fascia when indicated. Contrary to what happens in Europe and in Italy, lumpectomy is largely preferred in the United States because of the higher cosmetic result without the help of plastic remodelling. Quadrantectomy associated to axillary dissection with radiation therapy (QUART) or without it (QUAD), likely shows three advantages: 1) preservation of healthy breast with satisfying cosmetic appearance if reshaped by the plastic surgeon; 2) preservation of vascular supply and innervation of the nipple-areola complex except of central quadrantectomy; 3) maintenance of some average symmetry improvable with the reshaping reduction of the contralateral breast. Unfortunately many breast surgeons use to perform more lumpectomies rather than ask for plastic surgery aid in order to reshape a quadrantectomy. Disadvantages are given by the radiation effects on soft tissues and the long-term higher rate of local recurrences compared to mastectomy. May radiation be avoided in patients with DCIS? There are no extra-benefit for survival or distant metastases compared to excision alone; patients with high-grade DCIS lesions and positive margins benefited most from the addition of radiotherapy (Viani, 2007). Even if many trials suggest significant reduction of absolute local recurrence after radiation, many unicentric DCIS are conventionally treated by local excision alone. The unsolved problem remains how to identify subgroups of patients with DCIS with different rates of local recurrence incidence (Silverstein, 2006). Annual risk for in-breast recurrence is rated 1.97 per 100 patients even in the most favourable subgroup with clear margins and minimal amount of comedonecrosis without radiation (Fisher, 1995). At least clear margins of 1 cm for tumour size of $\leq$1.5 cm are considered wide excisions with a good Van Nuys Prognostic Index (Silverstein, 1996). Local control can be achieved without radiation therapy when margins widths of $\geq$1 cm are obtained, regardless of nuclear grade, comedonecrosis, or tumour size within 2.5 cm (Silverstein, 1999). It becomes mandatory marking all margins of the surgical specimen in order not to find positive margins. May DCIS of $\geq$3 cm be untreated by radiation therapy if clear margins should be more than 2cm with the same benefit? Avoiding radiation is fundamental for both the techniques and outcomes of plastic surgery. Reconstruction after BCT are more risky because of the damaged tissues of the breast. In addition the salvage mastectomy necessary in presence of further recurrence complicates the reconstructive chances and generates a worse psychological trauma in the patients more severely than a primary mastectomy with implant reconstruction.

End points of any breast-conserving treatment are: local control of disease and good cosmetic result. Based on our Institute's experience, successful BCT was always related to radical excision with wide clear margins along with expertise in mastopexy techniques. Medium and large breast-size can facilitate oncoplastic resections with optimal morphologic-cosmetic compliance. On the contrary in case of small breast, SSM or nipple-sparing mastectomy followed by reconstruction with expander or permanent silicone implant can give better perspectives concerning longer disease-free survival rate and more cosmetic results although the nipple will lose sensibility and the nipple-areola displacement could likely bring to asymmetry difficult to be corrected. The BCT reduction of a breast already small could become for many women inacceptable independently from the occurrence of permanent scarring deformity (Fig.1). The reconstruction after mastectomy can also permit to augment the contralateral breast according to the patient's wishes. Nowadays our rate of BCT reconstruction is decreasing because of the always earlier detection of smaller tumours and smaller resections as well as because of the increasing rate of nipple-sparing mastectomies especially for the younger patients with IDC, that are more exposed to a long-term relapse of disease.

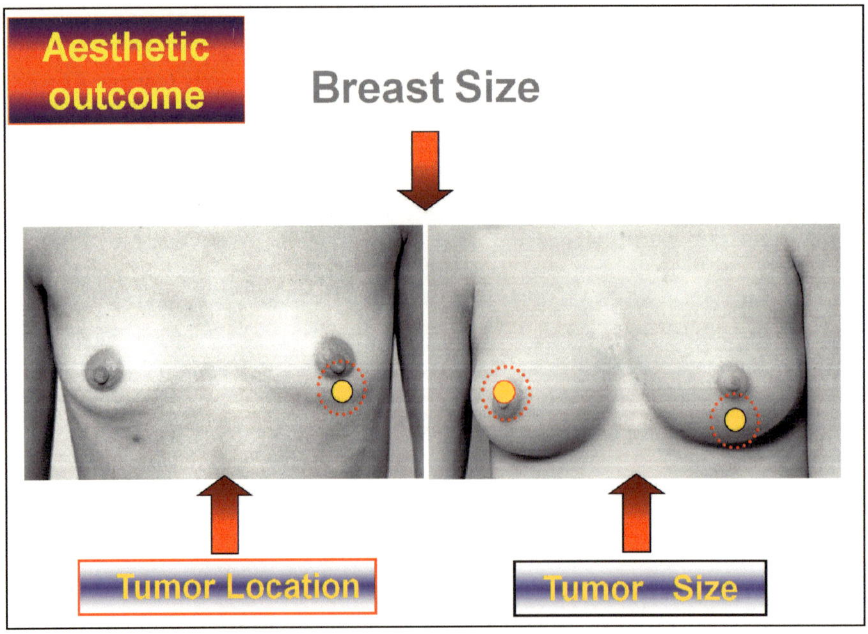

Fig. 1. Cancer localization and size related to the breast size

1.1 Historical focus on QUART

The idea of conserving the breast started forty years ago in our Institute (Fig.2): Milan Trial I (1973-1980; 701 patients; tumours up to 2-cm diameter; Halstedian mastectomy versus QUART). Disease-free and overall survival curves presented no difference between the two groups at 8 years: disease-free survival 77% for Halsted patients and 80% for the QUART patients, while overall survival was 83% and 85%, respectively (Veronesi, 1981-1986). The cumulative incidence of recurrences was 8.8 percent (QUART) versus 2.3 percent respectively, after a median follow-up of 20 years (Veronesi, 2002).

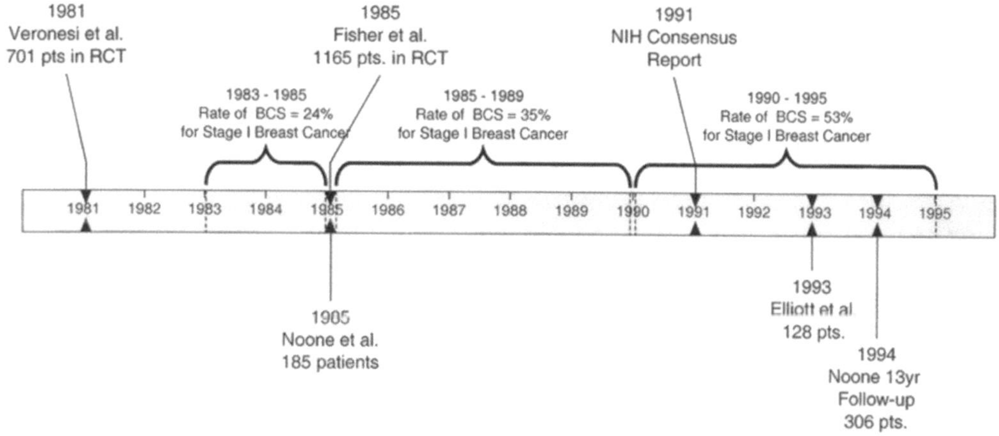

Fig. 2. Positive development of the breast-conserving treatment at the end of the last century. The first operations did use no techniques of plastic surgery and the contralateral breast was frequently reduced by a "mirror quadrantectomy" with evident scars. Plastic surgery was introduced earlier than 1985 through procedures of dermaglandular reshaping or silicone implant insertion, in the last two decades discontinued.

The Milan Trial II (1985-1987; 705 patients; tumours up to 2.5 cm; 345 TART - tumorectomy, axillary dissection, and radiation therapy - versus 360 QUART,) demonstrated higher frequency of local recurrences after tumorectomy (7.0 vs. 2.2%) (Veronesi, 1990). The importance of irradiation was supported by the Milan Trial III (1987-1989; 579 patients; tumours less than 2.5 cm; QUART (299) versus QUAD (280). After breast-conserving surgery, radiotherapy was indicated in all patients up to 55 years of age, in patients with positive axillary nodes, and in patients with extensive intraductal component at histology. The study suggested that irradiation may be avoided in patients older than 65, and be optional in women aged 56-65 years with negative nodes (Veronesi, 2001).

The oncological safety was confirmed by others studies: NSABP B-06 trial (Fisher, 1985). A total of 92.3 per cent of women treated with radiation remained free of breast tumor at five years. The BCT efficiency provided that the specimen margins were free of tumor and cosmetic outcome were acceptable (Fisher, 2002). After twenty-year follow-up, the cumulative incidence of recurrences in the ipsilateral breast was 14.3 percent.

The EORTC trial (Van Dongen, 1992) did show a significant difference about the rate of locoregional recurrence at 10 years: 12% of the mastectomy and 20% of the BCT patients. The locoregional recurrence rate for patients with a microscopically complete excision was

17.6% (95% CI = 11.2%–22.3%); for patients with microscopic margin involvement, it was 26.5.% (95% CI = 22.2%–33.0%). The locoregional recurrence rate progressively increased: the rate was 11.8% (95% CI = 8.5%–15.1%) at 5 years and 19.7% (95% CI = 15.4%–24.0%) at 10 years. After a median follow-up of 13.4 years, BCT and mastectomy still demonstrate similar survival rates for patients with tumors up to 5 cm (Joop - Van Dongen, 2000).

Even if the overall survival after QUART is equivalent to mastectomy, local recurrence rate is higher in the conserved breast. A significant predicting factor is young age of 40 years or less. Younger patients had a five-fold increased risk of developing a breast recurrence compared with patients older than 60 years (Arriagada, 2002; 717 patients treated by lumpectomy and breast irradiation and 1289 patients by total mastectomy for T up to 2.5 cm; most patients did not receive adjuvant chemotherapy or additive hormonal treatments; mean follow-up of 20 years).

BCT is still considered a valid choice for small tumors after meta-analysis of the main randomized controlled trials (Yang, 2008) despite the local recurrence rate not less than 1% per year and the early local recurrence (<5 years) associated with worse prognosis. Many relapses occur in the vicinity of the tumour bed, but the percentage of recurrences occurring in other quadrants increases over time and those after 10 years are considered new primary tumours. Open question remains how much is convenient to risk salvage mastectomy after irradiation to the aims of guaranteeing either the cosmetic result primarily fixed with BCT or the minor invasiveness of the elective reconstructive procedures.

1.2 Reconstruction after quadrantectomy

Glandular excision volume is the first element to determine the most appropriate oncoplastic treatment. This is the most predictive factor of surgical outcome and related breast deformity; if more than 20% of breast volume must be excised, risk for breast deformity becomes high.

The immediate and delayed reconstructions were developed after these trials performed in our Institute. The first Author coordinated a retrospective study of reconstructions after partial mastectomy, i.e. quadrantectomy. The first 100 patients' histories were detected in 1987 and 1992 (Table 1).

Patient number	100
Average age	50 (17-67)years
Tumor size	1.95 + 0.21 (0.4-2.7 cm)
Skin resection	4.5 x 3.0 cm
Breast glandular resection	6 x 5 x 4 cm
Adjuvant chemotherapy	10 patients
breast irradiation (50Gy+10Gy boost)	89 patients

Table 1. Clinical data per 100 patients

Tumours are IDC for the 45% (Table 2) and the most frequent sites of reconstruction are the upper-external and the central quadrants (Fig.3). The distribution per breast areas is different compared with the cancer incidence per site.

DIC	44
LIC	18
DIC + LIC	11
DISC	6
Paget	3
Paget + DISC	1
Paget + LIC	1
Adenocarcinoma	1
Sarcoma	2
Dysplasia	11

Table 2. Tumour hystology

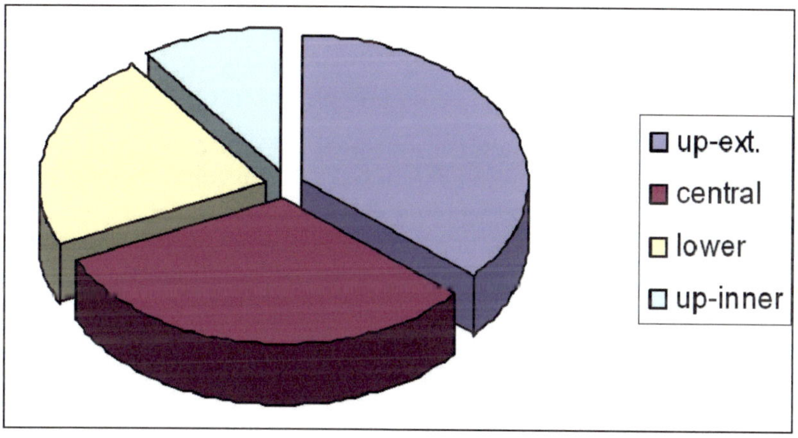

Fig. 3. Distribution of reconstruction per site of quadrantectomy

Even if the upper-external tumours show the larger incidence (50%), reconstructive procedures were applied in 35% of them, >20% immediate (Fig.4). On the contrary, the cancer centrally located occurs in 20% of the total breast cancer incidence, but the reconstructions are numerous and represents the 51% of the total, 1% is delayed. Immediate reconstructions are crucial: the 75% is immediate and 25% is delayed above all. Primary aim is the restitution of shape and symmetry to the breast before irradiation; for this reason the complimentary aid among general and breast surgeons is important. The 89% of patients with BCT reconstruction underwent radiotherapy. Hence immediate reconstruction should be furthermore increased. Delayed reconstructions are usually performed after three years from radiation therapy and must be carefully selected because of higher complication rate related to irradiated tissues.

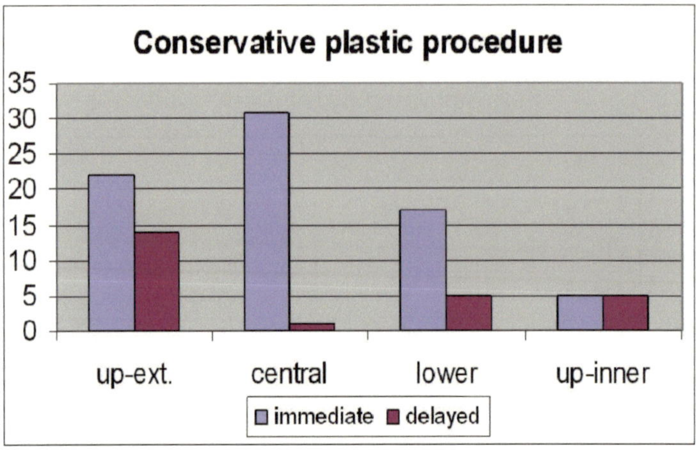

Fig. 4. Different distribution for immediate and delayed reconstructions

The choice for silicone implant is seriously disadvantageous after irradiation : 67% of severe capsular contracture and 55.5% of cases were surgically revised in our series. No significant differences were found in surgical timing, i.e. implant before or after radiotherapy.

The tissue loss generated by quadrantectomy can be immediately restored using a variety of mastopexy techiniques, mostly based on lower pedicle or round-block, with different skin incisions in relationship with the anatomical site of tumour excision, breast size, thorax length and breast ptosis (especially the jugulum-nipple distance).

In delayed steps, multiple z-plasty and/or areola-nipple replacement can be performed in the upper internal or external region of the breast. On the contrary, a defect at the mid-upper region is more difficult to be repaired especially when associated to areola-nipple cranial displacement. In the last condition, autologous tissue transfer can be indicated for the larger defects while fat injections can be preferred for middle/lower defects with minimal skin loss. Latissimus dorsi and TRAM flaps were mostly used, in a delayed time.

Before the end of the last century, the different rates of surgical procedures were: dermaglandular flaps, 68%; breast silicone implants 20%; autologous flaps, 12% (latissimus dorsi 10%, 2 with implants, TRAM 2%). Nowadays, implants were discontinued for irradiation complications and were substituted by lipofillings, after a 3-year follow-up and in patients at minor risk of recurrence. The autologous flaps are less necessary and then decreased due to: a) the major number of immediate dermaglandular remodelling and b) the preference for the removal of the remaining breast, before performing a composite flap, instead of retaining the higher risk of local recurrence and consequent salvage mastectomy and new flap reconstruction.

2. Immediate reconstruction

One crucial question is the decision about the timing of reconstruction following conservative treatment and successive radiotherapy. Ideally, reconstruction should be both immediate and definitive so as to avoid patients undergoing further surgery later. It is now generally considered, from an oncological point of view, that there are no contraindications to reconstruction, even if it is immediate, in that it does not interfere with the progress of the disease. In many cases it is only for organisational reasons (absence of a surgeon specialised in reconstruction, insufficient time, lack of material for reconstruction–prosthesis) that reconstructive surgery must be scheduled after the quadrantectomy time. From a surgical point of view it is "always" possible to carry out immediate reconstruction provided that the general conditions of the patient permit so, yet it might not always be opportune to do so. In most cases reconstruction must be immediate if we wish to restore by rotating local flaps. Extensive mobilization of the local flaps is indeed much more difficult and riskier when carried out at a secondary time after radiotherapy. Nowadays the gold standard is to use a fast technique which also assures a good final outcome. The tendency and general opinion regarding restoration timing following conservative treatment agree on performing immediate breast reconstruction in all cases where it is possible.

The cases of partial mastectomy are multifarious. This variability mainly depends on the extent of resection of the mammary volume, the quadrant involved, and then direction and length of the surgical incision. Moreover the results of quadrantectomy depend on the size of the tumour removed, on the effects of radiotherapy, on the administration of adjuvant chemotherapy and on the surgeon skill. The reconstructive technique is chosen on the basis of these factors.

The amount of breast tissue removed, which is conditioned by the size of the tumour, is the most important factor and the smaller the breast the more evident is its effect. The larger the breast, the better the final result will be in aesthetic terms.

Scarring, an important aesthetic issue, generally depends on the type of surgical incision, on the primary site of tumour, on the patient characteristics, on the radiotherapy and on any complications post-surgery (infections, hematoma). The main radial axis of the incision typically extends from the area of the areola to the periphery of the breast. Unless required by the lesion, the incision should not over-extend peripherally, towards the axilla, or arrive too closely to the nipple. For lesions behind the areola it is usually necessary to comprise areola and nipple. The tissue deficit depends on the amount removed, including skin, mammary gland and areola–nipple part.

Unless reconstructed at the same time as surgical removal, a quadrantectomy sums the above deficits to the damage caused by radiotherapy, which leads to alterations in the skin and glands of the breast treated. Irradiated tissue becomes fibrotic, and hence inelastic. In these cases it is often necessary to remove a further part of radio-damaged tissue, hence increasing the deficit. At this point it is necessary to resort to myocutaneous flaps.

Mammary prostheses can only be used in selected cases when other techniques (local reshaping, transfer of distance flaps or contralateral procedures) have been refused by the patient. Periprosthesic fibrosis in irradiated tissue can be highly aggressive and lead to serious distortion of the prosthesis. The presence of a prosthesis could interfere with instrumental examinations (mammography) and with the diagnosis of intramammary recurrences but the potential problem could be exist also for inner scars after reshaping.

A contralateral mammaplasty (pexy or reduction), that substitutes the old concept of "mirror quadrantectomy," is aimed to reach a good symmetry of the breast. It can be carried out both at the same time as the quadrantectomy or successively as the patient wishes or as oncoplastic reasons could suggest.

2.1 The reconstruction after upper quadrantectomy

Half of the breast tumours involved the upper-external zone where most defects do not require a particular reconstruction technique but simply undermining. Nevertheless the general surgeon must be conscious that some defects about tissue loss or scar will appear later, and very often after radiation (Fig. 5). It is often sufficient to mobilize slightly the dermoglandular flaps adjacent to the resection and to balance areola and nipple position. Aesthetic results are easily better in upper-external quadrant than in other quadrants.

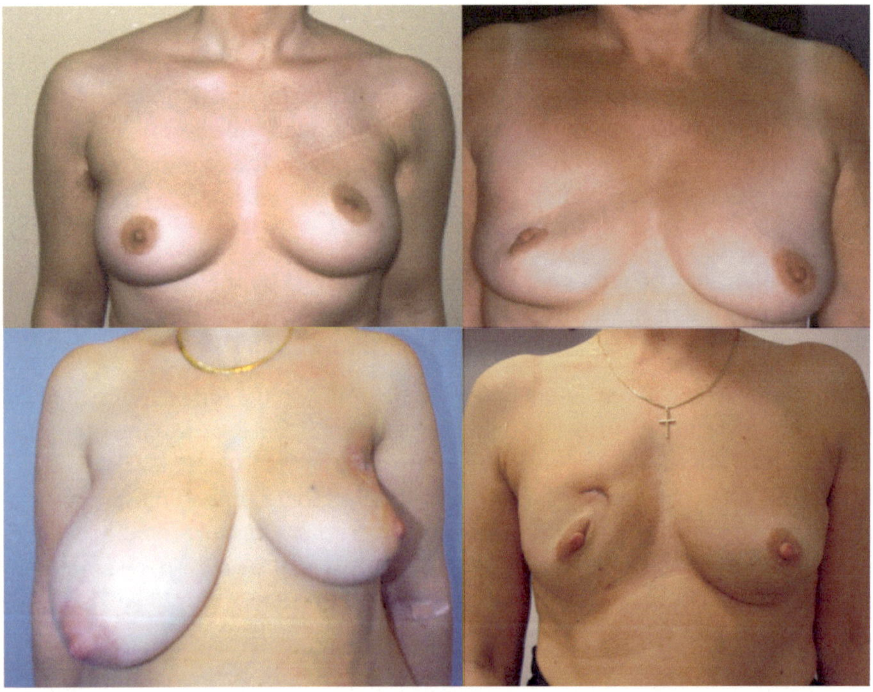

Fig. 5. Results after upper quadrantectomy without immediate reconstruction

Reconstruction is always advisable because of the volume loss of the mammary gland and the visibility of scarring, especially in case of upper-medial quadrantectomy. Local reshaping via dermaglandular flaps is the technique most frequently used except when the breast is small and without signs of ptosis. Areola upper edge cannot be placed at a length shorter than 16 cm from the sternal notch and 7-9 cm from the sternal midline because it can represent a severe cosmetic damage highly difficult to be solved. Upper-inner position of the nipple-areola complex cannot be displaced out of this zone, known as "no man's land", without further worse scars. It is much better repair the quadrantectomy defect using a linear suture rather than jeopardising the areola position. The figures 6a-b-c show the uppermost advancement that may be considered as acceptable, at least half centimetre less could be the optimum. When the preoperative plan is drawn it is basic to take into account some grade of post-op bottoming-out of the breast gland.

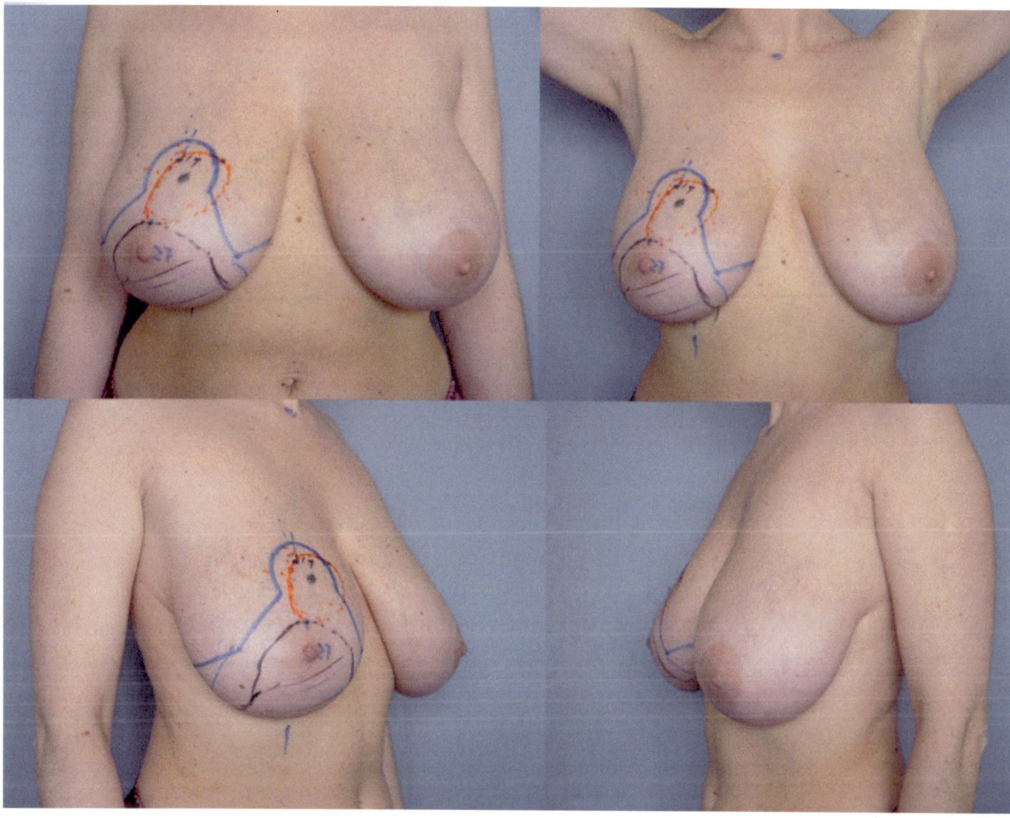

Fig. 6a. Preoperative marks of an inferior dermaglandular flap harvesting for right breast reshaping immediate to superior quadrantectomy. Above: Frontal view. Below: Lateral view

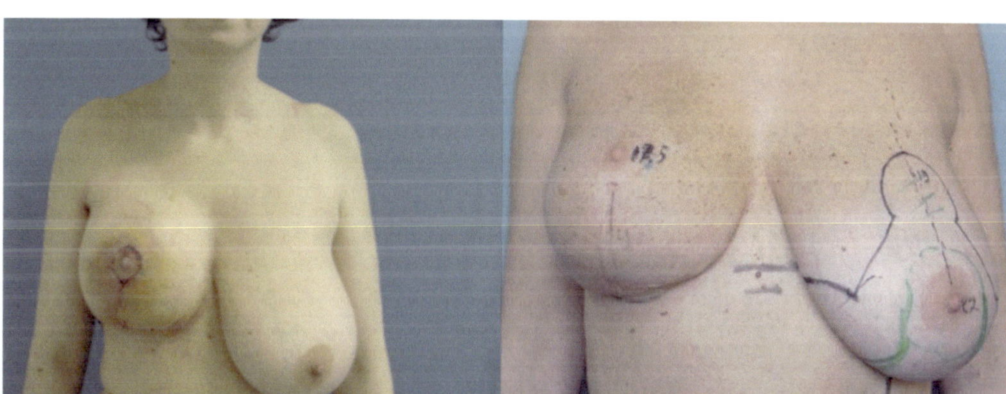

Fig. 6b. Inferior flap for right breast reshaping after superior quadrantectomy. Left : Result. Right: Preoperative marks for left breast mirror mammaplasty by similar inferior pedicle flap. Nipple was placed at 17.5 cm from the sternal notch; in the other breast, it was planned at 19 cm.

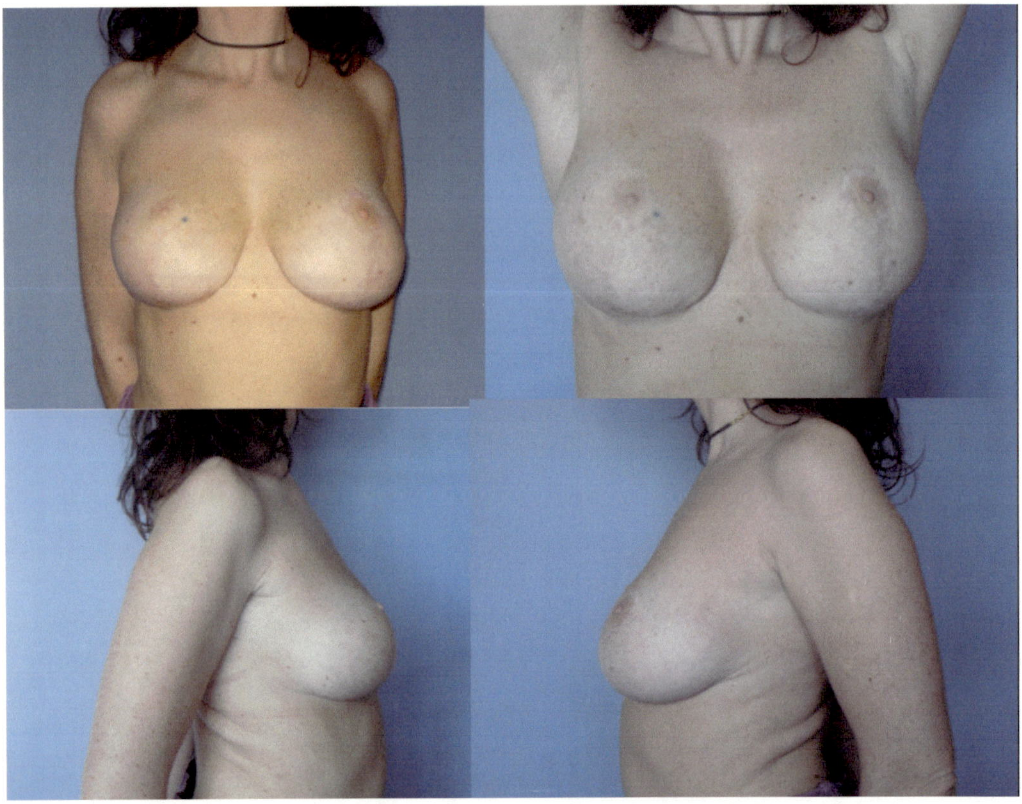

Fig. 6c. Final breast shape and symmetry after right upper quadrantectomy reshaping and left breast reduction after 2.9 years. Above: Frontal view. Below: Lateral view

2.1.1 Surgical techniques

The procedures are several depending on size and fine localization of resection (Fig. 7).

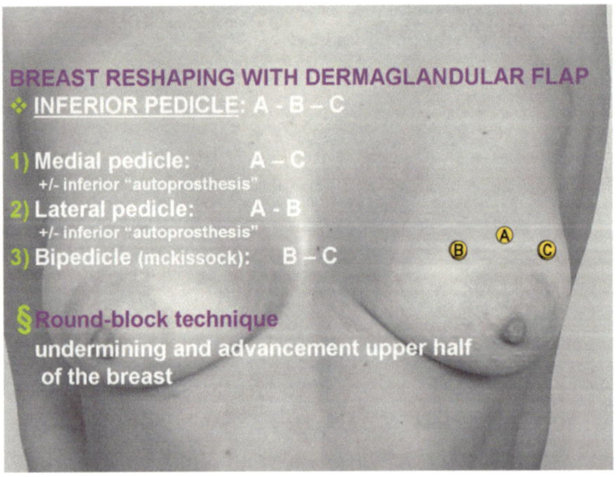

Fig. 7. Different techniques for upper quadrantectomy related to specific site (A. upper central, B. inner, C. external).

The most used technique includes the harvest of a dermagladular flap inferiorly-based to supply the nipple-areola complex (Fig. 8). The flap better fills a upper median tissue loss in a large and ptotic breast (Fig. 6). If the resection is placed in the "no man's land," it is prudently better associate minor cranial advancement of nipple-areola to a direct vertical closure of the uppermost part of resection (Fig. 9-10).

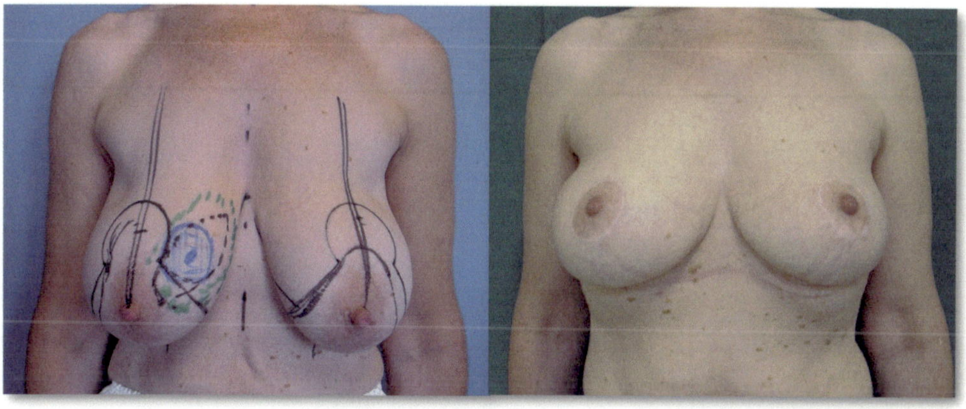

Fig. 8. Inferior dermaglandular flap for reshaping after superior inner quadrantectomy and mirror reduction mammoplasty. Left: Preoperative view. Right: Postoperative view after 2 years.

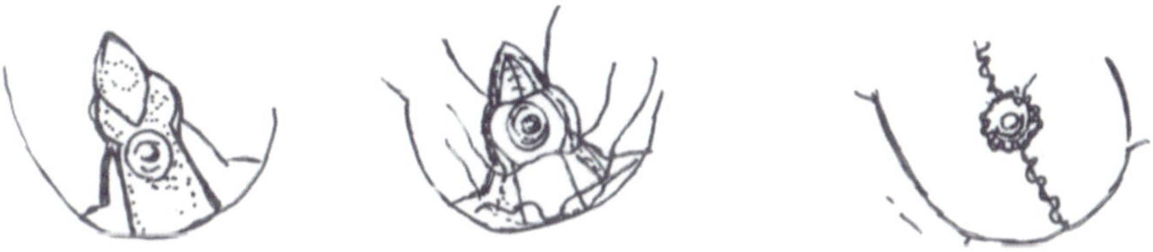

Fig. 9. Drawing of inferior dermaglandular flap with vertical direct closure upwards, in superior central quadrantectomy

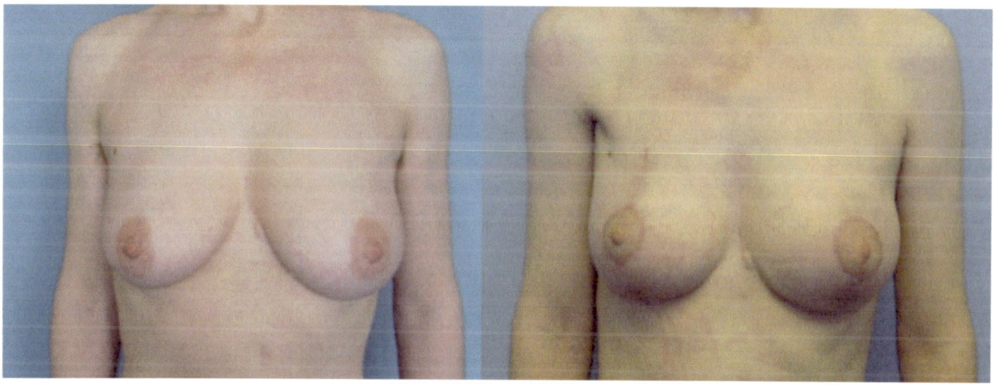

Fig. 10. Breast reshaping after superior central quadrantectomy with reconstructive technique illustrated in Fig, 9. Left: Preoperative view. Right: Postoperative view after right breast reshaping and left breast mirror mammaplasty.

In case of breast with no or moderate ptosis a round-block technique is advisable (Fig. 11a-b); a radial skin closure is associated to the periareolar pexy in smaller breast or with skin excision (Fig. 12). When the quadrantectomy is upper-medial or upper-lateral, a different technique at medial or lateral pedicle flap is preferred. These last procedures can be combined with an inferior dermaglandular flap inferiorly-based that fits the central deep part of the breast to give more projection (Fig. 13).

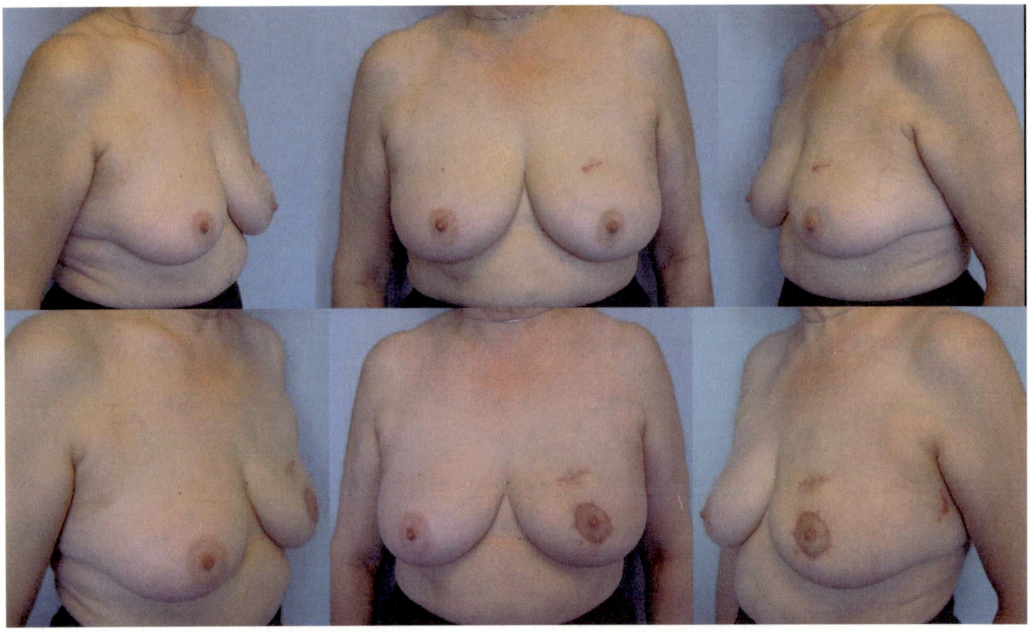

Fig. 11a. Breast reshaping after superior quadrantectomy using round-block pexy and harvesting of adjacent sliding flaps. Above: Preoperative view. Below: Postoperative view

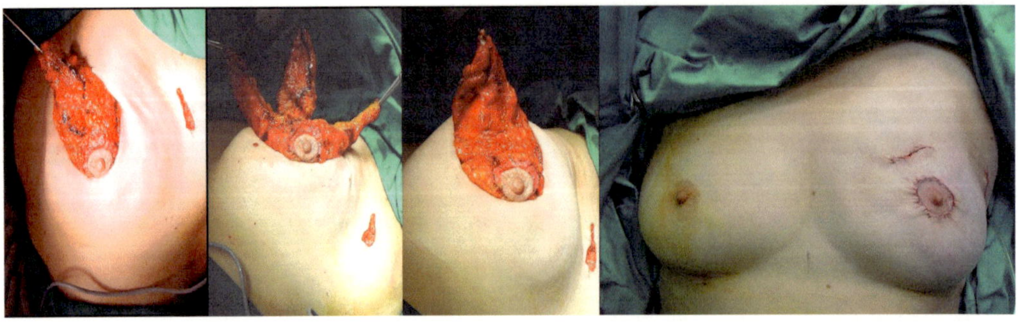

Fig. 11b. The same breast reshaping after superior quadrantectomy using round-block pexy and harvesting of adjacent sliding flaps. Intraoperative view

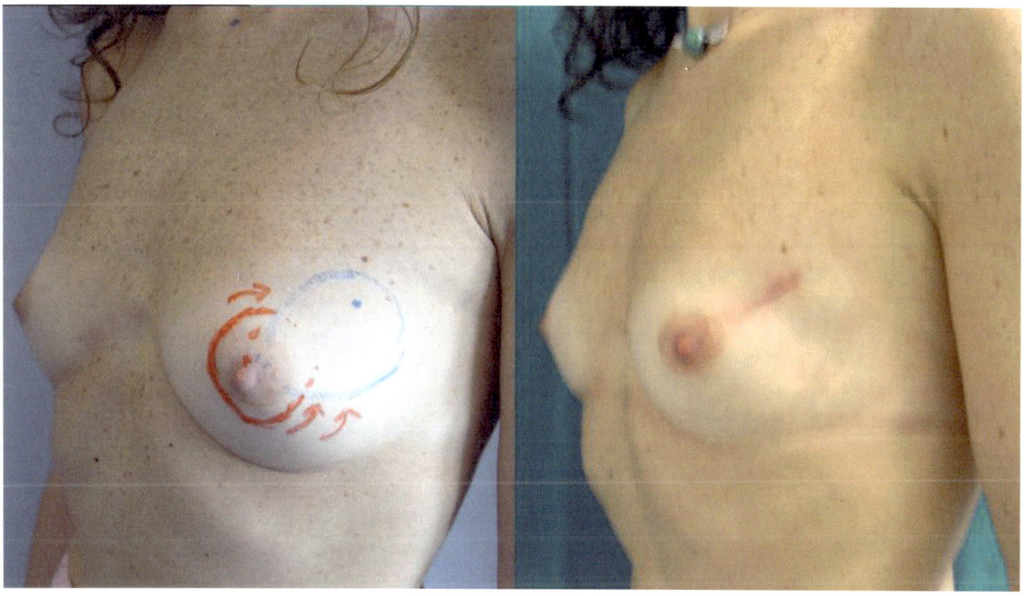

Fig. 12. Periareolar reshaping associated to radial skin closure, for upper lateral quadrantectomy. Left: Preoperative view. Right: Postoperative view

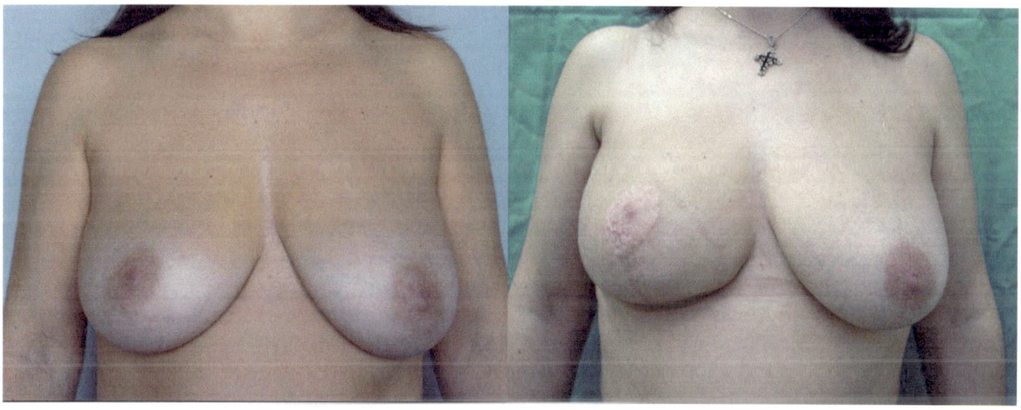

Fig. 13. Breast reshaping after superior quadrantectomy using lateral dermaglandular flap supporting nipple-areola and inferior pedicle as an endoprosthesis. Left: Preoperative view. Right: Postoperative view after 1 year

The reconstruction with dermaglandular flap inferiorly-based or with round-block technique can maintain the prior breast shape with a size moderately smaller. On the contrary, the reconstruction with dermaglandular flap medially- or laterally-based with endoprosthesis tries more frequently to modify shape, consistence and projection of the breast mould. Furthermore, these technique can be modulated to be used for very large resections (Fig. 14a-b) or for secondary surgery (Fig. 15).

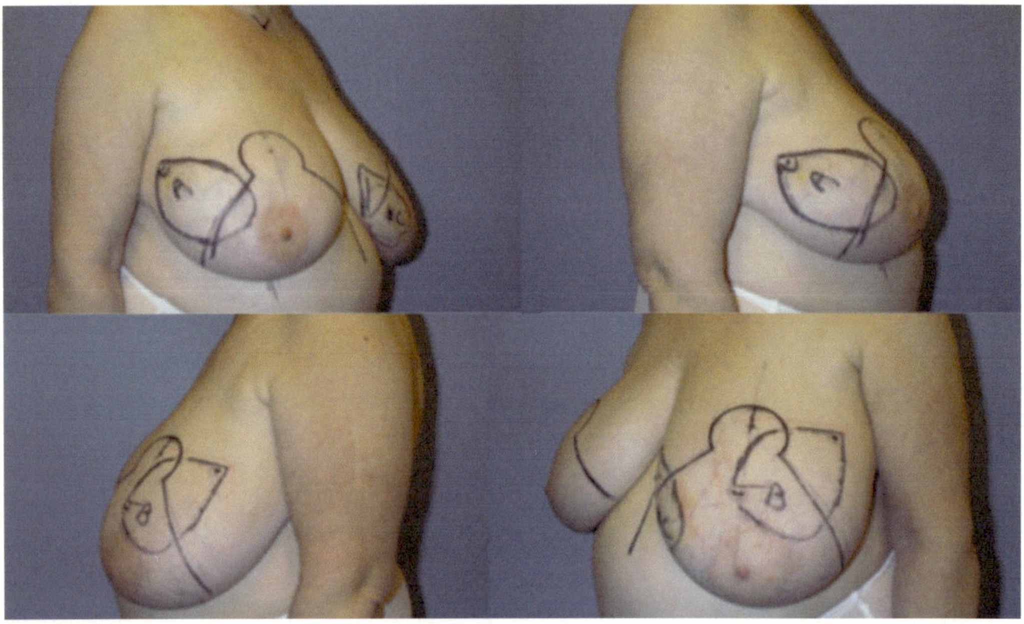

Fig. 14a. Breast reshaping after lateral quadrantectomy, on the right, and bifocal lateral-medial quadrantectomy, on the left: inferior pedicle flaps. Preoperative drawing. Above: right breast. Below: left breast

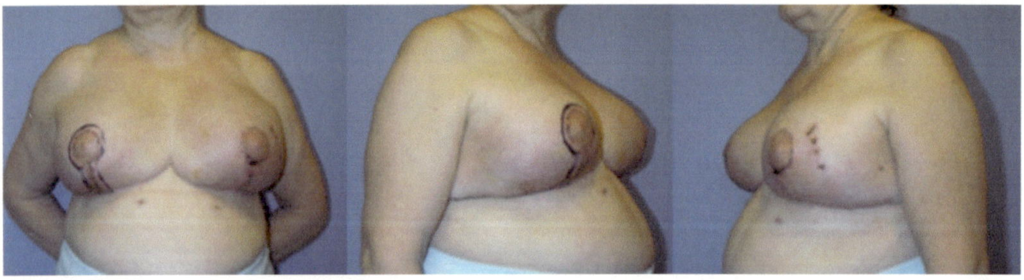

Fig. 14b. The same breast reshaping after extended quadrantectomies: immediate result. Left: Frontal view. Center: Right breast. Right: Left breast

2.2 The reconstruction after central quadrantectomy

Reconstruction of central quadrants is mandatory not only for the loss of the mammary gland but above all of the areola–nipple, generally involved in case of Paget and sub-areolar IDC/DCIS tumours. The only reason not to switch to a mastectomy is given by the chance of rebuilding a breast mould with nice shape and adequate volume. The breast seems to be amputated after central resection if no valid reconstruction is applied (Fig. 16). Otherwise it is better a skin-sparing mastectomy with implant. The reconstruction of the nipple is advisable to carry out immediately, or however before irradiation in order to reduce the risk of complications. The tattooing of the areola should be carried out after six months when the result may be considered definitive.

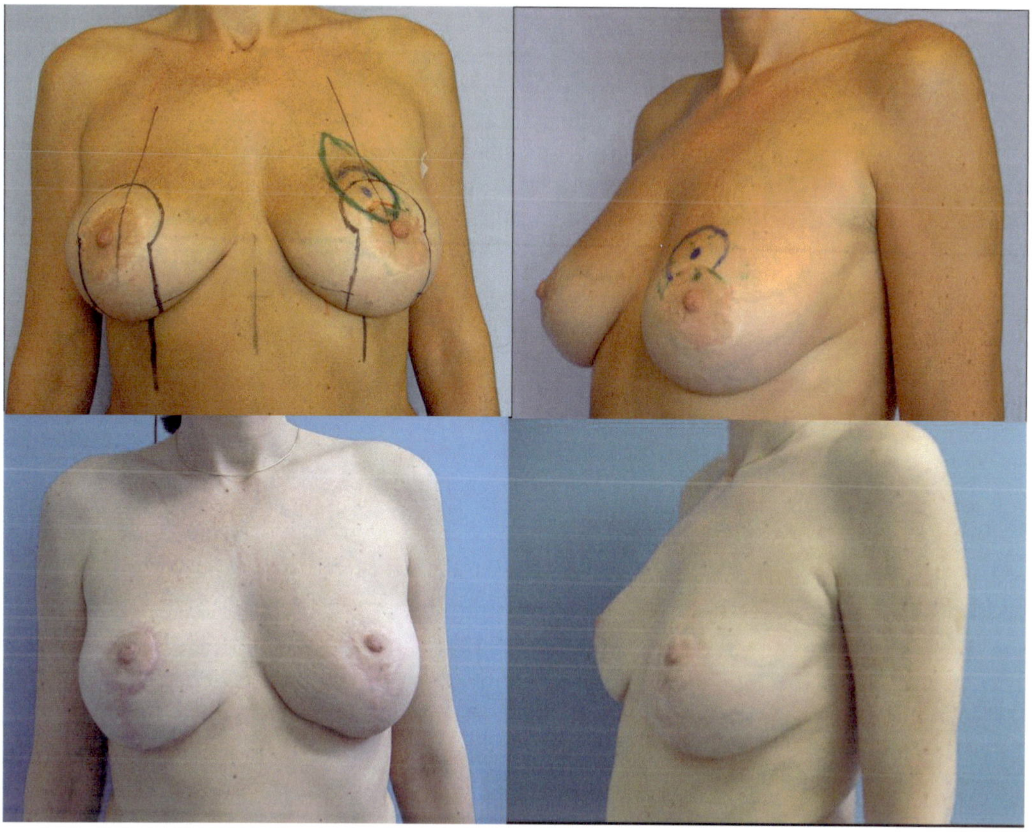

Fig. 15. Left breast reshaping for upper quadrantectomy after prior cosmetic bilateral mastopexy and contemporary contralateral pexy revision. Above: Preoperative view. Below: Postoperative view

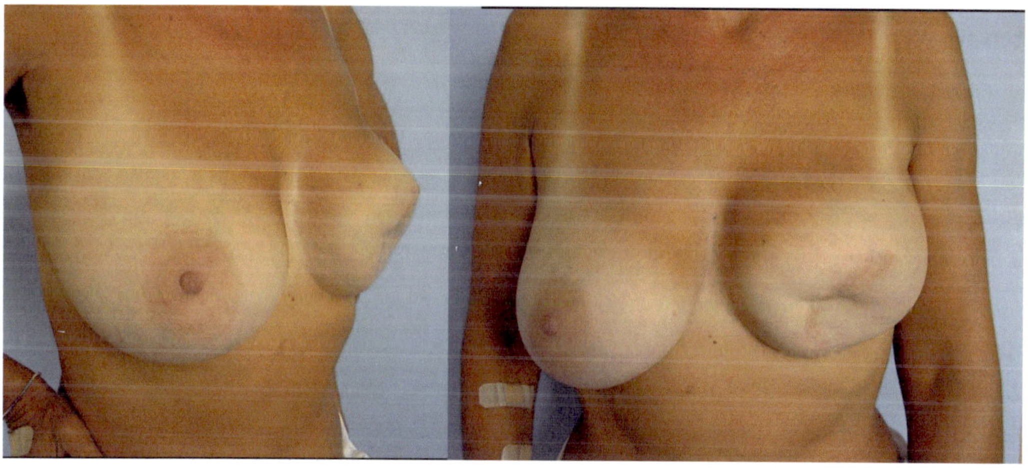

Fig. 16. Results after central quadrantectomy without immediate reconstruction

2.2.1 Surgical techniques

The gold standard technique is a mastopexy, with a B-pattern incision. The reshaping occurs through the rotation-advancement of the dermaglandular flap based on an inferior-lateral pedicle and conserving an island of integral skin for the areola (Fig. 17). The medial border of the deepithelialised flap is cut down to the fasciomuscular plane and the lateral dermoglandular flap along this plane is detached off and completely mobilized (Fig.18). This technique was firstly applied in our Institute (Grisotti, 1994). This has the following advantages compared to other techniques: minor reshaping, good maintenance of prior breast shape and ptosis, satisfactory symmetry (Fig.19-20).

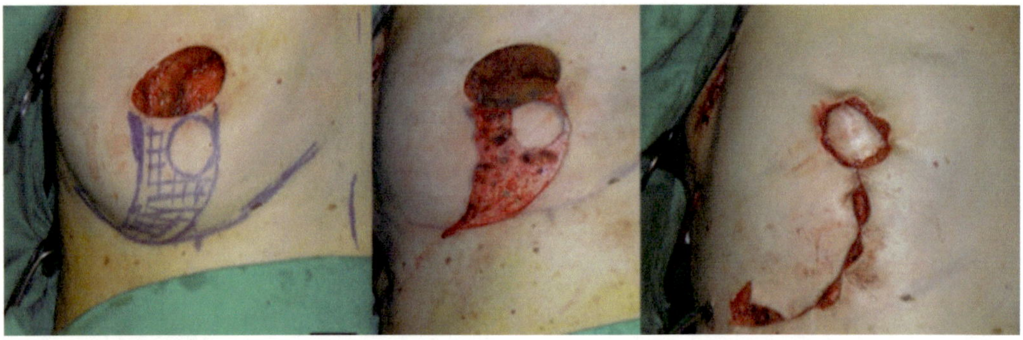

Fig. 17. Breast reshaping after central quadrantectomy. Left: Dermaglandular inferior-lateral flap marks. Center: Intraoperative harvesting of the flap with the skin island. Right: Intraoperative result.

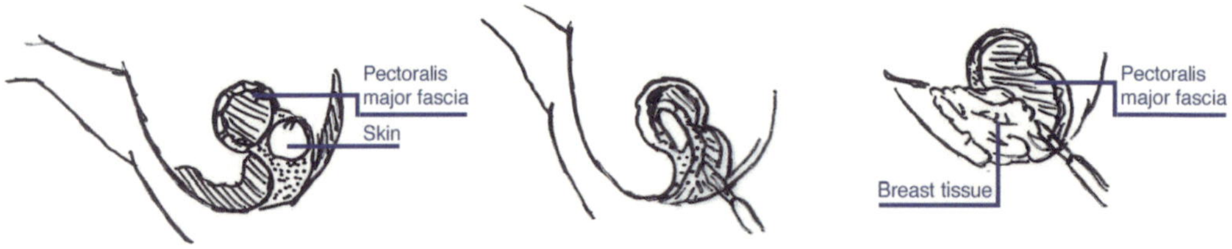

Fig. 18. Drawing of the dermaglandular inferior-lateral flap: Dissection and advancement.

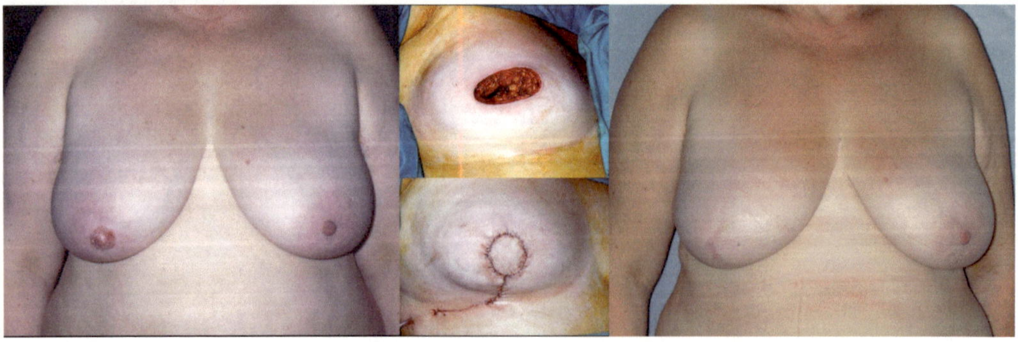

Fig. 19. Paget's disease. Reshaping of the breast after central quadrantectomy using the inferior-lateral pedicle with skin island pro areola. Left: Preoperative view. Center: Intraoperative result. Right: Result at long-term.

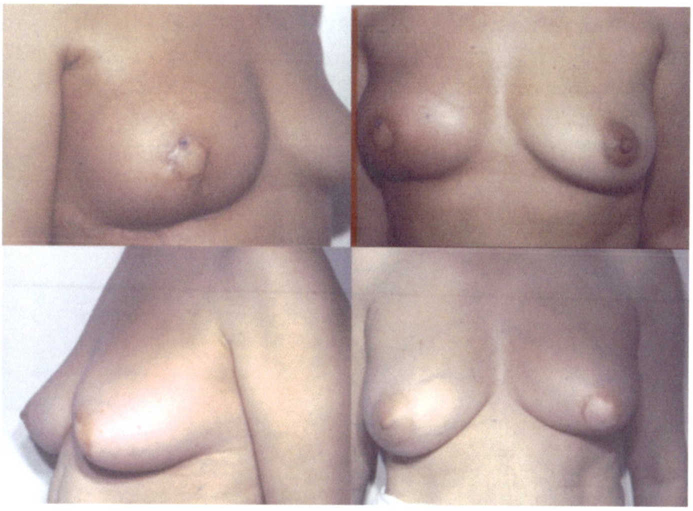

Fig. 20. Reshaping of the breast after central quadrantectomy with the same Grisotti's technique. Evident signs of radiodermitis. Above : Right breast central quadrantectomy and inferior skin glandular flap, postop. Below: Left breast central quadrantectomy and inferior skin glandular flap.

In large breasts, a technique similar to the reduction based inferiorly pedicle can facilitate the closure of the residual breast and make it possible concurrently to reconstruct the areola (Fig. 21). A personal (Riggio) variant consisted of an inferior-medial pedicle supporting an inferior-lateral skin island, that can be free of being transposed upwards (Fig. 22).

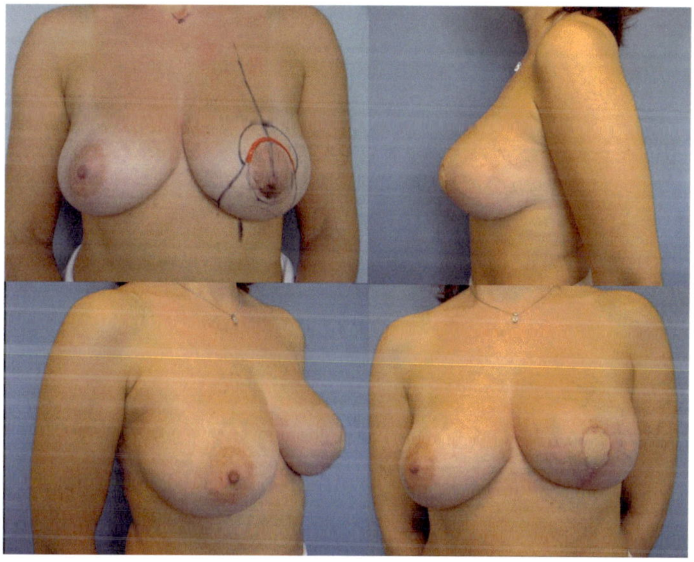

Fig. 21. Reshaping of the breast after central quadrantectomy using a standard dermaglandular flap pedicle supporting the skin island pro areola. Above, left: preoperative marks. Above, right: Lateral postoperative flap. Below: Lateral and frontal postoperative views.

Another type of dermaglandular reshaping, developed by Nava in our Institute, regards the use of a superior pedicle supporting the skin island and overlapped to an inferior flap placed deeply as an endoprosthesis that greatly increases breast projection (Fig.23a-b, 24). This technique better improve the aesthetic result and necessitates of a contralateral mirror mammaplasty using the same or different pedicled technique. In other cases, a similar procedure can be performed without skin island, with a linear T-inverted scar (Fig.25a-b centrale). The variants of techniques are several and can be customized for specific oncologic cases (Fig. 26).

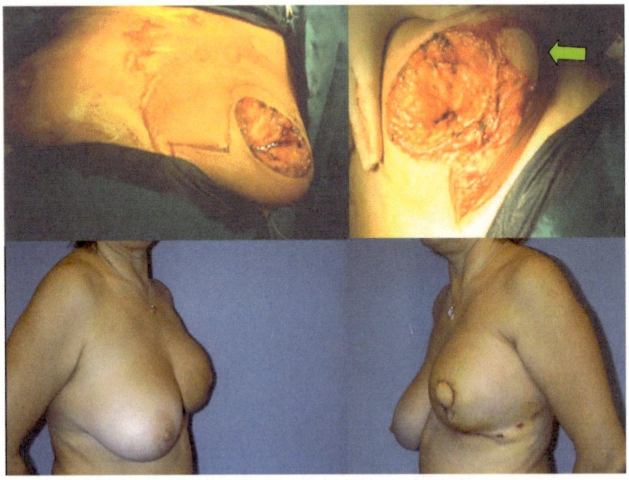

Fig. 22. Reshaping of the breast after central quadrantectomy by inferior-medial pedicle supporting an inferior-lateral skin island (see arrow). Above, Intraoperative view. Below, Postoperative view.

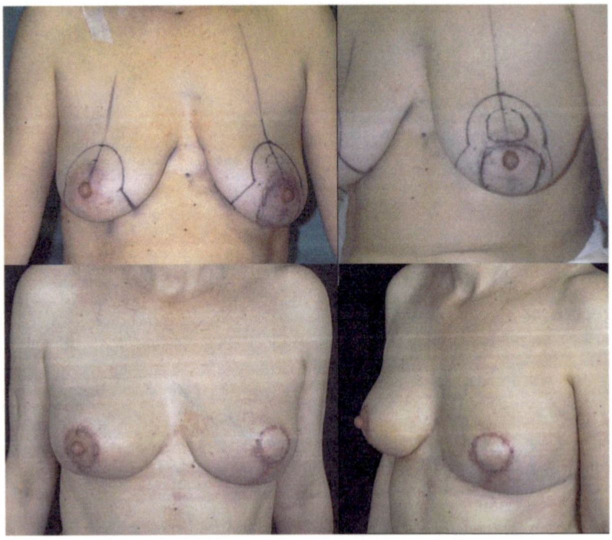

Fig. 23a. Reshaping of the left breast after central quadrantectomy using a superior pedicle supporting the skin island associated to an inferior flap as endoprosthesis; mirror mastopexy with similar technique. Above: Preoperative view. Below: Postoperative view.

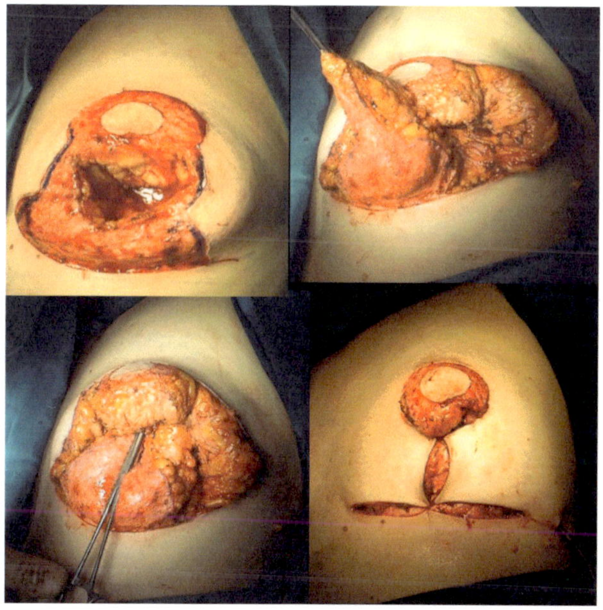

Fig. 23b. Reshaping of the left breast after central quadrantectomy using a superior pedicle supporting the skin island associated to an inferior flap as endoprosthesis. Above: Intraoperative view.

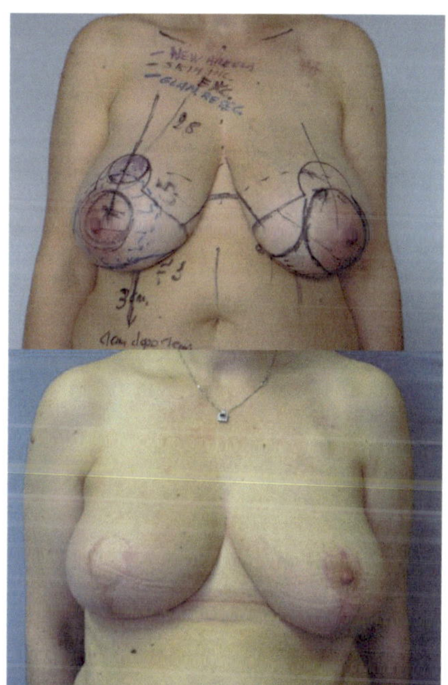

Fig. 24. Reshaping of the right breast after central quadrantectomy using a superior pedicle supporting the skin island associated to an inferior flap as endoprosthesis (introduced by Nava); mirror mammaplasty mastopexy with inferior pedicle flap. Above: Preoperative view. Below: Postoperative view.

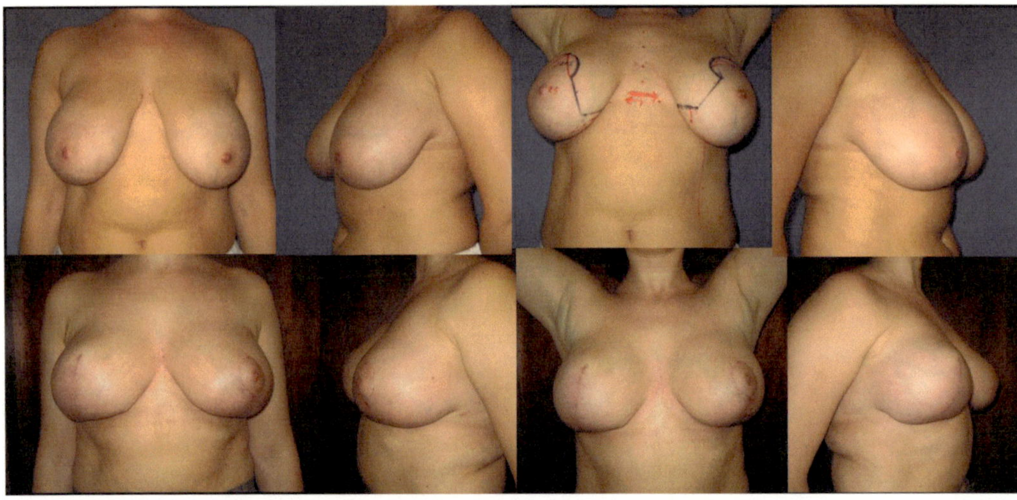

Fig. 25a. Reshaping of the right breast after central quadrantectomy using a superior pedicle without skin island, with a linear T-inverted, associated to an inferior flap as endoprosthesis; mirror mammaplasty mastopexy with medial-posterior pedicle flap, a variant of upper-medial flap designed by Riggio. Above: Preoperative view. Below: Postoperative view.

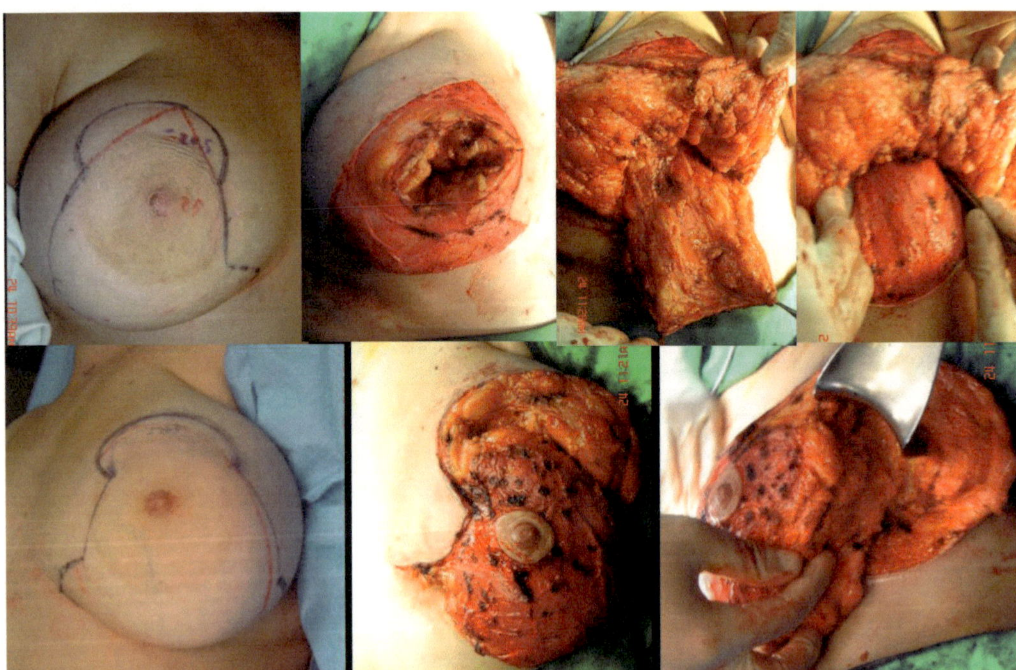

Fig. 25b. Reshaping of the right breast after central quadrantectomy using a superior pedicle without skin island, with a linear T-inverted, associated to an inferior flap as endoprosthesis; mirror mammaplasty mastopexy with the medial-posterior pedicle flap. Above: Intraoperative view of the right breast. Below: Intraoperative view of the left breast.

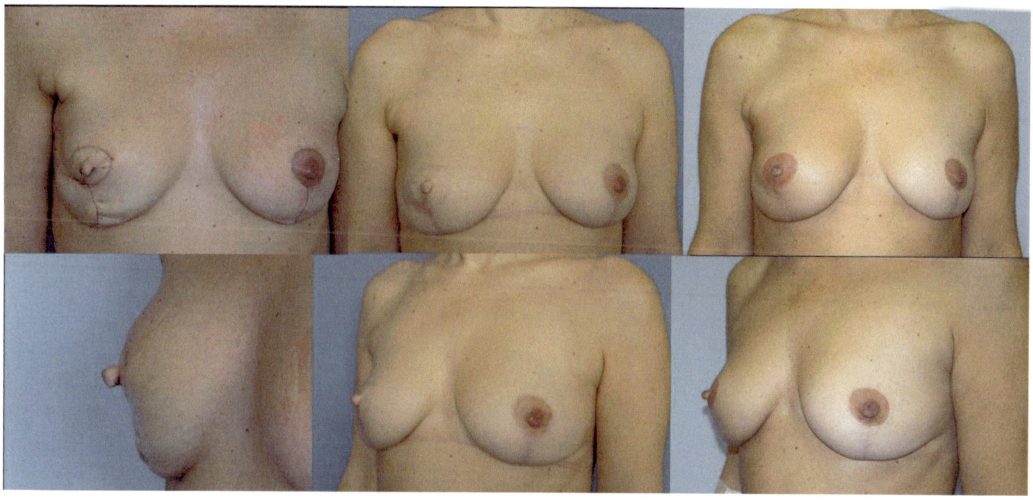

Fig. 26. Immediate right breast reshaping after bifocal central/upper-external quadrantectomy and nipple reconstruction; contralateral mirror mammaplasty. Left: short-term postoperative view. Center: medium-term postoperative view. Right: long-term postoperative view after areola tattoo.

2.3 The reconstruction after para-central inferior quadrantectomy

Tissue loss shows peculiar features at this level. There are both defects of areola skin and of the basement of nipple-areola complex. At least 7% of immediate reshaping involves this area. The retracting scar is a permanent cosmetic damage, if any correction is not immediately performed (Fig. 27).

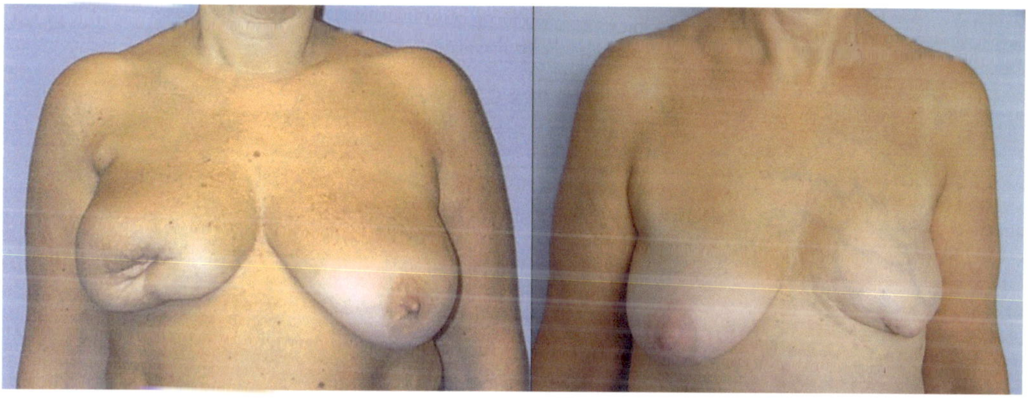

Fig. 27. Severe results after para-central/inferior quadrantectomy without immediate reconstruction. Collapse of nipple-areola complex.

2.3.1 Surgical techniques

The defect can be repaired with the same techniques used for central quadrant but with no or partial skin island. Fig. 28, 29, 30 demonstrate different applications.

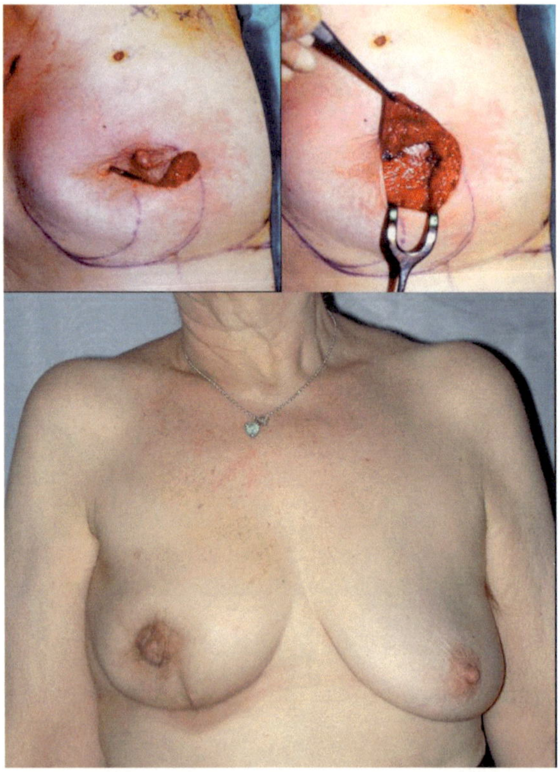

Fig. 28. Inferior-lateral pedicle flap according to Grisotti for reshaping after paracentral/inferior quadrantectomy. Above: Preoperative view. Below: Postoperative view

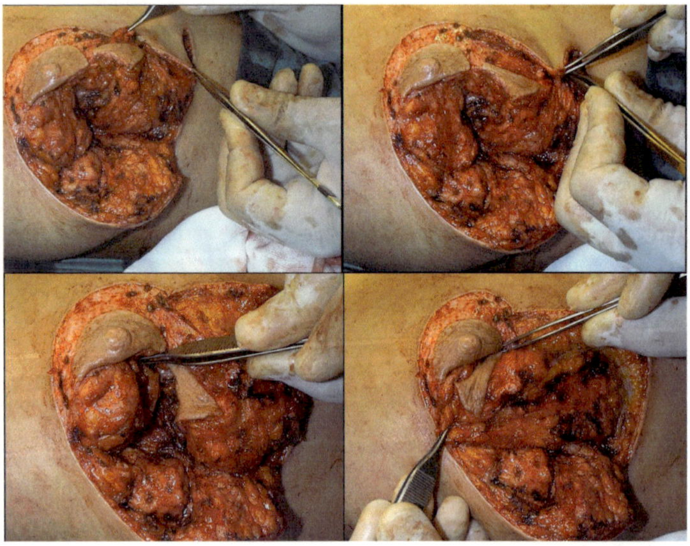

Fig. 29. Paracentral/inferior-external quadrantectomy repaired by superior dermaglandular pedicle combined to a small medial flap supporting partial skin island pro areola (special technique by Nava). Intraoperative view.

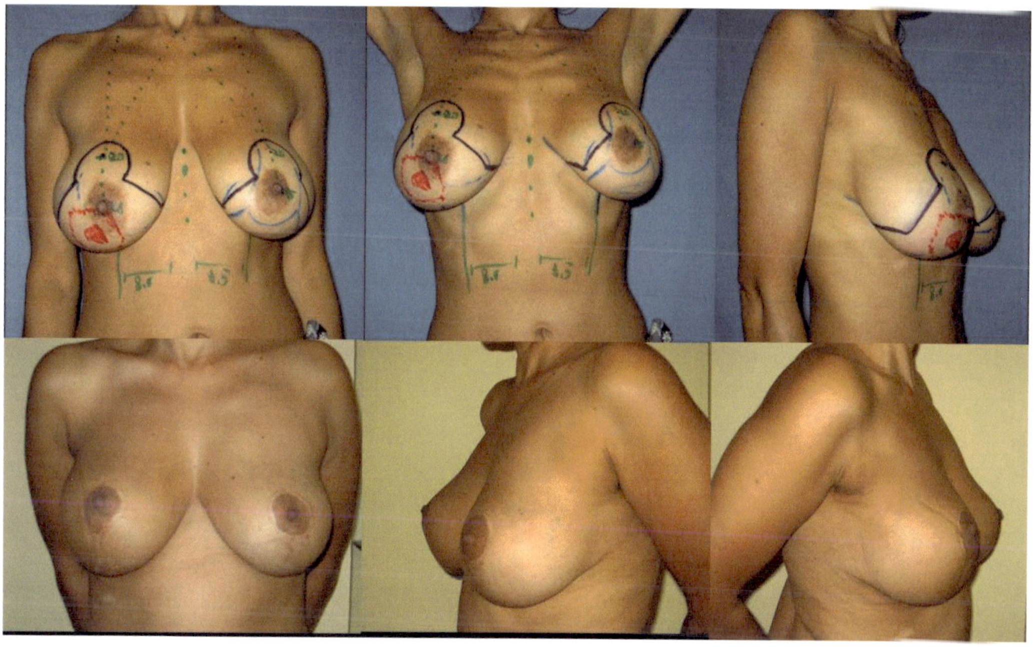

Fig. 30. Right breast paracentral/inferior-external quadrantectomy, with no areola skin excision, and reshaping by superior-medial dermaglandular pedicle combined to inferior pedicle as endoprosthesis. Contralateral mammaplasty using a superior pedicle combined to inferior endoprosthesis. Above: Pre-op view. Below: Post-op view at long-term.

2.4 The reconstruction after inferior quadrantectomy

After the central quadrant where the rate of immediate reconstruction overcomes the 95% in our experience, it is the inferior quadrant to have the highest rate of immediate reconstruction, at least 70% of total reconstructions including immediate and delayed. The inferior quadrantectomy produces a dramatic deformation if not reconstructed (Fig. 31).

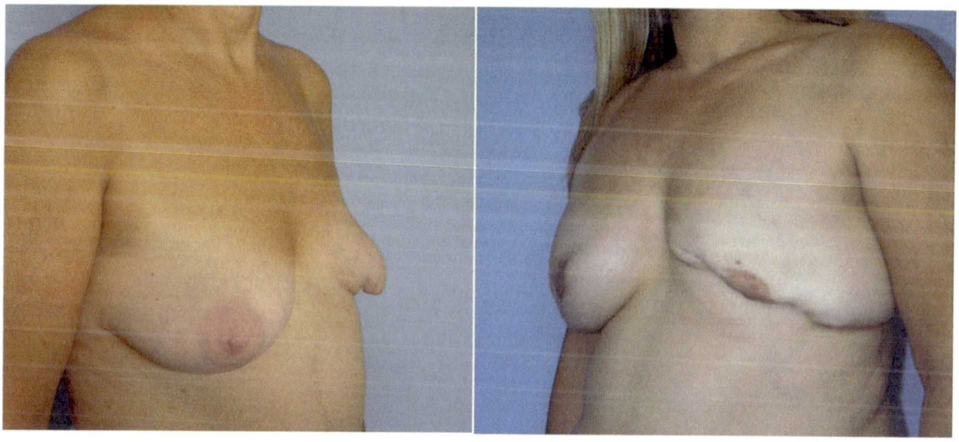

Fig. 31. Scar retraction and severe tissue loss in two patients after inferior quadrantectomy with no reconstruction.

2.4.1 Surgical techniques

The techniques are similar to those used in aesthetic surgery when a reduction mammaplasty is carried out through the resection of the inferior breast (Fig. 32). Nipple-areola is supported by a dermaglandular pedicle based superiorly.

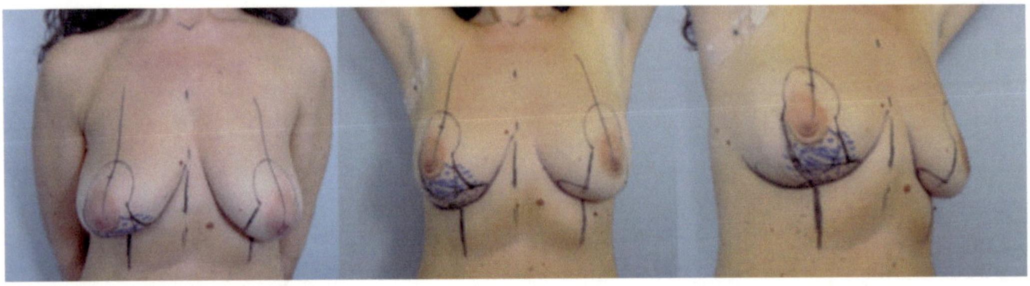

Fig. 32. Right breast reshaping deformities after inferior quadrantectomy using mastopexy at upper dermoglandular flap. Mirror mastopexy. Preoperative marks, details. Left: Frontal view. Center: Lifted arms. Right : Lateral Right view.

Skin incision can be as T-inverted or J or B; all the residual gland is dissected off the deep fascia and muscle plane and then mobilized(Fig. 33. 34, 35). The surgical difference consists of the direction of the wise-pattern that can be moved medially or laterally to include the cancer site (Fig. 36).

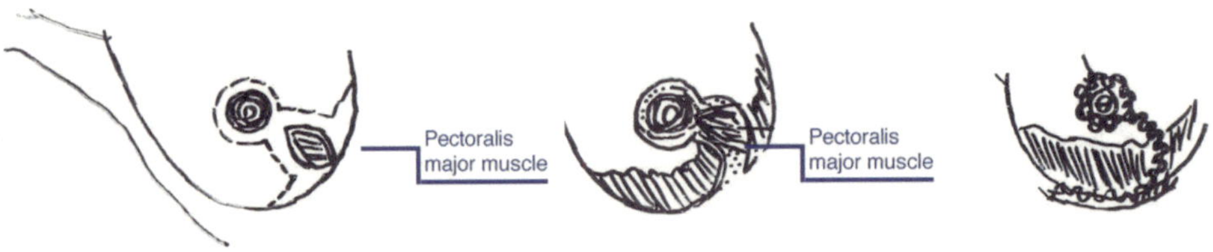

Fig. 33. Drawing of the flap harvesting for breast reshaping after inferior medial quadrantectomy. The incision pattern can be at T-inverted (Left) or at B (Center). All the residual gland is separated from the fascio-muscular plane and mobilized. The final scar must end alongside the inframammary fold (Right).

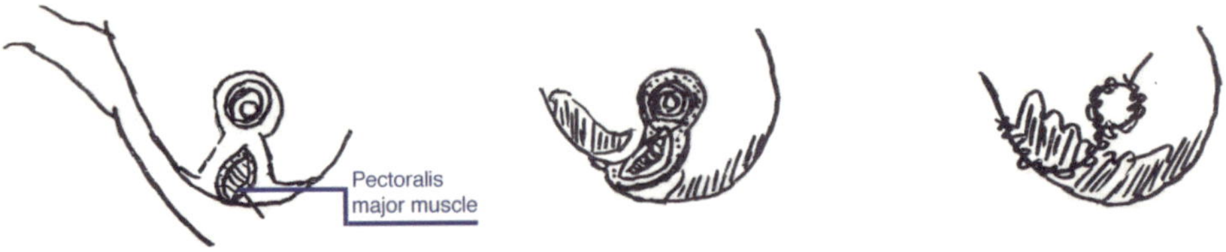

Fig. 34. Drawing of the flap harvesting for breast reshaping after inferior-lateral quadrantectomy

Another technical solution is given by the placement of the medial or lateral segment of the horizontal incision line from the inframmary fold to the tumour site (Fig. 37). This may occur in the clinical case where tumour is located more medially or laterally, overlying skin must be removed due to surgery or prior scar, or the breast is less ptotic and large.

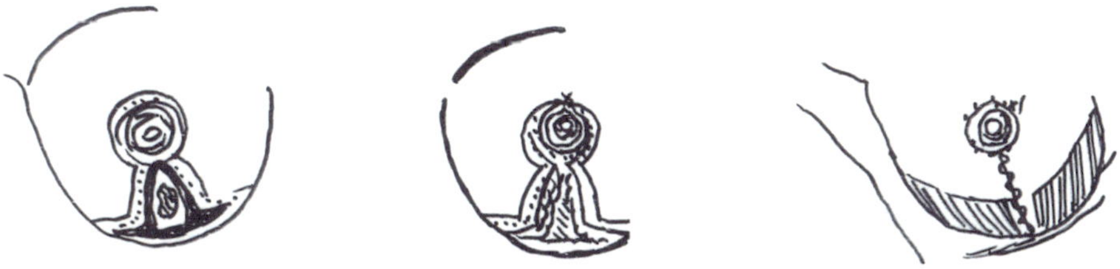

Fig. 35. Drawing of the flap harvesting for breast reshaping after inferior median quadrantectomy

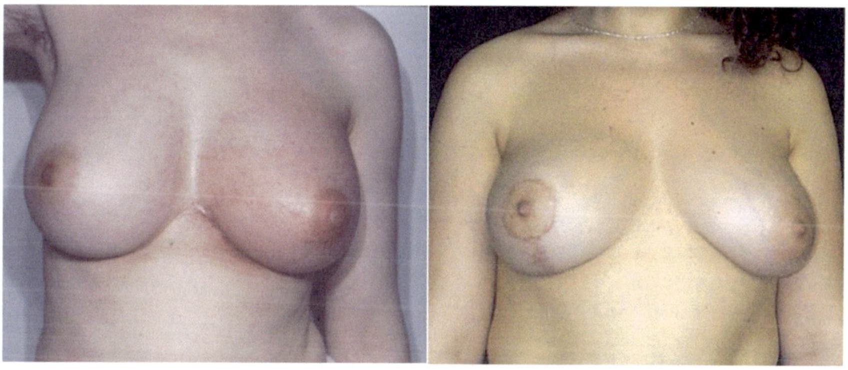

Fig. 36. Breast reshaping after inferior quadrantectomy using upper dermoglandular flap. Two final results different for cancer site. Left, inferior-medial quadrantectomy in the left breast with B-pattern. Right: inferior-median quadrantectomy in the right breast with T-inverted scar.

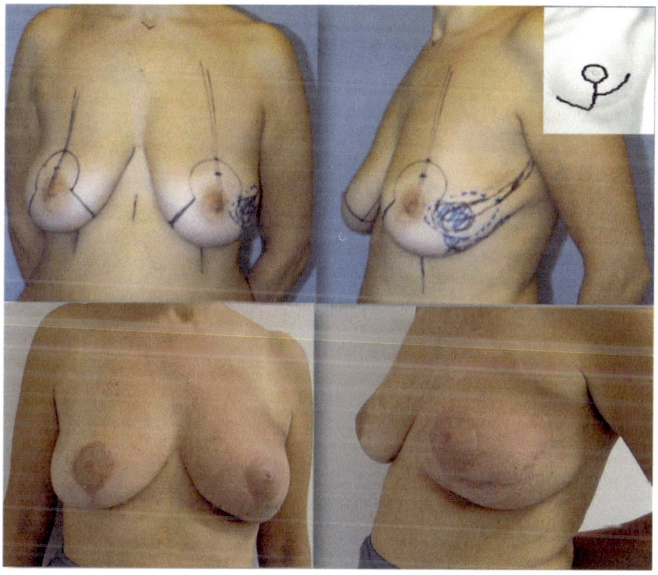

Fig. 37. Breast reshaping after inferior quadrantectomy using upper dermoglandular flap. Replacement of the lateral segment of horizontal incision line from the inframmary fold to the inframmary fold to the tumour site

As occurred in other quadrants, oncoplastic surgery can present operative situations outside the usual rules of aesthetic technique concerning breast reduction and pexy. There are items that can make breast reshaping much more difficult : deformities for prior tumorectomy and fibrotic retraction, or planning of wide skin excision. The first Author found a solution for the breast that needs for severe skin deformities to be repaired: an inferior skin-glandular flap to be transposed (Fig.38a, b, c).

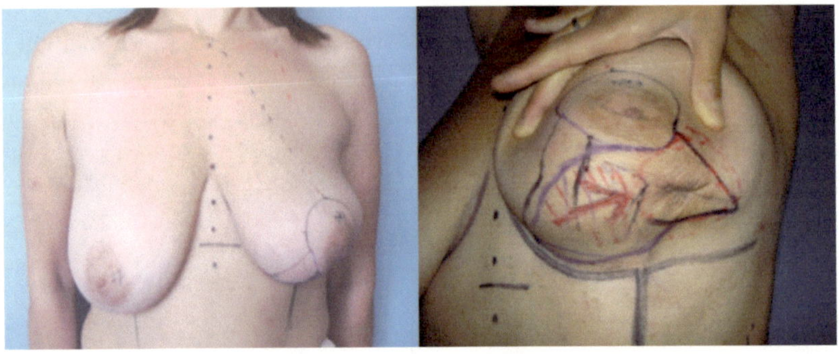

Fig. 38a. Inferior rotation skin-glandular flap, first performed by Riggio, for reshaping of deformities after inferior quadrantectomy, left breast. Left : Preoperative frontal view. Right: Preoperative close-up with marking details.

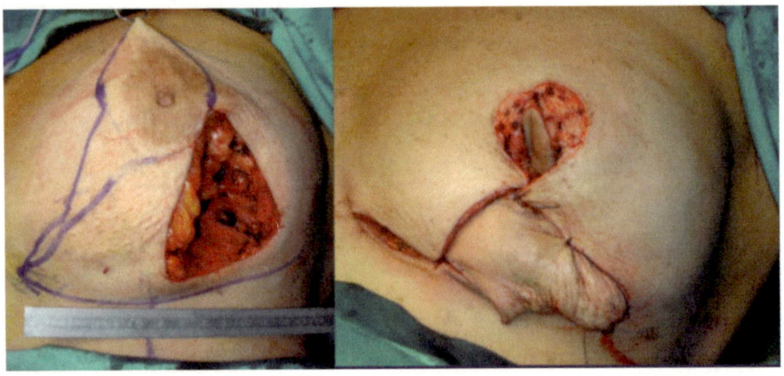

Fig. 38b. Inferior rotation skin-glandular flap, for reshaping of deformities after inferior quadrantectomy, left breast. Left: Intraoperative technical step. Right: Intraoperative result.

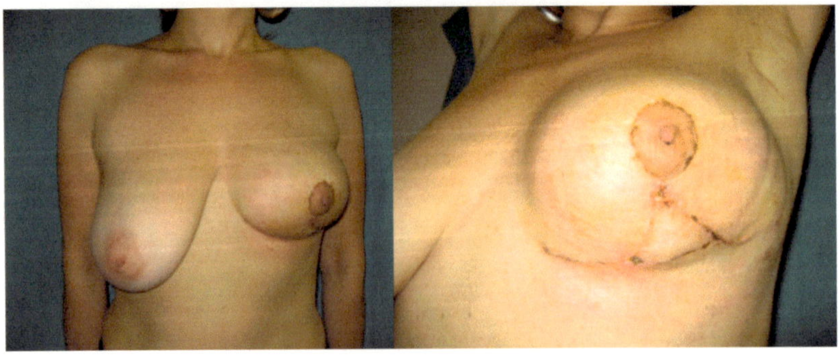

Fig. 38c. Inferior rotation skin-glandular flap, for reshaping of deformities after inferior quadrantectomy, left breast. Left : immediate result after surgery, frontal view. Right: Immediate result after surgery, close-up.

2.5 Reconstruction by prosthesis insertion

The experience started in the '80s of the last century - with round, semilunar, and tear-drop shapes and volume (range 40-400cc) - and suggested not to treat quadrantectomy defects using silicone implant, either immediately or secondarily. Result were mostly unsatisfactory. The 56% of capsular contracture (Baker 3-4) in all implant cases with/without irradiation) is to be compared with the 67% of severe contracture in the group of irradiated patients. Other complications were infection, seroma, and implant extrusion. Secondary surgery was necessary in the 55.5% of our series.

3. Delayed reconstruction

The analysis of the deformity should comprise: a) classification, b) surgical plan, c) reconstructive chance in case of recurrences . The type of previous surgery must be known: lumpectomy, extended tylectomy, partial mastectomy, quadrantectomy, and sectorial mastectomy.

The larger part of delayed reconstruction is consisted of autologous distant flaps (48%). Nevertheless this surgery finds minor indications for two reasons: 1) high rate of complication after breast irradiation; 2) increasing risk of local recurrence per year. The last issue leads to a dilemma in case of major reconstruction by distant or free flaps. Is it more advisable to preserve flap reconstruction in the case of future recurrences, if salvage mastectomy after QUART would require mandatory reconstruction with flap? Or else, to provide for a prophylactic mastectomy and consequent reconstruction by myocutaneous flap?

Most BCT deformities include partial breast resection and irradiation. Nearly 10% was excluded by radiotherapy due to the less malignant diagnosis (all severe dysplasia; a few carcinoma in situ). The breast not irradiated can be freely managed with secondary breast reshaping and implant augmentation with no increased risk for complications. Augmentation can be feasible and reliable in particular cases but requires higher skill in breast reconstruction as usual (Fig. 39).

Irradiated tissues (skin and parenchyma) requires extreme care to be surgically treated and is advisable to manage secondary corrections after three post-op years. Reshaping by pexy-technique is feasible for minor defects, but always risky for tissue necrosis. Reliable techniques utilise scar lengthening (multiple Z-plasty) and nipple-areola advancement to improve shape. As well, all the aesthetic procedures can be used in the contralateral breast in order to improve simmetry. Micro-fat injections, i.e. lipofilling, can be used for small tissue loss and skin scarring.

3.1 Autologous flap reconstruction

The prevalence of flap reconstruction is also decreased depending on the improvement of the general surgeon's care of cosmetic results and the higher rate of immediate plastic reshaping, but it still maintains a real capacity of sculpting an acquired deformity as no other can do it. Fig. 40 demonstrates how a latissimus dorsi flap - performed by the first Author - is able to be shaped and customized into the neighbouring scar tissues. In our experience, it is better isolate and cut the motor nerve of the muscle proximally. Irradiated tissues must be debrided, prudently dissected and carefully removed if necessary, in order to obtain optimal symmetry as volume and contouring. Breast perforators coming from the chest wall should be preserved as much as possible in order to reduce the risk for increased parenchyma post-surgical fibrosis or even necrosis.

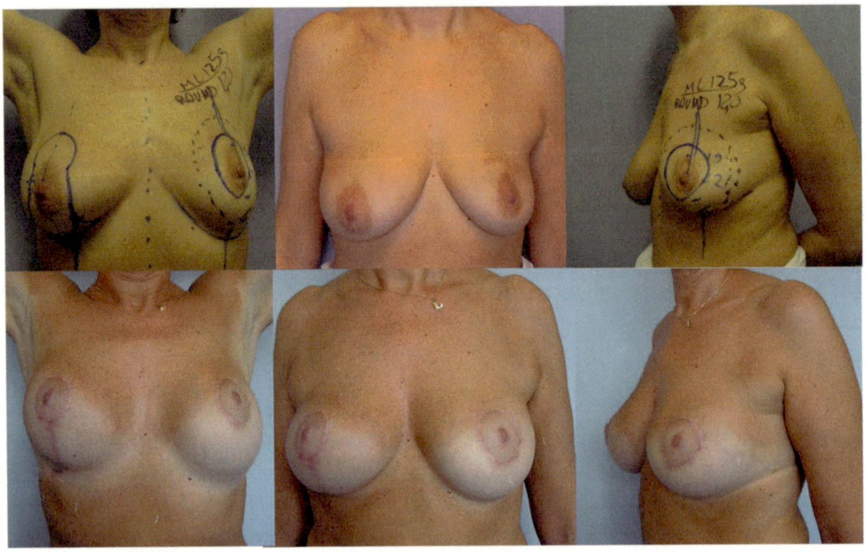

Fig. 39. Delayed left breast reconstruction after upper quadrantectomy, by anatomical implant (Allergan 410ML 125g) and round-block pexy. The previous scar was included in the deepithelialised area. The contralateral breast was corrected by a reshaping by upper pedicle flap. Above Left: Frontal view at lifted arms, preop marks. Center: Frontal view. Right: Lateral left view, preop marks. Below: corresponding postoperative views.

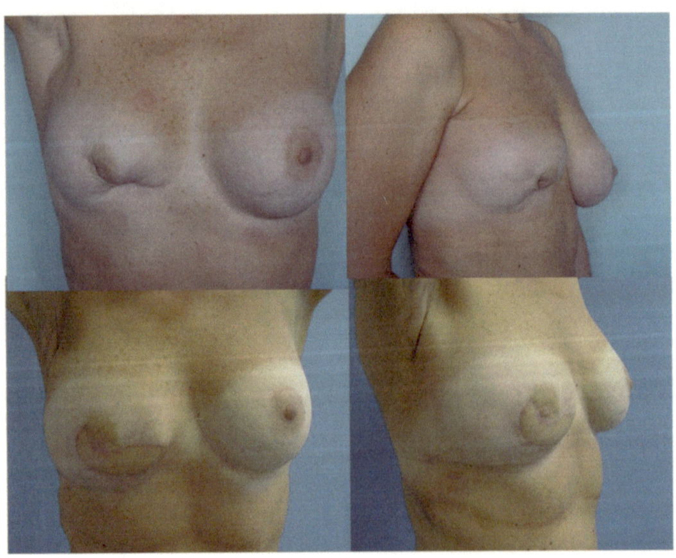

Fig. 40. Delayed reconstruction of the right breast after QUART using a latissimus dorsi myocutaneous flap. Above, Preoperative views, Left: frontal view at lifted arms. Right: lateral view. Below, Postperative views, Left: frontal view at lifted arms. Right: lateral view.

The preop analysis of the deformity after BCT must evaluate the balance between cutaneous and subcutaneous/glandular resection, that is the main factor which determines the type of deformity, The second consideration regards individual characteristics: a) size and shape of the operated breast; b) scar retraction; c) size and shape of the opposite healthy breast; d) patient body structure. Last of all, the donor area of the flap will be detected: a) distance from the recipient breast deformity; b) presence of scar; c) tissue thickness; d) skin elasticity/stiffness, texture, and pigmentation; e) the donor area sequels. Then, the fasciocutaneous or myocutaneous can be chosen. Our preference is towards the myocutaneous pedicled flaps for two reasons: 1) major mobilization and rotation grade to be accustomed into the defect; 2) no problem compared with free flap which needs for vascular dissection deeply to an irradiated breast tissue that cannot be easily cut or removed. According to our past experience, latissimus dorsi and TRAM flaps were respectively used in 10% and 2% of total reconstructive cases. Two latissimus dorsi flaps were augmented by implant. Nowadays, TRAM has been discontinued excepting the decision for a mastectomy. Different solutions have been taken into account as the perforator flaps (Tseng, 2010). The best of them is the parascapular flap as it regards BCT (Hamdi, 2004).

The latissimus dorsi flap requires correct preparation of the recipient site and planning of the skin island on the back, as first (Fig.41). The location of the skin island must suit the breast shape and perfectly harmonize the skin and parenchyma defects (Fig. 42).

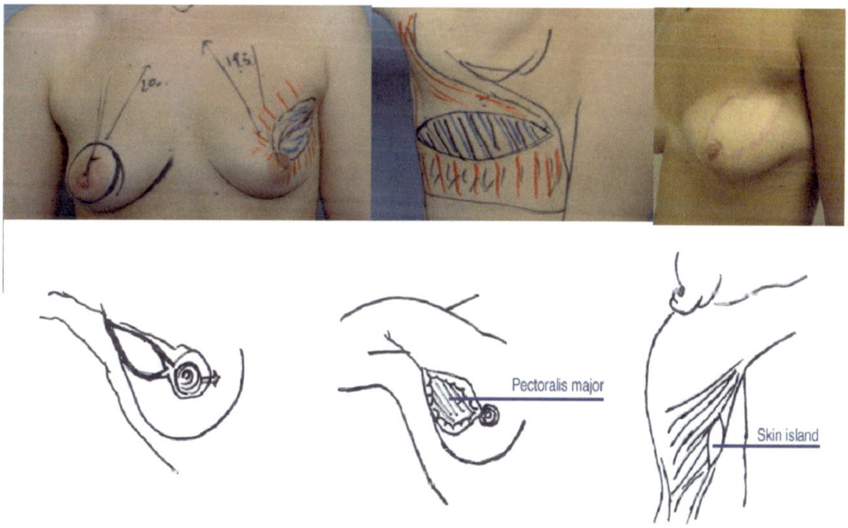

Fig. 41. Drawing of the latissimus dorsi flap for upper-external deformity. From left to right: dissection above the pectoralis maior muscle and removal of scar tissue, debridement and advancement of the nipple-areola complex, harvesting of skin island along with the muscular pedicle, result.

The TRAM flap must be limited to larger reconstruction (Fig.43). It was rarely used, and now indicated only for breast really amputated of the patients that decline the idea of a total mastectomy before the full-size reconstruction. Skin texture and subcutaneous thickness are less forgeable compared with latissimus dorsi flap, and hence the recipient site must be prepared with larger dissection and excision of fibrotic tissue.

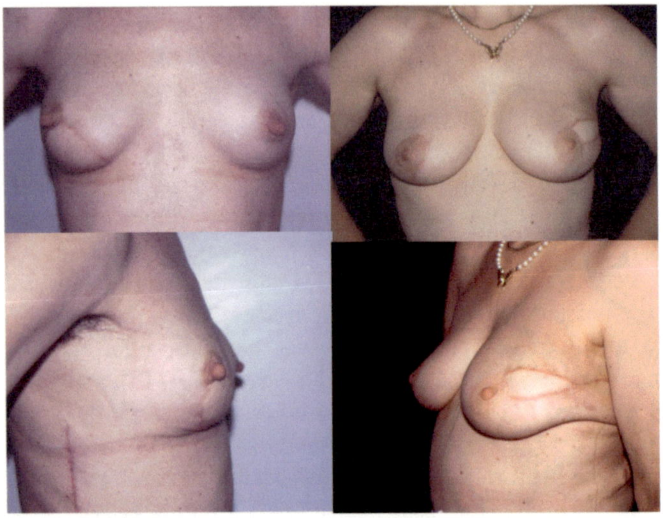

Fig. 42. Delayed breast reconstruction after QUART using latissimus dorsi myocutaneous flap. Left: Result after inferior resection, frontal and lateral views. Right: Result after lateral resection, frontal and lateral views.

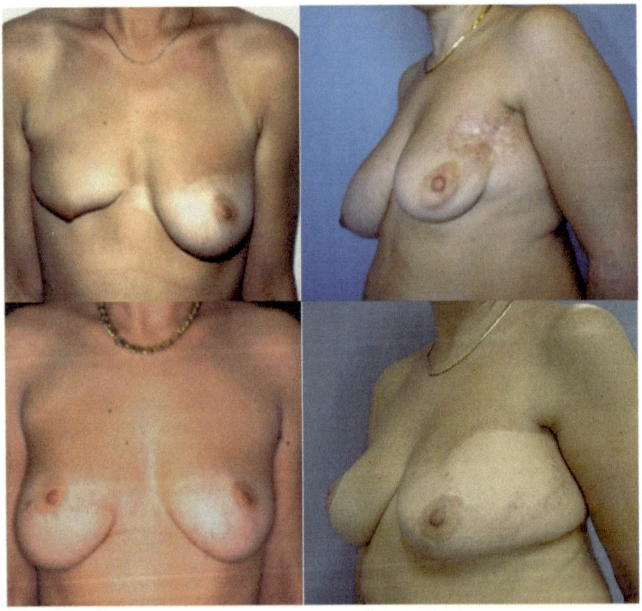

Fig. 43. Delayed breast reconstruction after QUART using TRAM flap. Left: Result after inferior resection, frontal view; above: preop, below: postop. Right: Result after lateral resection, lateral view; above: preop, below: postop.

4. Oncoplastic results

Reconstruction procedures must be considered as an integral part of the breast conservative treatment. Breast surgeon still thinks to manage many partial mastectomies without the aid of some plastic aesthetic surgeon. Many authors were interested of this item in the past as well as recently, and we have reported a series of up-to-date references.

Immediate reshaping specifically needs for skill in cosmetic mastopexy and reduction to be successful in addition to the reconstructive and oncological expertise. Cosmetic results without reconstruction show low rates of appraisal, nearly 35% of them is poor. In the institutional series (Fig. 44), the results of BCT with immediate reconstruction were satisfactory in almost the 70% after 13.5 years of follow-up. Shape satisfaction reached the 75% of appraisals. On the other hand, symmetry was a little more satisfactory in the delayed group of reconstructions (>60%). However immediate reshaping remains the primary option for the best result. Also the contralateral mammaplasty improves symmetry even if contemporary. According to the patient wishes, mirror mammaplasty is better to be carried out immediately. Only 37% of cases underwent contralateral aesthetic surgery. Half of them consisted of breast reduction with upper dermaglandular flap, secondarily reduction with inferior flap; all mastopexis overcame the 20%.

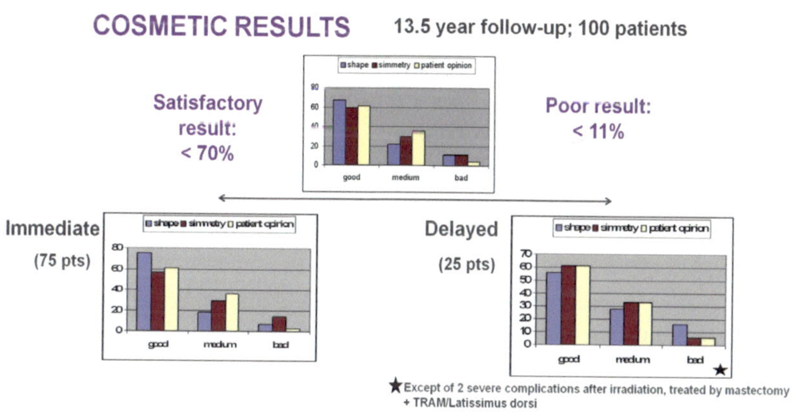

Fig. 44. Diagram of cosmetic results after BCT reconstruction in a pilot-study of 100 patients.

The oncological follow-up was 15 years in our pilot-study (Table 3):	
Time free of disease	2-11 yrs
Local recurrences	12/89
- Recurrences treated by further BCT	7
- Recurrences treated by salvage mastectomy (4 TRAM)	5
Contralateral cancer incidence	11
- Breast conservative treatment and dermaglandular reshape	5
- Patey mastectomy and breast reconstruction: 4 implants and 1 TRAM	6
Sporadic finding of controlateral cancer during surgery	0
Metastatic cancer	8
Patient survival after 15 years	95/100

Table 3. Oncological results (T<2.5cm; N0 out of N1 in 10 pts.; M0)

Above all, 13.5% of local recurrences, 9% of distant metastases, and 95% of survival rate reflect the literature data positively, and moreover demonstrate the comprehensive efficacy of the historical experience of our Cancer Institute.

5. References

Viani, GA., Stefano, EG., Afonso SL., De Fendi, LI., Soares, FV., Leon, PG., Guimaraes, FS., (2007)Breast-conserving surgery with or without radiotherapy in women with ductal carcinoma in situ: a meta-analysis of randomized trials. *Radiat Oncol.*, Vol. 2, (Aug 2007), pp. 2-28.

Silvertein, MJ. (2006). Ductal carcinoma in situ: basics, treatment controversies, and an oncoplastic approach, In: *Surgery of the Breast: Principles and Art*. Vol. 1, Spear SL (ed.), 2nd ed., pp. 512-534, Lippincott Williams and Wilkins, Philadelphia.

Fisher, ER., Costantino, J., Fisher, B., Palekar, AS., Redmond, C., Mamounas, E., (1995) Pathologic findings from the National Surgical Adjuvant Breast Project (NSABP) Protocol B-17. Intraductal carcinoma (ductal carcinoma in situ). The National Surgical Adjuvant Breast and Bowel Project Collaborating Investigators. *Cancer,* Vol. 15, No.75, 6, (Mar 1995), pp. 1310-9.

Silverstein, MJ., Lagios MD., Craig, PH., &al., (1996) A prognostic index for ductal carcinoma of the breast in situ. *Cancer,* Vol.77, (1996), pp.2267-2274

Veronesi, U., Bonadonna, G., Zurrida, S., Galimberti, V.Greco, M., Brambilla, C., Luini, A., Andreola, S.Rilke, F., Raselli, R.&al., (1995) Conservation surgery after primary chemotherapy in large carcinomas of the breast.*Ann Surg*., Vol.222, No.5, (Nov 1995), pp.612-8.

Veronesi, U., Saccozzi, F., Del Vecchio, M., &al., (1981) Comparing radical mastectomy with quadrantectomy, axillary dissection, and radiotherapy in patients with small cancers of the breast. *N Engl J Med,* Vol.305, (1981), pp.6-11

Veronesi, U., Banfi, A., Del Vecchio M., Saccozzi, R., Clemente, C. Greco, M., Luini, A., Marubini, E., Muscolino, G., Rilke, F., & al., (1986) Comparison of Halsted mastectomy with quadrantectomy, axillary dissection, and radiotherapy in early breast cancer: long-term results. *Eur J Cancer Clin Oncol.*, Vol.22, No.9, (Sept 1986), pp. 1085–1089.

Veronesi, U., Volterrani, F., Luini, A., &al.(1990) Quadrantectomy versus lumpectomy for small size breast cancer. *Eur J Cancer*, Vol.26, (1990), pp. 671-673

Veronesi, U., Cascinelli, N., Mariani, L., Greco, M., Saccozzi, R., Luini, A., Aguilar, M., (2001)Radiotherapy after breast-conserving surgery in small breast carcinoma: long-term results of a randomized trial.*Ann Oncol.,* Vol.12, No.7, (Jul 2001), pp.997-1003.

Veronesi, U., Cascinelli, N., Mariani, L., Greco, M., Saccozzi, R., Luini, A., Aguilar, M., Marubini, E., (2002)Twenty-year follow-up of a randomized study comparing breast-conserving surgery with radical mastectomy for early breast cancer.*N Engl J Med.*, Vol.17, No.347(16) pp.1227-32.

Fisher, B., Bauer, M., Margolese, R., Piosson, R., Pilch, Y., Redmond, C., Fisher, E., Wolmark, N., Deutsh, M., Montague, E., &al.(1985) Five-year results of a randomized clinical trial comparing total mastectomy and segmental mastectomy with or without radiation in the treatment of breast cancer.*N Engl J Med.*, Vol.14, No.312(11), (1985), pp.665-73

Fisher, B., Anderson, S., Bryant, J., Margolese, RG., Deutsch, M., Fisher, ER., Jeong, JH., Wolmark, N., (2002)Twenty-year follow-up of a randomized trial comparing total mastectomy, lumpectomy, and lumpectomy plus irradiation for the treatment of invasive breast cancer. *N Engl J Med.*Vol.17, No.347(16)(Oct 2002), pp.1233-41.

Joop, A. van Dongen, Adri, C.Voodg, Ian, S. Fentiman, Catherine Legrand, Richard J.Sylvester, David Tong, Emmanuel, van der Shueren, Peter A., Helle, Kobus van Zijl and Harry Bartelink, (2000) Long-Term Results of a Randomized Trial Comparing Breast-Conserving Therapy With Mastectomy: European Organization for Research and Treatment of Cancer 10801Trial. *J Natl Cancer Inst* ., Vol.92, No.14, (2000)pp. 1143-1150.

Arriagada, R., Le, MG., Contesso, G., Guinebrètiere, JM, Rochard, F., Spielmann, M., (2002) Predictive factors for local recurrence in 2006 patients with surgically resected small breast cancer.*Ann Oncol.*Vol.13, No.9(2002)pp.1404-13.

Yang, SH., Yang, KH., Li, YP., Zhang YC, He XD., Song, AL., Tian JH., Jiang, L., Bai ZG., He, LF., Liu, YL., Ma, B., (2008).Breast conservation therapy for stage I or stage II breast cancer: a meta-analysis of randomized controlled trials. *Ann Oncol* ., Vol.19 (2008)pp.1039–1044.

Grisotti, A., (1994)Immediate reconstruction after partial mastectomy.*Oper. Techn. Plast Reconstr.Surg.*, Vol.1, No.1, (1994)pp.1-12.

Tseng, CY., Lipa, JE., (2010) Perforator flaps in breast reconstruction. *Clin Plast Surg.*, Vol.37, No.4(Oct 2010), pp.641-54 vi-ii.

Hamdi, M. Van Landuyt, K., Monstrey, S., Blondeel, P., (2004)Pedicled perforator flaps in breast reconstruction: a new concept. *Br J Plast Surg.* Vol.57, No.6, (Sept 2004)pp.531-9

De Lorenzi, F.(2010) Oncoplastic surgery : the evolution of breast cancer treatment. *Breast J.*, Vol.16, Suppl 1, (Sept-Oct 2010), pp.S 20-1.

Perez, CA.(2010)Breast conservation therapy in patients with stage T1-T2 breast: current challenges and opportunities. *Am J ClinOncol.*, Vol.33, No.5, (Oct 2010), pp.500-10.

Fitoucci, AD., B erry MG., Famà, F., Falcou, MC., Curnier, A., Couturaud, B., Reyal, F., Salmon, RJ., (2010)Oncoplastic breast surgery for cancer:analysis of 540 consecutiva cases. *Plast Reconstr Surg.*, Vol.125, No.2, (Feb 2010), pp.454-62.

Hernanz, F. Regaño, S., Vega, A., Gómez Fleitas, M., (2010)Reduction mammoplasty: an advantageous option for breast conserving surgery for large breasted patients. *Surg.Oncol.*, Vol.19, No.4, (Dec 2010), pp. e95-e102.Epub 2009 Aug 27. Review

Berry, MG., Fitoussi, AD., Curnier, A., Couturaud, B., Salmon, RJ., (2010)Oncoplastic breast surgery: a rewiew and systematic approach. *J Plast Reconst Aesthet Surg.*, Vol.63, No.8, (Aug 2010), pp.1233-43 Epub 2009 Jun 25. Review

Hoffmann, J. Wallwiener, D., (2009)Classifying breast cancer surgery:a novel, complexity-based system for oncological, oncoplastic and reconstructive procedure, and proof of principle by analysis of 1225 operations in 1166 patients. *BMC Cancer*, Vol.8, No.9, (Apr2009), p.108.

Franceschini, G., Terribile, D., Fabbri, C., Magno, S., D'Alba, P., Chiesa, F., Di Leone, A., Masetti, R., (2008)Progress in treatment of early breast cancer. A mini- review *Annal Ital Chir*, Vol.79, No.1, (Jan-Feb 2008), pp.17-22.

Franceschini, G. Magno, S., Fabbri, C., Chiesa, F., Di Leone, A., Moschella, F., Scafetta, I., Scaldaferri, A., Fragomeni, S., Adesi Barone, L., Terribile, D., Salgarello M, Masetti,

R., (2008) Conservative and radical oncoplastic approaches in the surgical treatment of breast cancer. *Eur Rev Med Pharmacol Sci.*, Vol.12, No.6, (Nov- Dec 2008), pp.387-96.Review

Rietjens, M., Urban, CA., Rey, PC., Mazzarol, G., Maisonneuve, P., Garusi, C., Intra, M., Yamaguchi, S., Kaur, N., De Lorenzi, F., Matthes, AG., Zurrida, S., Petit, JY., (2007) Long term oncological results of breast conservative treatment with oncoplastic surgery. *Breast,* Vol.16, No.4(Aug 2007), pp. 387-95.Epub 2007 Mar 26.

Vallejo da Silva, A., Destro, C., Torres, W., (2007)Oncoplastic surgery of the breast: rationale and experience of 30 cases. *Breast,* Vol.16, No.4(Aug2007), pp.411-9.Epub 207 Mar 19

Luini, A. Gatti, G., Galimberti, V., Zurrida, S., Intra, M., Gentilini, O., Paganelli, G., Viale, G., Orecchia, R., Veronesi, P, Veronesi, U., (2005) Conservative treatment of breast cancer: its evolution. *Breast Cancer Res Treat.*, Vol.94, No.3, (Dec2005)pp.195-8 Review